Early-Stage Breast Cancer: New Developments and Controversies

Guest Editor

ELEFTHERIOS P. MAMOUNAS, MD, MPH

SURGICAL ONCOLOGY
CLINICS OF NORTH AMERICA

www.surgonc.theclinics.com

Consulting Editor
NICHOLAS J. PETRELLI, MD

July 2010 • Volume 19 • Number 3

SAUNDERS an imprint of ELSEVIER, Inc.

W.B. SAUNDERS COMPANY
A Division of Elsevier Inc.

1600 John F. Kennedy Boulevard ● Suite 1800 ● Philadelphia, PA 19103-2899

http://www.theclinics.com

SURGICAL ONCOLOGY CLINICS OF NORTH AMERICA Volume 19, Number 3
July 2010 ISSN 1055-3207, ISBN-13: 978-1-4377-2617-6

Editor: Catherine Bewick
Developmental Editor: Theresa Collier

Surgical Oncology Clinics of North America (ISSN 1055-3207) is published quarterly by Elsevier Inc., 360 Park Avenue South, New York, NY 10010-1710. Months of publication are January, April, July, and October. Business and Editorial Offices: 1600 John F. Kennedy Blvd., Ste. 1800, Philadelphia, PA 19103-2899. Customer Service Office: 3251 Riverport Lane, Maryland Heights, MO 63043. Periodicals postage paid at New York, NY and additional mailing offices. Subscription prices are $225.00 per year (US individuals), $340.00 (US institutions) $113.00 (US student/resident), $259.00 (Canadian individuals), $423.00 (Canadian institutions), $163.00 (Canadian student/resident), $323.00 (foreign individuals), $423.00 (foreign institutions), and $163.00 (foreign student/resident). Foreign air speed delivery is included in all *Clinics* subscription prices. All prices are subject to change without notice. **POSTMASTER**: Send address changes to *Surgical Oncology Clinics of North America*, Elsevier Health Science Division, Subscription Customer Service, 3251 Riverport Lane, Maryland Heights, MO 63043. **Customer Service: 1-800-654-2452 (US and Canada). 314-447-8871 (outside U.S. and Canada). Fax: 314-447-8029. E-mail: journalscustomerservice-usa@elsevier.com** (for print support); **journalsonline support-usa@elsevier.com** (for online support).

Reprints. For copies of 100 or more, of articles in this publication, please contact the Commercial Reprints Department, Elsevier Inc., 360 Park Avenue South, New York, New York 10010-1710. Tel. 212-633-3813; Fax: 212-462-1935; E-mail: reprints@elsevier.com.

Surgical Oncology Clinics of North America is covered in *MEDLINE/PubMed (Index Medicus)* and *EMBASE/ Excerpta Medica, Current Contents/Clinical Medicine,* and *ISI/BIOMED.*

Printed and bound in the United Kingdom
Transferred to Digital Print 2011

Contributors

CONSULTING EDITOR

NICHOLAS J. PETRELLI, MD
Bank of America Endowed Medical Director, Helen F. Graham Cancer Center at Christiana Care Health System, Newark, Delaware; Professor of Surgery, Thomas Jefferson University, Philadelphia, Pennsylvania

GUEST EDITOR

ELEFTHERIOS P. MAMOUNAS, MD, MPH, FACS
Medical Director, Aultman Cancer Center, Canton; Professor of Surgery, Northeastern Ohio Universities College of Medicine, Rootstown, Ohio

AUTHORS

BIJAN ANSARI, MD
Breast Surgery Fellow, Department of Surgery, Mayo Clinic, Rochester, Minnesota

HARRY D. BEAR, MD, PhD
Professor of Surgery and Microbiology and the Walter Lawrence Jr Distinguished Professor of Oncology, Division of Surgical Oncology, Department of Surgery, Massey Cancer Center, Virginia Commonwealth University, Richmond, Virginia

PATRICK IVAN BORGEN, MD
Director, Brooklyn Breast Cancer Project; Chairman, Department of Surgery, Maimonides Medical Center, Brooklyn, New York

JUDY C. BOUGHEY, MD
Associate Professor of Surgery, Department of Surgery, Mayo Clinic, Rochester, Minnesota

HAROLD J. BURSTEIN, MD, PhD
Associate Professor of Medicine, Breast Oncology Center, Dana-Farber Cancer Institute, Harvard Medical School, Boston, Massachusetts

ANEES B. CHAGPAR, MD, MA, MSc, MPH, FRCSC, FACS
Associate Professor, Department of Surgery, University of Louisville; Director, Multidisciplinary Breast Program, James Graham Brown Cancer Center; Academic Advisory Dean, University of Louisville School of Medicine, Louisville, Kentucky

JANE S. CHAWLA, MD
Division of Oncology, Department of Medicine, Washington University, St Louis, Missouri

HIRAM S. CODY III, MD
Attending Surgeon, Breast Service, Department of Surgery, Memorial Sloan-Kettering Cancer Center; Professor of Clinical Surgery, Weill Cornell Medical College, New York, New York

MATTHEW J. ELLIS, MB, BChir, PhD
Division of Oncology, Department of Medicine; Siteman Cancer Center, Washington University, St Louis, Missouri

MELISSA FAZZARI, PhD
Department of Epidemiology and Population Health, Albert Einstein College of Medicine, Bronx, New York

JENNIFER J. GRIGGS, MD, MPH
Associate Professor, Hematology and Oncology Division, Department of Internal Medicine; Associate Professor, Department of Health Management and Policy; Director, Breast Cancer Survivorship Program, Comprehensive Cancer Center, University of Michigan, Ann Arbor, Michigan

AMAR GUPTA, MD
Department of Surgery, Mount Sinai Hospital, University of Toronto, Toronto, Canada

GABRIEL N. HORTOBAGYI, MD, FACP
Professor and Chairman, Department of Breast Medical Oncology, University of Texas M.D. Anderson Cancer Center, Houston, Texas

APARNA C. JOTWANI, MD
Indiana University Simon Cancer Center, Indianapolis, Indiana

CATHERINE M. KELLY, MD, MSc (ClinEpi)
Susan G. Komen Interdisciplinary Breast Fellow, Department of Breast Medical Oncology, University of Texas M.D. Anderson Cancer Center, Houston, Texas

PARAIC A. KENNY, PhD
Department of Development and Molecular Biology, Albert Einstein College of Medicine, Bronx, New York

GAIL S. LEBOVIC, MA, MD, FACS
President, American Society of Breast Disease, Frisco, Texas

CYNTHIA X. MA, MD, PhD
Division of Oncology, Department of Medicine; Siteman Cancer Center, Washington University, St Louis, Missouri

LIDA MINA, MD
Indiana University Simon Cancer Center, Indianapolis, Indiana

MONICA MORROW, MD
Chief, Breast Service, Department of Surgery; Anne Burnett Windfohr Chair of Clinical Oncology, Memorial Sloan-Kettering Cancer Center, Evelyn H. Lauder Breast Center; Professor of Surgery, Weill Medical College of Cornell University, New York, New York

MICHAEL S. SABEL, MD
Associate Professor of Surgery, Department of Surgery, University of Michigan Comprehensive Cancer Center, Ann Arbor, Michigan

GEORGE W. SLEDGE Jr, MD
Indiana University Simon Cancer Center, Indianapolis, Indiana

JOSEPH A. SPARANO, MD
Department of Medicine and Oncology, Albert Einstein College of Medicine; Montefiore Medical Center, Bronx, New York

D. LAWRENCE WICKERHAM, MD
Associate Chairman, National Surgical Adjuvant Breast and Bowel Project (NSABP); Chief, Section of Cancer Genetics and Prevention, Allegheny General Hospital; Associate Professor of Human Oncology, Drexel University School of Medicine, Pittsburgh, Pennsylvania

Contents

Foreword   xiii

Nicholas J. Petrelli

Preface   xv

Eleftherios P. Mamounas

Erratum   xvii

Breast Cancer Chemoprevention: Progress and Controversy   463

D. Lawrence Wickerham

> The chemoprevention of breast cancer using pharmacologic agents has had substantial clinical success. Randomized clinical trials evaluating selective estrogen-receptor modulators (SERMs) have shown that these agents reduce the incidence of breast cancer by up to 50% in healthy women at increased risk for the development of the disease. SERMs have been of particular value in women with biopsy-proven risk factors, including atypical hyperplasia or lobular carcinoma in situ of the breast. The agents of established value are important options for women today, and efforts are under way to identify additional more effective therapies.

Magnetic Resonance Imaging for Screening, Diagnosis, and Eligibility for Breast-conserving Surgery: Promises and Pitfalls   475

Monica Morrow

> Magnetic resonance imaging (MRI) is able to visualize small tumor deposits that previously could only be identified on pathologic examination. MRI is most valuable in areas in which patient management has been problematic, including screening women with known or suspected BRCA 1 and 2 mutations, and identification of the primary tumor site in patients presenting with axillary adenopathy. The role of MRI in the patient with newly diagnosed breast cancer remains controversial. Success rates for patients selected for breast-conserving therapy without MRI are high, and rates of ipsilateral breast tumor recurrence are low. Future efforts to improve the local therapy for breast cancer must acknowledge the heterogeneity of the disease and tailor approaches to the biology of individual subsets. This goal can only be accomplished through a multidisciplinary approach that examines the applications of newer diagnostic modalities such as MRI.

Clinical Significance of Minimal Sentinel Node Involvement and Management Options   493

Anees B. Chagpar

> Since its introduction in the mid-1990s, sentinel lymph node (SLN) biopsy has revolutionized the management of breast cancer patients, allowing for

a minimally invasive method to accurately stage the axilla without the need for axillary lymph node dissection and its concomitant morbidity in node-negative patients. The ability to identify the lymph nodes most likely to harbor metastases has allowed for increased scrutiny of these lymph nodes, often finding minimal disease in the SLNs. The relevance of such minute disease has been controversial, and there has been considerable debate as to how best to manage such patients.

Clinical Significance and Management of Extra-Axillary Sentinel Lymph Nodes: Worthwhile or Irrelevant?   507

Hiram S. Cody III

Nonaxillary drainage is demonstrable by lymphoscintigraphy in up to one-third of breast cancer patients, and nonaxillary sentinel lymph node (SLN) biopsy (most frequently of the internal mammary nodes) is the subject of a growing body of literature. It is not yet clear that the identification of non-axillary SLN significantly affects treatment or outcome in patients with primary operable disease. The greatest future potential for nonaxillary SLNs biopsy is in the management of patients with ipsilateral breast tumor recurrence, where prior axillary surgery may have unpredictably altered the lymphatic drainage of the breast.

Sentinel Lymph Node Biopsy Before or After Neoadjuvant Chemotherapy: Pros and Cons   519

Michael S. Sabel

This article summarizes the relative pros and cons surrounding the timing of sentinel lymph node (SLN) biopsy in patients undergoing neoadjuvant chemotherapy. Several institutions initiated prospective trials of SLN biopsy performed after neoadjuvant chemotherapy in conjunction with a completion axillary lymph node dissection, with the goal of ultimately showing that SLN biopsy could be safely and accurately performed after the patient completed systemic therapy. Other institutions adopted a policy of performing SLN biopsy before initiation of chemotherapy. This avoided the issue surrounding the accuracy of SLN biopsy after chemotherapy and potentially provided information that might influence adjuvant therapy decisions. This article addresses the clinical questions regarding the 2 approaches including the accuracy of the procedure and the prognostic information gleaned.

Sentinel Lymph Node Surgery in Uncommon Clinical Circumstances   539

Bijan Ansari and Judy C. Boughey

Sentinel lymph node (SLN) surgery has largely replaced axillary dissection for nodal staging in clinically node negative breast cancer patients. However, in patients with previous breast and/or axillary surgery, pregnant patients, male patients, multifocal/multicentric breast tumors, DCIS, and patients receiving neoadjuvant chemotherapy, the use of SLN surgery is more controversial. Lymphoscintigraphy is important in patients with prior surgery to evaluate for drainage to extra-axillary sites.

Total Skin Sparing (Nipple Sparing) Mastectomy: What is the Evidence?   555

Amar Gupta and Patrick Ivan Borgen

The surgical treatment of breast cancer has evolved from radical mastectomy with routine removal of the nipple-areolar complex (NAC) to breast conservative therapy with preservation of the breast and NAC. Each step along this evolutionary process was met with criticism, skepticism, controversy, anger, emotion, and often bitter and impassioned debate. Today we find ourselves at yet another therapeutic decision point: the management of the skin of the nipple-areolar complex in mastectomy. Enhanced understanding of the pathogenesis of breast cancer coupled with rising interest in improved cosmesis has led to the investigation of the skin-sparing and nipple-sparing mastectomy as potential modifications to conventional mastectomy.

Oncoplastic Surgery: A Creative Approach to Breast Cancer Management   567

Gail S. Lebovic

Oncoplastic surgery combines the principles of surgical oncology with those of plastic and reconstructive surgery. The intent is to use established techniques from each field in order to provide adequate tumor resection without compromise while optimizing aesthetic outcomes. This patient-centered approach requires a multidisciplinary preoperative evaluation in order to devise a comprehensive surgical plan and coordinate adjuvant treatment as needed. This article provides a historical perspective as well as insight into various creative techniques for breast cancer surgery.

Clinical Application of Gene Expression Profiling in Breast Cancer   581

Joseph A. Sparano, Melissa Fazzari, and Paraic A. Kenny

Breast cancer is a heterogeneous disease associated with variable clinical outcomes and response to therapy. Classic clinicopathologic factors associated with outcome include anatomic features associated with prognosis (eg, tumor size, number of positive regional lymph nodes) and biologic features associated with prognosis and/or predictive of response to specific therapies, usually by evaluating protein expression by immunohistochemistry (eg, estrogen and/or progesterone receptors) or amplification of a single gene (eg, HER2/neu). Gene expression profiling evaluating thousands of genes is now feasible, and has facilitated the development of multiparameter assays that may identify breast cancer subtypes associated with distinct clinical outcomes that were not previously recognized, or provide more accurate information about prognosis or response to specific therapies than may be provided by classic clinicopathologic features alone. Several multiparameter gene expression assays are commercially available, and additional assays are being developed that will facilitate more accurate therapeutic individualization.

Neoadjuvant Chemotherapy for Operable Breast Cancer: Individualizing Locoregional and Systemic Therapy   607

Harry D. Bear

Neoadjuvant chemotherapy (NAC) is being used with increasing frequency in the multidisciplinary care of women with breast cancer. NAC can increase the chances for successful breast conservation and may decrease the need for axillary node dissection in selected patients. Some patients with chemoresistant tumors may benefit more from hormonal neoadjuvant therapy. The greatest potential for this approach is to predict responses of different breast cancers to therapy based on molecular profiles. This will accelerate better understanding of breast cancer biology and progress toward improved and more individualized therapy.

Neoadjuvant Endocrine Therapy for Breast Cancer   627

Jane S. Chawla, Cynthia X. Ma, and Matthew J. Ellis

Neoadjuvant endocrine therapy improves surgical outcomes for postmenopausal women with bulky hormone receptor–positive breast cancer. Recent studies indicate that this approach may also be used in the management of smaller tumors with the hope of predicting outcomes from adjuvant endocrine manipulation. Neoadjuvant endocrine therapy provides a unique opportunity to identify molecular predictors of endocrine responsiveness and agents that can be used in combination with endocrine therapy to improve tumor response and overcome endocrine resistance.

Adjuvant Hormonal Therapy for Early-Stage Breast Cancer   639

Harold J. Burstein and Jennifer J. Griggs

Adjuvant endocrine treatment is an essential component in therapy for hormone receptor–positive breast cancer. Among postmenopausal patients, options include tamoxifen, aromatase inhibitors, or a sequence of these agents. Tamoxifen and aromatase inhibitors have distinctive side-effect profiles. Among premenopausal women, tamoxifen remains the standard treatment. The role of ovarian suppression in addition to tamoxifen is under investigation. Questions about the duration of adjuvant endocrine therapy, the use of biomarkers for treatment selection and prognosis, and the management of side effects of adjuvant endocrine therapy remain key areas of investigation.

Adjuvant Chemotherapy in Early-Stage Breast Cancer: What, When, and for Whom?   649

Catherine M. Kelly and Gabriel N. Hortobagyi

Adjuvant chemotherapy is effective in reducing the risk of recurrence and death from breast cancer. Tumor stage and biologic characteristics are important when making decisions about who should receive chemotherapy and what chemotherapy to give. The results of ongoing clinical trials will establish whether more precise determination of prognosis and populations most likely and least likely to benefit from specific therapies can improve the efficacy and reduce the toxicity of systemic treatments. As individual tumors are molecularly characterized and molecularly targeted therapies are clinically validated, "personalized" adjuvant therapy will become a reality in the not too distant future.

Targeted Therapies in Early-Stage Breast Cancer: Achievements and Promises   669

George W. Sledge Jr, Aparna C. Jotwani, and Lida Mina

One of the most impressive changes in the therapeutic landscape of breast cancer in the past decade has been the advent of targeted therapies for specific subtypes. This article discusses the meaning of targeted therapy and examines the genomic basis for targeted therapy as it has emerged over the past decade. Human epidermal growth factor receptor 2 (HER2)–targeted therapy, the principle example of targeted therapy to enter the adjuvant arena in the past decade, is described in depth. Novel targeted therapies under development, many currently being examined in the adjuvant setting, are also explored, including anti–vascular endothelial growth factor therapy, poly (ADP ribose) polymerase (PARP) inhibition for triple-negative breast cancers, and agents targeting site-specific metastasis to the bone (receptor activator of NF-kB [RANK] ligand inhibition). Chemotherapy, the epitome of nonspecific anticancer therapy, is in the process of becoming targeted therapy as understanding of breast cancer biology improves.

Index   681

FORTHCOMING ISSUES

October 2010
Colorectal Cancer
Jose Guillem, MD, *Guest Editor*

January 2011
Melanoma
Jeffrey Gershenwald, MD, *Guest Editor*

RECENT ISSUES

April 2010
Pancreatic Cancer: Current Concepts
in Treatment and Research
Andrew M. Lowy, MD, *Guest Editor*

January 2010
Randomized Clinical Trials in Surgical
Oncology
Adam C. Yopp, MD, and
Ronald P. DeMatteo, MD,
Guest Editors

October 2009
Hereditary Colorectal Cancer
Steven Gallinger, MD, *Guest Editor*

RELATED INTEREST

PET Clinics, July 2009 (Vol. 4, Issue 3)
Breast Cancer Imaging I
Rakesh Kumar, MD, Sandip Basu, MD, and Abass Alavi, MD, *Guest Editors*

THE CLINICS ARE NOW AVAILABLE ONLINE!

Access your subscription at:
www.theclinics.com

Foreword

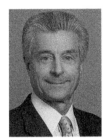

Nicholas J. Petrelli, MD
Consulting Editor

This issue of the *Surgical Oncology Clinics of North America* is devoted to breast cancer. The last edition of the *Clinics* on breast cancer was in 2005; hence, it is time for an update. The Guest Editor for this edition is Eleftherios Mamounas, MD, MPH, FACS, professor of surgery at Northeastern Ohio University College of Medicine in Rootstown, Ohio. Dr Mamounas is also medical director of the Aultman Cancer Center in Canton, Ohio, and chair of the Breast Committee of the National Surgical Adjuvant Breast and Bowel Project. He has held this latter position since 1997. Perhaps the best way to describe Dr Mamounas is by a direct quotation from the last National Surgical Adjuvant Breast and Bowel Project cooperative group National Cancer Institute site report, which described Dr Mamounas as a "strong, extremely knowledgeable and capable surgical oncologist...who does an impressive job with coordinating a very powerful cadre of other surgeons and medical oncologists that serve on this committee."

This edition of the *Surgical Oncology Clinics of North America* contains 14 articles. It covers many areas, including the role of MRI for screening, diagnosis, and eligibility for breast-conserving surgery, as discussed by Dr Monica Morrow from Memorial Sloan-Kettering Cancer Center, to neoadjuvant chemotherapy for operable breast cancer by Dr Harry Bear from Virginia Commonwealth University. Additional areas discussed are sentinel node biopsy before or after neoadjuvant chemotherapy by Dr Michael Sabel from the University of Michigan and targeted therapies in early-stage breast cancer by Dr George Sledge and associates from Indiana University's Simon Cancer Center.

Dr Mamounas discusses in his preface the reasons that since the mid-1980s there has been a worldwide steady decline in breast cancer mortality that has persisted to date without any evidence of a slow down. According to the American Cancer Society, breast cancer rates have risen approximately 30% in the past 25 years in Western countries, the reason in part due to increased screening discovering the cancer in its earliest stages. In the United States, breast cancer rates decreased by 10% between 2000 and 2004 due in part to a reduction in the use of hormone replacement therapy. Although breast cancer rates are rising in many Western countries, deaths from the

Surg Oncol Clin N Am 19 (2010) xiii–xiv
doi:10.1016/j.soc.2010.04.008
surgonc.theclinics.com
1055-3207/10/$ – see front matter © 2010 Elsevier Inc. All rights reserved.

disease have decreased in many countries as a result of improved screening and treatment.

Dr Mamounas and his colleagues continue to research surrogate endpoint biomarkers to serve as early indicators of treatment effectiveness along with developing better breast imaging and other technologies for the diagnosis of breast cancer. Together with research in the academic centers and the National Cancer Institute cooperative groups clinical trials process, we will continue to advance in the prevention, early diagnosis, and treatment of breast cancer.

I would like to thank Dr Mamounas and his colleagues for this edition of the *Surgical Oncology Clinics of North America*, which can serve as a practical resource for physicians and individuals in training.

Nicholas J. Petrelli, MD
Helen F. Graham Cancer Center
4701 Ogletown-Stanton Road, Suite 1213
Newark, DE 19713, USA

E-mail address:
npetrelli@christianacare.org

Preface

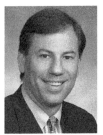

Eleftherios P. Mamounas, MD, MPH
Guest Editor

To say that our understanding of the biology of early-stage breast cancer and the management of this disease underwent significant evolution in the last quarter of the twentieth century is an understatement. During that time, the postulation of an alternative hypothesis of tumor dissemination challenged the previously accepted Halstedian principles and eventually led to the establishment of breast-conserving surgery and adjuvant systemic therapy as accepted standards of care. In addition, the introduction and widespread use of screening mammography and an increased awareness of breast cancer in the general public dramatically changed the landscape of disease presentation, allowing considerably more options for patients. As a result of these developments, since the mid-1980s there has been a worldwide, steady decline in breast cancer mortality that has persisted to date without evidence of a slowdown.

Over the past decade, there have been extraordinary developments in breast cancer research and clinical management. The introduction of molecular classification of breast cancer and the subsequent clinical application of genomic profiling in patients with early-stage disease; the adoption of sentinel node biopsy as the standard of care for staging the axilla; and the successful introduction of targeted biologic therapies, such as trastuzumab, lapatinib, and bevacizumab, in the clinic represent significant milestones in the fight against breast cancer. Improvements in imaging modalities, adjuvant endocrine therapy, and adjuvant chemotherapy have also played a major role in the continuing improvement in breast cancer outcomes.

Some of these remarkable changes have come with considerable controversy as we continue to work toward their integration into everyday clinical practice. This issue of the *Surgical Oncology Clinics of North America* is devoted primarily to the review and discussion of some of these new developments and areas of debate. D. Lawrence Wickerham discusses the recent advancements and remaining areas of controversy in breast cancer chemoprevention. Monica Morrow reviews promises and pitfalls with the application of MRI for screening, diagnosis, and eligibility for breast-conserving surgery. Several articles address controversial and timely topics surrounding sentinel node biopsy. Anees Chagpar discusses the clinical significance

Surg Oncol Clin N Am 19 (2010) xv–xvi
doi:10.1016/j.soc.2010.04.007
1055-3207/10/$ – see front matter
surgonc.theclinics.com

of minimal sentinel node involvement and appropriate management options, a topic that clinicians are being confronted with at tumor board conferences on a daily basis. Hiram Cody addresses controversies over the clinical significance and management of extra-axillary sentinel lymph nodes. Michael Sabel thoroughly reviews and discusses the controversial topic of timing of sentinel lymph node biopsy in patients treated with neoadjuvant chemotherapy. Bijan Ansari and Judy Boughey review current knowledge of the use of sentinel lymph node biopsy in uncommon clinical circumstances. The last two surgical articles, by Amar Gupta/Patrick Borgen and Gail Lebovic, address two areas in primary breast cancer surgery that have attracted considerable attention in the past few years, namely the role of total skin-sparing (nipple-sparing) mastectomy and the role of oncoplastic surgery.

Following the theme of treatment individualization, Joseph Sparano and his colleagues provide an excellent assessment of the current status and clinical application of gene expression profiling in early-stage breast cancer, a development that has dramatically changed how breast cancer is viewed and treated today. Subsequently, Harry Bear discusses the topic of neoadjuvant chemotherapy as a way to individualize locoregional and systemic therapy, and Matthew Ellis and colleagues address the emerging field of neoadjuvant endocrine therapy, a topic that has gained importance as the biology of breast cancer subtypes becomes better defined. Harold Burstein and Jennifer Griggs review recent developments in adjuvant endocrine therapy, one of the most successful treatments in breast cancer, and Catherine Kelly and Gabriel Hortobagyi address new developments in adjuvant chemotherapy, such as the incorporation of taxanes and the use of genomic classifiers to select appropriate chemotherapy candidates. Last but not least, George Sledge and colleagues present an outstanding discussion on the achievements and promises of biologic targeted therapies in early-stage breast cancer.

A common theme with all these articles—whether or not they address surgical or adjuvant therapy questions or prognostic and predictive markers—is that of treatment tailoring and the use of clinical and biologic parameters to help match the right patient to the right treatment. This approach promises not only to increase the efficacy of existing and new therapies but also to eliminate unnecessary toxicity for patients who would not benefit.

I would like to express my gratitude to all the authors for their enthusiastic support of this issue. They are all dedicated clinicians and scientists and their high-quality articles serve as yet another testimony to their knowledge, expertise, and leadership in the field of breast cancer. My sincere thanks also go to Catherine Bewick for her dedication in seeing this work completed in a timely fashion.

I hope that the readers enjoy this issue and find the articles thought provoking and a good reference source for everyday practice.

Eleftherios P. Mamounas, MD, MPH
Aultman Cancer Center
2600 6th Street, SW
Canton, OH 44710, USA

Northeastern Ohio Universities College of Medicine
Rootstown, OH, USA

E-mail address:
tmamounas@aultman.com

Erratum

A typographical error appeared within a table in the article, "Status of Neoadjuvant Therapy for Resectable Pancreatic Cancer," by Dr John P. Hoffman, published in the April 2010 issue of the *Surgical Oncology Clinics of North America*. In Table 1, the last two words in the top row of the first column should have been "portal vein." The Publisher apologizes for this error.

Refers to: Status of Neoadjuvant Therapy for Resectable Pancreatic Cancer, Volume 19, Issue 2, April 2010, Pages 411–418, John P. Hoffman, MD.

Surg Oncol Clin N Am 19 (2010) xvii
doi:10.1016/j.soc.2010.04.009
1055-3207/10/$ – see front matter © 2010 Elsevier Inc. All rights reserved.

Breast Cancer Chemoprevention: Progress and Controversy

D. Lawrence Wickerham, MD[a,b,c,*]

KEYWORDS

• Breast cancer • Chemoprevention • Tamoxifen • Raloxifene

Despite newer, more effective treatments and improvements in detection, there were more than 42,000 deaths from breast cancer in the United States in 2009, according to the American Cancer Society.[1] Because breast cancer is a major health problem for all women, the concept of preventing the disease is an attractive addition to the established roles of screening and treatment. Prophylactic mastectomy is an effective approach that reduces the risk of developing a breast cancer by an estimated 90% or more.[2] However, it is a drastic and irreversible choice that is perhaps best reserved for women with high risk of the disease, such as those with known deleterious BRCA1 or 2 mutations. This article focuses on nonsurgical approaches to reducing breast cancer risk.

Some of the risk factors associated with breast cancer are modifiable, such as postmenopausal obesity, alcohol intake, and dietary fat. Reducing weight, exercising, low-fat diets, and moderation of alcohol intake are healthy behaviors. Such lifestyle modifications for breast cancer risk reduction remain an active area of research but are not yet of established value. The factors that place a woman at greatest risk (gender, age, and family history) are not amenable to lifestyle modifications.

Hong and Sporn[3] have defined chemoprevention as "the use of pharmacologic or natural agents that inhibit the development of invasive breast cancer either by

This work was supported by Grant Nos. U10CA37377and U10CA69974 from the National Institutes of Health.
Dr Wickerham is a consultant to Eli Lilly and Company and has received honoraria from AstraZeneca.

a National Surgical Adjuvant Breast and Bowel Project (NSABP), Four Allegheny Center – 5th Floor, Pittsburgh, PA 15212, USA
b Section of Cancer Genetics and Prevention, Allegheny General Hospital, Pittsburgh, PA, USA
c Pittsburgh Campus, Drexel University School of Medicine, Pittsburgh, PA, USA
* National Surgical Adjuvant Breast and Bowel Project (NSABP), Four Allegheny Center – 5th Floor, Pittsburgh, PA 15212.
E-mail address: larry.wickerham@nsabp.org

Surg Oncol Clin N Am 19 (2010) 463–473
doi:10.1016/j.soc.2010.03.005
1055-3207/10/$ – see front matter © 2010 Elsevier Inc. All rights reserved.

blocking the DNA damage that initiates carcinogenesis or by arresting or reversing the progression of premalignant cells in which such damage has already occurred."

SELECTED ESTROGEN RECEPTOR MODULATORS

Although the precise mechanism or mechanisms that cause a breast cancer are not fully established, hormones play a significant role in a large percentage of cases, and current chemoprevention strategies have targeted hormonally responsive breast cancers. The selective estrogen receptor modulators (SERMs) are the group of agents that have been evaluated the most, and the best known of these drugs is tamoxifen. Tamoxifen is a well-established adjuvant therapy for receptor-positive breast cancer that has been shown repeatedly to reduce the risk of recurrence and death from this disease.[4] In the large trials that showed tamoxifen to be an effective adjuvant treatment, there was also a substantial reduction in new primary cancers of the opposite breast. The duration of tamoxifen therapy in these studies varied from 1 to 5 years, but the reduction in opposite breast cancer persisted through at least 15 years of follow-up, showing this to be a durable, if not lifelong, benefit.

TAMOXIFEN CHEMOPREVENTION TRIALS

The findings from the adjuvant trials, combined with extensive laboratory data documenting the potential of tamoxifen as a chemoprevention agent, led to the initial randomized breast cancer chemoprevention trials. The largest of these trials was the National Surgical Adjuvant Breast and Bowel Project (NSABP) Breast Cancer Prevention Trial, P-1, which randomized more than 13,000 healthy women from centers in North America to receive 20 mg of tamoxifen daily or placebo for a 5-year period (**Fig. 1A**).[5,6]

Eligible participants for the trial were at increased risk for breast cancer, which was defined as having 5-year projected invasive breast cancer risk of at least 1.66% as determined by the modified Gail model or having a history of lobular carcinoma in situ (LCIS) treated by local excision alone, or being at least 60 years of age. Women were not eligible for the trial if they had a history of deep vein thrombosis (DVT), a pulmonary embolus (PE), or if they had taken hormone therapy, oral contraceptives, or androgens within 3 months before random assignment into the trial. Estrogen or combinations of estrogen-progestin therapy were not permitted during the course

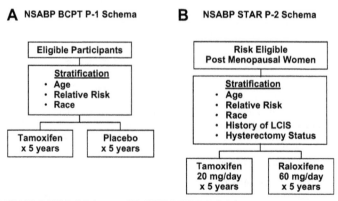

Fig. 1. (A) NSABP BCPT P-1 Schema. (B) NSABP STAR P-2 Schema.

of the study. The primary end point of the trial was the incidence of invasive breast cancer. Secondary end points included all other invasive cancers, noninvasive breast cancers, osteoporotic bone fracture, cardiac events, quality of life measurements, and death from any cause.

The initial results were published in 1998, with an average follow-up of approximately 4 years, and showed a highly significant 49% reduction in invasive breast cancer in favor of the tamoxifen-treated women (relative risk [RR] = 0.51, 95% confidence interval [CI] 0.39–0.66).[5] The rate of noninvasive breast cancers (ductal carcinoma in situ [DCIS] and LCIS combined) was reduced by a similar magnitude. The reduction of invasive breast cancer appeared to be only in estrogen-receptor (ER)-positive cases, with a 69% reduction in incidence; there was no difference between the treatment groups in terms of the incidence of ER-negative disease.

Evaluation of secondary end points showed a 45% reduction in the number of osteoporotic fractures with tamoxifen (79 in the placebo group and 49 in the tamoxifen group). Tamoxifen was known to reduce blood lipids, but there was no reduction in the risk of myocardial infarction, severe angina, or acute ischemic syndrome noted in the tamoxifen-treated group compared with the placebo group. There were 28 cases of myocardial infarction in the placebo group and 39 in the tamoxifen-treated group (RR = 1.11; 95% CI 0.65–1.92). There were no significant statistical differences in the other 2 cardiac end points.

The toxicity associated with tamoxifen has been well documented in the treatment trials for invasive breast cancer and includes increases in the risk of endometrial cancer and thromboembolic events. Both of these toxicities were identified in the P-1 trial as well: the RR of endometrial adenocarcinoma was 2.53 (95% CI 1.35–4.97), with 15 cases occurring in the placebo group compared with 36 in the tamoxifen group. No excess of endometrial cancer was noted in the women younger than the age of 50 years, primarily a premenopausal group, at the time of random assignment. Thromboembolic events were also associated with tamoxifen use, and the magnitude of risk seems to be similar to that for postmenopausal women who take estrogen-replacement therapy. There was a 60% increase in the risk of DVT (RR = 1.60; 95% CI 0.91–2.86), with 22 cases occurring in the placebo group and 35 in the tamoxifen group. The risk of pulmonary embolism was also increased 3-fold (RR = 3.10; 95% CI 1.15–9.27), with 6 cases occurring in the placebo group and 18 in the tamoxifen group. There was a slight increase in strokes among women on tamoxifen, although it did not reach statistical significance. As with the endometrial cancer data, the increase in thromboembolic events appeared predominantly in women older than 50 years at the time they entered the trial.

The data for the use of tamoxifen in women with BRCA1 or BRCA2 inherited mutations are limited, and definitive statements about the effectiveness of tamoxifen in such patients are not available. In the P-1 trial, King and colleagues[7] identified only 18 women with inherited BRCA1 or BRCA2 mutations. Although tamoxifen reduced breast cancer incidence among BRCA2 carriers by 62%, this reduction was not statistically significant given the small numbers of patients out of the 13,000-plus women who entered the trial. Patients with BRCA2 frequently develop ER-positive breast cancers, although not uniformly. In the patients with BRCA1 noted in the P-1 trial, there was also no significant benefit from tamoxifen; there were numerically more cancers in the tamoxifen group. Narod and colleagues[8] published a matched case-control study that reported significant protection from contralateral breast cancer in women with BRCA1 mutations who developed an invasive breast cancer and were treated with tamoxifen. A lesser effect was seen in women with BRCA2 mutations. That report and the P-1 data suggest that women with BRCA1 or BRCA2 mutations who have or will develop ER-positive breast cancer are potential candidates for tamoxifen therapy, but at the present time it is not possible to determine which women with BRCA1 or BRCA2 mutations will develop ER-positive disease.

All the various subgroups of women in the P-1 trial appeared to benefit from the use of tamoxifen, including pre- and postmenopausal women as well as those with Gail scores ranging from 1.66% to more than 5%. The group that seems to have the greatest benefit is those women with a biopsy-proven history of LCIS or atypical hyperplasia. Such women are known to have a risk of subsequent invasive breast cancer that is 4- to 10-fold greater. In the P-1 trial, the annual breast cancer rate per 1000 women in the placebo arm with a history of LCIS at the time of entry was 12.99, and for those with a prior history of atypical hyperplasia, 10.11 (**Fig. 2**A). Both groups showed a substantial benefit from tamoxifen, with a 56% reduction in invasive breast cancer in women with LCIS and an 86% reduction in those with atypical hyperplasia.

ADDITIONAL TAMOXIFEN BREAST CANCER PREVENTION TRIALS

Several additional tamoxifen breast cancer prevention trials have been performed with different designs and sample sizes, and as a result have produced somewhat variable results. The International Breast Cancer Intervention Study (IBIS I) evaluated 7145 women, aged 35 to 70 years, who were at increased risk for breast cancer and randomly assigned them to receive either 20 mg of tamoxifen or placebo for a 5-year period. The initial results published in 2002 with 49 months of median follow-up reported that tamoxifen reduced the risk of ER-positive breast cancer by 31%, and the updated results showed that these benefits persisted with 12 years of follow-up.[9,10]

The Royal Marsden Trial began as a pilot study in 1986 to evaluate the feasibility of conducting tamoxifen prevention trials. In a 10-year period, 2471 participants entered the study and were assigned either tamoxifen, 20 mg per day, or placebo for an 8-year period. The initial analysis was published in 1998 and reported no reduction in breast cancer incidence.[11] However, a more recent paper with a median follow-up of 13 years shows a statistically significant reduction in ER-positive breast cancer.[12]

The Italian Tamoxifen Prevention Study enrolled 5408 women, aged 35 to 70 years, to receive either tamoxifen or placebo, but the study was not restricted to women at increased risk for breast cancer. The initial results of this trial failed to show an overall benefit of tamoxifen, but in a subset of 1580 women who had used estrogen-replacement therapy at some point during the trial, there were 23 breast cancers (17 in the placebo group and 6 in the tamoxifen group).[13] This finding led to the Hormone-Replacement Therapy (HRT) Opposed to Tamoxifen (HOT) Study to evaluate tamoxifen, 5 mg per day, in women taking HRT.

An overview of the tamoxifen prevention trials was released in 2003 and reported a 37% decrease in invasive breast cancer in a combined tamoxifen treatment group.[14] An update of this overview is currently being analyzed but has not yet been published.

RALOXIFENE STUDIES

Raloxifene is a second-generation SERM that was originally developed as a breast cancer treatment for receptor-positive tumor. The results of the initial trial showed limited effectiveness, and further examination for its use in breast cancer treatment was discontinued. Raloxifene has well-established favorable effects on bone metabolism in postmenopausal women, and the pivotal raloxifene study that led to its approval by the US Food and Drug Administration for the treatment of osteoporosis was the Multiple Outcomes of Raloxifene Evaluation (MORE) study.[15] The MORE

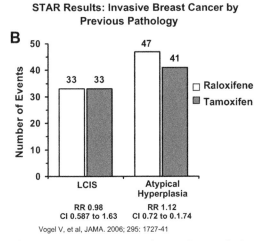

Fig. 2. (A) BCPT Results: Invasive Breast Cancer by Previous Pathology. (B) STAR Results: Invasive Breast Cancer by Previous Pathology (*Data from* Fisher B, Costantino J, Wickerham DL, et al. Tamoxifen for the prevention of breast cancer: current status of the National Surgical Adjuvant Breast and Bowel Project P-1 study. J Natl Cancer Inst 2005;97:1652–62; and Vogel VG, Costantino JP, Wickerham DL, et al. Effects of tamoxifen vs raloxifene on the risk of developing invasive breast cancer and other disease outcomes: the NSABP study of tamoxifen and raloxifene (STAR) P-2 trial. JAMA 2006;295:2727–41.).

trial randomly assigned 7705 postmenopausal women with osteoporosis to receive raloxifene, 60 mg per day or 120 mg per day, compared with placebo. The participants received the study drug daily for up to 4 years. The primary objective of this multicenter international trial was to evaluate the effects of raloxifene compared with placebo on the incidence of osteoporotic fracture and bone mineral density in this population of women. Breast cancer was a secondary end point, and participants were not selected or prospectively evaluated for their breast cancer risk. The initial

MORE results reported a significant reduction in vertebral fractures in the raloxifene-treated women, but the incidence of nonvertebral fractures was not significantly different. In the raloxifene-treated group, the risk of invasive breast cancer was significantly reduced after 4 years by 72% (RR = 0.28; 95% CI 0.17–0.46). As was noted in the tamoxifen trial, the benefits appeared to be specific to receptor-positive invasive breast cancer. An increased risk in thromboembolic events, including DVT and pulmonary embolism, was identified (RR = 3.1; 95% CI 1.5–6.2), but unlike what occurs with tamoxifen, there was no difference in the incidence of endometrial carcinoma. The Continuing Outcomes Relevant to Evista (CORE) trial was a double-blind, placebo-controlled study that evaluated the efficacy of an additional 4 years of raloxifene compared with placebo in reducing the risk of invasive breast cancer in women who had participated in the MORE trial.[16] The primary breast cancer analysis included 3996 patients who had completed MORE and agreed to enter CORE, and data from an additional 1217 patients who were still participating in MORE when CORE began. The incidence of invasive breast cancer was reduced by 59% (hazard ratio [HR] = 0.41; 95% CI 0.24–0.71) in women in the raloxifene-treated group compared with those in the placebo group. During 8 years of both trials, the incidence of invasive breast cancer was reduced by 66% (HR = 0.34; 95% CI 0.22–0.50); no new safety concerns related to raloxifene were identified.

THE STUDY OF TAMOXIFEN AND RALOXIFENE TRIAL, NSABP P-2

The initial results of the NSABP tamoxifen-versus-placebo trial, P-1, were published in 1998 and reported that tamoxifen could reduce the incidence of breast cancer by up to almost 50% in a population of healthy women at increased risk for the future development of breast cancer. The raloxifene studies reported a reduction in breast cancer incidence in an unselected population, making the Study of Tamoxifen and Raloxifene (STAR) trial the next logical step. This study was a double-blind and randomized clinical trial that entered 19,747 postmenopausal women who were at least 35 years of age and had a history of LCIS treated by local incision alone or a modified Gail score showing a 5-year risk for invasive breast cancer of at least 1.66% (see **Fig. 1B**).[17] Women were randomly assigned to take either tamoxifen, 20 mg per day, plus a placebo, or raloxifene, 60 mg per day, plus a placebo, for a 5-year period. The primary end point of the trial was the development of biopsy-proven invasive breast cancer. The secondary end points included noninvasive breast cancer, uterine malignancies, thromboembolic events, fractures, cataracts, quality of life, and death from any cause. To minimize the risk of stroke or thromboembolic events, eligible participants could not have a history of cerebral vascular accidents, transient ischemic attack (TIA), pulmonary embolism, DVT, uncontrolled diabetes, uncontrolled hypertension, or atrial fibrillation. The median 5-year risk of developing invasive breast cancer based on the modified Gail score was 4.03%, and the projected lifetime risk for these women to age 80 years was 14%. Seven percent of the women entering the trial had 1 or more first-degree relatives with breast cancer, and more than 9% had a history of LCIS. More than 22% had had a breast biopsy before enrollment that showed either atypical ductal or atypical lobular hyperplasia. Slightly more than 6% of the participants had undergone a hysterectomy, with or without oopherectomy, before random assignment.

The initial results from the STAR trial showed there was no difference in the effects in tamoxifen or raloxifene on the incidence of invasive breast cancer: 163 of the women assigned tamoxifen and 168 of those assigned raloxifene developed an invasive breast cancer. The rate per 1000 woman years was 4.3 in the tamoxifen group and 4.4 in the raloxifene group (RR = 1.02; 95% CI 0.82–1.28). Although there was no placebo-alone group in the trial, the Gail model scores of the women who entered the trial allow us to estimate the number of invasive breast cancers that would have occurred in the untreated group and showed that there was a 47% reduction in the incidence of invasive breast cancer. The characteristics of the invasive breast cancers showed no differences between the treatment groups with regard to distribution by tumor size, nodal status, or ER level.

Raloxifene did not seem to be as effective as tamoxifen in reducing the incidence of noninvasive breast cancers (LCIS or DCIS), although the difference did not reach statistical significance. There were 57 cases of noninvasive breast cancer among the women assigned to tamoxifen and 80 among those who took raloxifene (RR = 1.40; 95% CI 0.98–2.00).

More uterine malignancies occurred in STAR in the tamoxifen-treated women than in those treated with raloxifene, but the difference was not statistically significant at the time of the original analysis. There were 36 cases in the tamoxifen group and 23 in the raloxifene group, with an annual incidence rate of 1.99 per 1000 and 1.25 per 1000, respectively (RR = 0.63; 95% CI 0.35–1.08). Uterine hyperplasia with and without atypia was significantly less common in the raloxifene-treated group. There were also significantly fewer hysterectomies performed for nonmalignant indications in the raloxifene group (244 tamoxifen; 111 raloxifene [RR = 0.29; 95% CI 0.30–0.50]). There was no statistically significant difference between the groups in regard to other malignancies.

No statistically significant differences were noted between the 2 groups relative to the incidence of ischemic heart disease, TIA, stroke, or fracture; however, there were significantly fewer thromboembolic events (DVT or PE) in the raloxifene-treated group. Fewer women on raloxifene developed cataracts during treatment, and fewer underwent surgical removal of those cataracts. Mortality within the 2 groups was similar, with 101 deaths in those assigned to tamoxifen and 96 deaths in those assigned to raloxifene (RR = 0.94; 95% CI 0.71–1.26). The distribution by cause of death did not differ by treatment.

Data from the STAR trial and the other raloxifene/placebo trial resulted in the approval of raloxifene by the US Food and Drug Administration for a reduction in the risk of invasive breast cancer in postmenopausal women with osteoporosis and reduction in risk of invasive breast cancer in postmenopausal women at high risk of invasive breast cancer. No data are currently available on the use of raloxifene in patients with BRCA1 or BRCA2 mutations, nor was raloxifene approved for women with a previous invasive breast cancer or for the treatment of invasive breast cancer. However, the approval of raloxifene gives an important new option to postmenopausal women beyond that of tamoxifen, one that avoids an excess of endometrial cancers and reduces the risk of thromboembolic events. The optimum duration of raloxifene therapy for breast cancer prevention has not been established. The drug was used for a period of 5 years in the STAR trial based on the standard 5-year duration of treatment with tamoxifen. The MORE/CORE combined results of 8 years of treatment reported a continued benefit of breast cancer risk reduction as well as risk reduction in bone fractures without increased or new toxicities being identified. In the MORE trial, the number needed to treat to prevent 1 invasive breast cancer in the population of postmenopausal women with osteoporosis was 91, which compares favorably with the number needed to prevent a myocardial infarction with a statin.

There continues to be a concern that raloxifene does not seem to be as effective as tamoxifen in preventing the development of noninvasive breast cancer; this is different from saying there is no effect. At the time of the initial STAR publication, the difference between tamoxifen and raloxifene was not quite statistically significant. A mechanism to explain the difference in noninvasive breast cancer incidence is unknown, but long-term follow-up results for the STAR trial may result in additional information regarding this issue.

ADDITIONAL SERMS

At least 2 additional SERMs are in development and may prove to be of value in breast cancer chemoprevention. The first is lasofoxifene. At the 2008 San Antonio Breast Cancer Symposium, the results of the Postmenopausal Evaluation and Risk Reduction with Lasofoxifene (PEARL) Study were presented.[18] This trial included 8556 postmenopausal women with osteoporosis randomly assigned to receive either a placebo or lasofoxifene 0.5 mg per day or 0.25 mg per day. Lasofoxifene reduced the incidence of vertebral and nonvertebral fracture, but there was an increased risk of thromboembolic events. The results showed a significant reduction in invasive breast cancers in the group that received lasofoxifene 0.5 mg per day (HR = 0.15; 95% CI 0.04–0.50). The other SERM being studied is arzoxifene. A large multicenter, placebo-controlled double-blind trial, the Generations Trial, compared arzoxifene, 20 mg per day, versus placebo in 9254 postmenopausal women with osteoporosis or low bone mass.[19] A total 75 breast cancers were identified, 53 in the placebo group and 22 in the arzoxifene group (HR = 0.14; 95% CI 0.25–0.68, $P<.001$). As with the other SERMs, the reduction in breast cancer was primarily in receptor-positive disease. There was a significant reduction in vertebral fractures in favor of the arzoxifene-treated individuals but no significant reduction in nonvertebral fractures.

AROMATASE INHIBITORS

High circulatory estrogen levels, as well as high aromatase levels in breast tissue, have been known to increase breast cancer risk.[20] In postmenopausal women, aromatase inhibitors (AIs) block the production of estrogens in extragonadal peripheral tissues. Circulatory estrogen levels are dramatically reduced, and aromatase activity in the breast may also be influenced. The development of third-generation selective AIs has had a profound effect on the adjuvant treatment of postmenopausal women with receptor-positive breast cancer. In adjuvant trials of various designs, these AIs have resulted in improved disease-free survival and are associated with fewer life-threatening side effects than is tamoxifen.[21–25] Women in these adjuvant trials who received AIs had a decrease in new primary breast cancers of the opposite breast when compared with those who received tamoxifen, which we know to be effective in reducing risk compared with no treatment. A 35% to 50% decrease in opposite breast cancer in AI trials reported to date provides strong clinical evidence that these agents may be superior to tamoxifen in breast cancer chemoprevention.

The adjuvant trial results reporting a reduction in opposite breast cancers in AI-treated women has led to 2 primary prevention trials evaluating AIs in healthy persons at increased risk for the development of breast cancer. The first of these studies is the IBIS II trial, which will randomize 6000 postmenopausal women to receive anastrozole, 1 mg per day, or placebo. The primary end point of the study is the development of breast cancer. Other cancers, toxicities, cognition, and bone effects will also be evaluated. The IBIS II trial is being conducted in 40 centers in the United Kingdom and around the world. The second trial, the MAP-3 study being led by the National Cancer Institute of Canada Clinical Trials Group, will enter 4560 postmenopausal women assigned to receive exemestane, 25 mg per day, or placebo for a 5-year period. Eligible women are those at increased risk for breast cancer, which is defined as being older than 60 years of age or having a Gail score greater than 1.65%, or having a previous breast biopsy documenting atypical hyperplasia of the breast, or LCIS. Also eligible are women who were treated with mastectomy for DCIS. The main objective of this trial is to compare the incidence of breast cancer in the 2 groups. Data will also be collected on bone fractures, cardiovascular events, tolerability and safety, and the incidence of other malignancies.

The IBIS II and MAP-3 trials have placebo-alone control groups. Although this design is scientifically compelling, a direct comparison of either tamoxifen or raloxifene would allow a better risk/benefit evaluation. The IBIS II study does have a separate component for DCIS patients that compares anastrozole with tamoxifen and should allow some insight into the risk/benefit issues. The NSABP has already completed accrual of 3000 patients in the B-35 study, which also evaluates anastrozole and tamoxifen in ER-positive DCIS. The primary study end points of the B-35 trial include ipsilateral and contralateral invasive and noninvasive breast cancers. The B-35 results may be available before those from IBIS II or the MAP-3 prevention trials.

2009 AMERICAN SOCIETY OF CLINICAL ONCOLOGY CLINICAL PRACTICE GUIDELINES ON THE USE OF PHARMACOLOGIC INTERVENTION, INCLUDING TAMOXIFEN, RALOXIFENE, AND AIS, FOR BREAST CANCER RISK REDUCTION

The American Society of Clinical Oncology updated its Clinical Practice Guidelines regarding breast cancer risk reduction in 2009.[26] The original 1999 guidelines and the 2002 update suggest women at increased risk for breast cancer may be offered tamoxifen (20 mg per day for 5 years) to reduce the risk of invasive ER-positive breast cancer, with benefits that persist for at least 10 years.[27,28] Since the publication of the STAR results, the guidelines have been updated and state that for postmenopausal women raloxifene at 60 mg per day may be considered as an additional option. A discussion of risks and benefits by health care providers is believed to be critical to a patient's decision making. The use of AIs and other potential chemopreventive agents is not recommended outside clinical trials.

SUMMARY

Compared with breast cancer screening and treatment, the chemoprevention of this disease is in its infancy. However, SERMs have shown substantial clinical benefit in several large, well-conducted randomized clinical trials. For women with LCIS or atypical hyperplasia of the breast, tamoxifen, and to a lesser degree, raloxifene, are highly effective in reducing the risk of subsequent invasive breast cancer (see **Fig. 2**B). Thus the option of SERM therapy should be considered for these women.

The history of medicine has shown us that the greatest advances in care are often through prevention of disease as opposed to treatment. Although there are issues with the current breast cancer chemoprevention agents, such as side effects, costs, and the identification of proper candidates for use, these are not insurmountable barriers, and efforts are under way to address them. Over the years, cardiologists have recognized and refined the role of disease prevention in their practices; they can serve as a model. The oncology community has always been supportive of cancer prevention strategies, and chemoprevention offers an opportunity to expand those strategies beyond behavior and lifestyle modifications.

REFERENCES

1. Jemal A, Siegel R, Ward E, et al. Cancer statistics, 2009. CA Cancer J Clin 2009; 59:225–49.
2. Hartmann LC, Schaid DJ, Woods JE, et al. Efficacy of bilateral prophylactic mastectomy in women with a family history of breast cancer. N Engl J Med 1999;340:77–84.
3. Hong WK, Sporn MB. Recent advances in chemoprevention of cancer. Science 1997;278:1073–7.
4. Tamoxifen for early breast cancer: an overview of the randomised trials. Early Breast Cancer Trialists' Collaborative Group. Lancet 1998;351:1451–67.
5. Fisher B, Costantino JP, Wickerham DL, et al. Tamoxifen for prevention of breast cancer: report of the National Surgical Adjuvant Breast and Bowel Project P-1 study. J Natl Cancer Inst 1998;90:1371–8.
6. Fisher B, Costantino J, Wickerham DL, et al. Tamoxifen for the prevention of breast cancer: current status of the National Surgical Adjuvant Breast and Bowel Project P-1 study. J Natl Cancer Inst 2005;97:1652–62.
7. King MC, Wieand S, Hale K, et al. Tamoxifen and breast cancer incidence among women with inherited mutations in BRCA1 and BRCA2: National Surgical Adjuvant Breast and Bowel Project (NSABP P-1) breast cancer prevention trial. JAMA 2001;286:2251–6.
8. Narod SA, Brunet JS, Ghadirian P, et al. Tamoxifen and risk of contralateral breast cancer in BRCA1 and BRCA2 mutation carriers: a case-control study. Hereditary Breast Cancer Clinical Study Group. Lancet 2000;356:1876–81.
9. Cuzick J, Forbes J, Edwards R, et al. First results from the International Breast Cancer Intervention Study (IBIS-I): a randomised prevention trial. Lancet 2002; 360:817–24.
10. Cuzick J, Forbes JF, Sestak I, et al. Long-term results of tamoxifen prophylaxis for breast cancer–96-month follow-up of the randomized IBIS-I trial. J Natl Cancer Inst 2007;99:272–82.
11. Powles T, Eeles R, Ashley S, et al. Interim analysis of the incidence of breast cancer in the Royal Marsden Hospital tamoxifen randomised chemoprevention trial. Lancet 1998;352:98–101.
12. Powles TJ, Ashley S, Tidy A, et al. Twenty-year follow-up of the Royal Marsden randomized, double-blinded tamoxifen breast cancer prevention trial. J Natl Cancer Inst 2007;99:283–90.
13. Veronesi U, Maisonneuve P, Rotmensz N, et al. Italian randomized trial among women with hysterectomy: tamoxifen and hormone-dependent breast cancer in high-risk women. J Natl Cancer Inst 2003;95:160–5.
14. Cuzick J, Powles T, Veronesi U, et al. Overview of the main outcomes in breast-cancer prevention trials. Lancet 2003;361:296–300.
15. Cummings SR, Eckert S, Krueger KA, et al. The effect of raloxifene on risk of breast cancer in postmenopausal women: results from the MORE randomized trial. Multiple Outcomes of Raloxifene Evaluation. JAMA 1999;281: 2189–97.
16. Martino S, Cauley JA, Barrett-Connor E, et al. Continuing Outcomes Relevant to Evista: breast cancer incidence in postmenopausal osteoporotic women in a randomized trial of raloxifene. J Natl Cancer Inst 2004;96:1751–61.
17. Vogel VG, Costantino JP, Wickerham DL, et al. Effects of tamoxifen vs raloxifene on the risk of developing invasive breast cancer and other disease outcomes: the

NSABP Study of Tamoxifen and Raloxifene (STAR) P-2 trial. JAMA 2006;295: 2727–41.

18. LaCroix AZ, Cummings SR, Delmas P, et al. Effects of 5 years of treatment with lasofoxifene on incidence of breast cancer in older women [abstract 11]. San Antonio Breast Cancer Symposium. San Antonio (TX), December 11, 2008, General Session I. Cancer Res 2009;69:11.

19. Powles T, Diem S, Wickerham L, et al. Effects of arzoxifene on breast cancer incidence in postmenopausal women with osteoporosis or with low bone mass [abstract 51]. San Antonio Breast Cancer Symposium. San Antonio (TX), December 11, 2009, General Session IV.

20. Goss PE, Strasser K. Aromatase inhibitors in the treatment and prevention of breast cancer. J Clin Oncol 2001;19:881–94.

21. Thüerlimann B. Adjuvant hormonal therapy for breast cancer: an evolving process (archived web conference). Presented at Primary Therapy of Early Breast Cancer 9th International Conference. St Gallen (Switzerland), January 26–29, 2005. Available at: http://www.medscape.com/viewprogram/3800_pnt. Accessed February 12, 2010.

22. Jakesz R, on behalf of the ABCSG and the GABG. Benefits of switching postmenopausal women with hormone-sensitive early breast cancer to anastrozole after 2 years adjuvant tamoxifen: combined results from 3,123 women enrolled in the ABCSG Trial 8 and the ARNO 95 Trial [abstract 2]. San Antonio Breast Cancer Symposium. San Antonio (TX), December 8–11, 2004. Breast Cancer Res Treat 2004;88(Suppl 1):S1–265.

23. Goss PE, Ingle JN, Martino S, et al. A randomized trial of letrozole in postmenopausal women after five years of tamoxifen therapy for early-stage breast cancer. N Engl J Med 2003;349:1793–802.

24. Coombes RC, Hall E, Gibson LJ, et al. A randomized trial of exemestane after two to three years of tamoxifen therapy in postmenopausal women with primary breast cancer. N Engl J Med 2004;350:1081–92.

25. Baum M, Buzdar AU, Cuzick J, et al. Anastrozole alone or in combination with tamoxifen versus tamoxifen alone for adjuvant treatment of postmenopausal women with early breast cancer: first results of the ATAC randomised trial. Lancet 2002;359:2131–9.

26. Visvanathan K, Chlebowski RT, Hurley P, et al. American Society of Clinical Oncology Clinical Practice Guideline update on the use of pharmacologic interventions including tamoxifen, raloxifene, and aromatase inhibition for breast cancer risk reduction. J Clin Oncol 2009;27:3235–58.

27. Chlebowski RT, Collyar DE, Somerfield MR, et al. American Society of Clinical Oncology technology assessment on breast cancer risk reduction strategies: tamoxifen and raloxifene. J Clin Oncol 1999;17:1939–55.

28. Chelbowski RT, Col N, Winer EP, et al. American Society of Clinical Oncology technology assessment of pharmacologic interventions for breast cancer risk reduction including tamoxifen, raloxifene, and aromatase inhibition. J Clin Oncol 2002;20:3328–43.

Magnetic Resonance Imaging for Screening, Diagnosis, and Eligibility for Breast-conserving Surgery: Promises and Pitfalls

Monica Morrow, MD[a,b,*]

KEYWORDS

- Magnetic resonance imaging • Breast-conserving therapy
- Local recurrence • Occult cancer

Breast cancer mortality in the United States, as well as in other parts of the world, has decreased in recent years, a finding that is attributable in part to the use of screening mammography and in part to improved treatment, particularly the use of adjuvant endocrine therapy and chemotherapy.[1] Although randomized trials have shown that screening mammography reduces breast cancer mortality, it fails to detect some cancer, and its application in women less than 40 years of age remains controversial. In the cancer patient, disease burden has traditionally been the major consideration in selecting local therapy. In patients treated with breast-conserving therapy (BCT) consisting of excision of the tumor and whole-breast irradiation, randomized trials have shown that failure to reduce the tumor burden in the breast to a subclinical level is associated with an increased risk of local recurrence.[2,3] This failure has resulted in multicentric cancer and margins that cannot be cleared of cancer cells being accepted as indications for mastectomy.[4,5] As experience with BCT has been gained, local recurrence rates have steadily decreased.[6,7]

Magnetic resonance imaging (MRI) is capable of detecting small foci of cancer in the breast that were previously only evident on detailed pathology evaluation. MRI has

[a] Breast Service, Department of Surgery, Memorial Sloan-Kettering Cancer Center, Evelyn H. Lauder Breast Center, 300 East 66th Street, New York, NY 10065, USA
[b] Weill Medical College of Cornell University, 300 East 66th Street, New York, NY 10065, USA
* Breast Service, Department of Surgery, Memorial Sloan-Kettering Cancer Center, Evelyn H. Lauder Breast Center, 300 East 66th Street, New York, NY 10065.
E-mail address: morrowm@mskcc.org

Surg Oncol Clin N Am 19 (2010) 475–492
doi:10.1016/j.soc.2010.03.003
1055-3207/10/$ – see front matter © 2010 Elsevier Inc. All rights reserved.

been applied in the screening setting and in the selection of local therapy for patients with known cancer. This article considers the available data on the effect of MRI on breast cancer screening in women at high risk, as well its effect on short- and long-term outcomes of surgical treatment of operable breast cancer.

MRI FOR SCREENING

Mammography is the proven standard of care for breast cancer screening throughout the world. After the implementation of a national mammographic screening program, a greater than 1% per year decline in breast cancer mortality was observed in the Netherlands,[8] and the uptake of screening mammography has also been credited with up to half of the observed reduction in breast cancer mortality in the United States.[1] Although mammography is a successful screening tool, with a documented effect on patient outcomes, approximately 10% to 15% of cancers are not visible mammographically. In particular, mammography has a lower sensitivity for cancers occurring in dense breast tissue,[9] and misses up to 22% of invasive breast cancers in women less than 50 years of age, compared with 10% in women more than 50 years of age.[10] Mammographic sensitivity also seems to be decreased in BRCA mutation carriers, with a high percentage of cancer being identified in the interval between annual mammograms.[11,12] This is likely a consequence of the more aggressive nature of BRCA1-related cancers, which have been shown to have higher mitotic counts and are more commonly estrogen receptor (ER) negative, progesterone receptor (PR) negative, and HER2 negative than sporadic cancers. In addition, BRCA-related cancers frequently occur in younger women with dense breast tissue.[13] These limitations have led to a search for alternate methods of screening in younger women at high risk.

Compared with mammography, MRI, which relies on the increased vascularity of neoplasms, has been found to have a higher sensitivity for the detection of breast cancer, and the sensitivity is not altered by breast density.[14] Because of the high cost of the examination, initial limited availability, and early limitations in sampling lesions visible only on MRI, screening studies to date have been performed in patients at high risk. Although there have been no prospective randomized trials of MRI screening, a systematic review from Warner and colleagues[15] in 2008 identified 11 prospective studies of MRI screening. These included a mix of single- and multi-institutional studies with varying entry criteria. For example, the proportion of known BRCA mutation carriers varied from 8% in the study by Kuhl and colleagues[12] to 100% in the study by Warner and colleagues[16] In addition, all but the studies of Kreige and colleagues[17] and Leach and colleagues[18] included women with a prior history of breast cancer. Although all studies compared the outcome of screening with MRI to that of screening with mammography, there was variation in the number of screening rounds and the use of additional studies, such as ultrasound between studies. The sensitivity of mammography varied from 14% to 59% when a positive mammogram was defined as a Breast Imaging Reporting and Data System (BI-RADS) 4 or 5 score, whereas the sensitivity of MRI ranged from 51% to 100%. Characteristics of the largest studies included in the meta-analysis are summarized in **Table 1**.[12,16–19] In the meta-analysis,[15] the sensitivity of mammography was 32% (95% confidence interval [CI], 23–41), and that of MRI was 75% (95% CI, 62–88). Combining the 2 procedures increased the sensitivity to 84% (95% CI, 70–97). Although all studies reported a higher sensitivity for MRI for the detection of invasive cancer, results were conflicting regarding its sensitivity for the detection of ductal carcinoma in situ (DCIS). In the studies by Kreige and colleagues[17] and Leach and colleagues,[18] the

Table 1
Studies of MRI screening in women at high risk

	Kriege et al[17]	Leach et al[18]	Warner et al[16]	Kuhl et al[12]	Hagen et al[19]
No. of patients	1909	649	236	529	491
Risk criteria	≥15%	≥25%	BRCA carrier	≥20%	BRCA carrier
Proven mutation carriers	19%	19%	100%	8%	100%
No. of cancers	50	22	35	43	25
Sensitivity MRI	80%	77%	77%	91%	68%

sensitivity of mammography was superior to that of MRI for the detection of DCIS. In contrast, Kuhl and colleagues[20] reported a high sensitivity for the detection of DCIS with MRI. In all the studies in the meta-analysis, except that by Kuhl and colleagues,[20] the specificity of mammography was higher than the specificity of MRI. The specificity of MRI ranged from 75% to 98%, with a meta-analysis value of 96.1% (95% CI, 94.8–97.4), and increased with subsequent screens in studies that provided these data. There was a decreased specificity of MRI (81%) in the United Kingdom study compared with the other studies.[18] This was a multi-institutional study involving 22 centers across the United Kingdom, and the results may be more reflective of outcomes of MRI screening in the community than results from single-institution studies in which high volumes of MRI are performed and read by radiologists with substantial expertise in the field.

The lack of specificity of MRI results in the need for additional testing. In the study by Kriege and colleagues,[17] the recall rate for additional imaging was 10.7% compared with 3.9% for mammography, and biopsy rates were 3.1% for MRI and 1.3% for mammography. This result may be an acceptable trade-off in patients at high risk, but the additional testing and high false-positive rates are a concern in applying MRI screening to the general population. The need for additional testing has a potential negative psychological effect and may influence compliance with future screening rounds. In a subset of the United Kingdom MRI screening study,[18] 47% reported intrusive thoughts about the MRI examination 6 weeks later, and 4% found the MRI extremely distressing.

Although MRI screening of women at high risk clearly identifies cancers not found by mammography, whether this conveys a survival advantage is uncertain. In the trials using screening MRI, lymph node involvement was present in 14% to 26% of women at diagnosis. This finding may be a reflection of the unfavorable biologic characteristics of tumors that occur in BRCA 1 mutation carriers (ER, PR, HER2 negative), but is an important point when counseling these women at high risk regarding the benefits and risks of surveillance and intervention strategies. Although it seems unlikely that a prospective randomized trial with a survival end point will be conducted, further follow-up of the studies conducted to date should provide additional information relevant to this question.

There are few data on the outcomes of MRI screening in women who are at an increased risk of breast cancer due to factors other than a family history. Patients with diagnoses of lobular carcinoma in situ (LCIS) or atypical ductal hyperplasia (ADH) were studied retrospectively by Port and colleagues.[21] Those patients undergoing MRI screening were younger and had stronger family histories of breast cancer. Cancer was only identified in 1% of the 478 MRI scans performed. However, of the patients undergoing MRI, 25% were recommended to have a biopsy (most solely because of MRI findings), and almost half had at least 1 MRI requiring short-term follow-up. The sensitivity and specificity of MRI was similar to that previously reported at 75% and 92%, respectively, but clear evidence of benefit for MRI screening was not found. A potential reason that the favorable results of screening with MRI in women at genetic risk may not be duplicated in other risk groups is related to the young age of onset of cancer in BRCA mutation carriers, as well as the infrequent occurrence of DCIS in this patient group, so caution should be used when extrapolating the benefits of screening known or suspected BRCA mutation carriers to other high-risk groups.

The American Cancer Society convened a group of experts to develop guidelines for annual MRI screening that were published in 2007. The only groups for which sufficient evidence to justify the use of MRI screening was felt to be present were women proven to be BRCA mutation carriers, untested first-degree relatives of mutation carriers, and women with a lifetime risk of breast cancer development of 20% or greater as determined by models based on a family history of breast cancer.[22] The committee considered that MRI screening was justified based on expert consensus in women at high risk due to radiation exposure at a young age and less common genetic syndromes associated with an increased risk of breast cancer. For a larger group of women at increased risk of breast cancer development, including those with a personal history of breast cancer, dense breasts, atypical hyperplasia, or LCIS, the committee considered that there was insufficient evidence to recommend for or against MRI screening (**Table 2**). When screening with MRI was indicated, the committee recommended that mammographic screening also be performed.

Table 2 American Cancer Society screening guidelines	
Recommend annual MRI screening (based on evidence[a])	• *BRCA* mutation • Untested first-degree relative of *BRCA* carrier • Lifetime breast cancer risk ~20%–25% or greater, as defined by models that are largely dependent on family history
Recommend annual MRI screening (based on expert consensus opinion[b])	• Radiation to chest between age 10 and 30 years • Li-Fraumeni syndrome and first-degree relatives • Cowden syndrome and first-degree relatives
Insufficient evidence to recommend for or against MRI screening	• Lifetime risk 15%–20%, as defined by models that are largely dependent on family history • LCIS or atypical lobular hyperplasia (ALH) • ADH • Heterogeneously or extremely dense breast on mammography • Women with a personal history of breast cancer, including DCIS
Recommend against MRI screening (based on expert consensus opinion)	• Women at <15% lifetime risk

[a] Evidence from nonrandomized screening trials and observational studies.
[b] Based on evidence of lifetime risk for breast cancer.

MRI FOR TREATMENT SELECTION

Current guidelines for the use of BCT cite multicentric cancer as an indication for mastectomy.[5] Clinically and radiographically, breast cancer is usually a unicentric lesion, with multicentric carcinoma identified by physical examination or mammography in fewer than 10% of cases.[23] However, pathology studies using serial subgross sectioning of mastectomy specimens have documented that additional tumor foci are present in 21% to 63% of cases,[24–26] in the same quadrant (multifocal) or other quadrants (multicentric), of a breast with what seems to be a clinically unicentric tumor. In 1 such study, Holland and colleagues[24] evaluated mastectomy specimens of 282 patients with unicentric cancers 5 cm or smaller in size and found additional tumor foci in 63%. In 20% of cases, the additional tumor was identified within 2 cm of the index tumor, and, in the remaining 43%, at a greater distance from the primary site, although usually within 4 cm. The likelihood of identifying additional tumor foci was not related to the size of the primary tumor,[24] and a 44% incidence of additional tumor was seen in patients with mammographically detected lesions. Such studies were initially used to argue that the treatment of breast cancer with approaches that did not remove the entire breast was inappropriate and would result in high rates of local recurrence. Extensive clinical experience, including multiple prospective randomized trials, has since shown that survival after BCT is equal to survival after mastectomy. In the current era of the routine use of adjuvant systemic therapy, 10-year rates of local recurrence after BCT are less than 10%,[27,28] which is considerably lower than the incidence of multifocality/multicentricity seen in pathology studies. These findings indicate that, although subclinical tumor foci are present in significant numbers of women with clinically localized breast cancer, most of these subclinical tumor foci are controlled with radiotherapy (RT), and this paradox lies at the heart of the debate about the benefit of MRI for cancer staging and treatment selection.

In women with breast cancer, MRI identifies additional cancer foci that are not evident on clinical examination, mammogram, or ultrasound. In a meta-analysis of 19 studies, including 2610 breast cancer patients, Houssami and colleagues[29] reported that additional cancer was identified by MRI in 16% of patients (with a range of 6%–34%). In a meta-analysis of MRI restricted to patients with lobular carcinoma reported by Mann and colleagues,[30] which included 18 studies and 450 cancers, additional disease was detected with MRI in 32% of cases (95% CI, 22%–44%). The usefulness of MRI in DCIS is unclear. Sardanelli and colleagues[14] observed a sensitivity of only 40% for the detection of DCIS by MRI when the results of serial subgross sectioning were used as the standard. In contrast, Kuhl and colleagues[20] reported that MRI was significantly more sensitive than mammography for the detection of DCIS using conventional pathologic evaluation as the comparator. Of 167 women with DCIS who had undergone mammography and MRI preoperatively, DCIS was diagnosed by mammography in 56% of cases, and by MRI in 98%, with the superior performance of MRI particularly evident in high-grade DCIS.

It seems that MRI identifies some, but not all, of the tumor foci identified by pathologists using serial subgross sectioning. This question was most directly addressed by Sardanelli and colleagues,[14] who performed MRI on 90 patients before mastectomy, then processed the mastectomy specimens with serial subgross sectioning and correlated the pathologic tumor location with the findings of the preoperative MRI. The overall sensitivity of MRI for the detection of tumor was 81%: 89% for invasive carcinoma and 40% for DCIS. In the 90 breasts studied, MRI failed to identify microscopic multifocal or multicentric disease in 19, and incorrectly indicated additional disease in

30, whereas it correctly identified the extent of tumor in 50. The mean diameter of malignant lesions not seen by MRI was 5 mm, and ranged from 0.5 mm to 15 mm.

Indirect evidence also suggests that the same tumor is identified with both techniques. Berg and colleagues[31] observed that in 40 of 46 breasts with additional tumor foci detected with MRI, the tumor foci were within 4 cm of the index lesion. Liberman and colleagues[32] also noted that most of the additional tumors detected were in the same quadrant as the index lesion. These findings correspond well with the observations of Holland and colleagues[24] that 96% of pathologically detected tumor foci were within 4 cm of the index tumor.

Until recently, it has been assumed that the finding of additional cancer on MRI was clearly of benefit to the patient. In the meta-analyses by Houssami and colleagues,[29] the results of the MRI examination changed surgical therapy in 7.8% to 33.3% of cases in individual studies, and virtually always in the direction of more extensive surgery, such as a wider excision or a mastectomy that would not otherwise have been performed. In a study of 5405 patients treated at the Mayo Clinic, Rochester, Minnesota, the use of MRI increased from 10% of newly diagnosed breast cancers in 2003 to 26% in 2006. A significant increase in the mastectomy rate was also observed during this period, and, after adjustment for age, stage, and the presence of contralateral carcinoma, women who had MRI were 1.7 times more likely to undergo mastectomy than their counterparts who did not have the examination.[33] If the more extensive surgery that occurs as a result of MRI findings is truly beneficial to patients, it should result in improvement in short-term outcomes of surgery, such as the improved ability to identify patients requiring a mastectomy preoperatively, or an increased likelihood of achieving negative margins with a single operative procedure. Alternatively, the benefit of MRI may be to improve long-term outcomes by decreasing the incidence of local recurrence after BCT or allowing the synchronous detection of contralateral breast cancer.

The Effect of MRI on Short-term Surgical Outcomes

The identification of patients who are appropriate candidates for BCT is not a major problem. Contraindications to the procedure[5] are reliably identified with a history, physical examination, and diagnostic mammography. Morrow and colleagues[34] reported that of 263 consecutive patients selected for BCT between 1989 and 1993 using a history, physical examination, and diagnostic mammography, conversion to mastectomy was necessary in only 2.9%. In a population-based sample of 800 women from the Los Angeles and Detroit Surveillance Epidemiology and End Results (SEER) registry sites attempting BCT between June 2005 and May 2006, 12% required conversion to mastectomy, although in 8% mastectomy occurred after a single attempt at BCT.[35] Two retrospective studies[36,37] and 1 prospective randomized trial[38] have examined whether the use of MRI reduces the need for mastectomy in patients attempting BCT. Bleicher and colleagues[36] retrospectively reviewed 290 patients attempting BCT between July 2004 and December 2006 after multidisciplinary preoperative evaluation and found no significant difference in the likelihood of requiring conversion from BCT to mastectomy on the basis of a preoperative MRI. Pengel and colleagues[37] compared outcomes with and without MRI among 355 women treated at a single institution. Those who had MRI were part of a study evaluating the procedure, and the control group consisted of patients who declined to enter the study. Again, no significant differences in the rate of unanticipated conversion to mastectomy were noted (**Table 3**).[36–38]

The most robust data addressing this question come from the Comparative Effectiveness of MRI in Breast Cancer (COMICE) trial, a prospective randomized study

Table 3
Effect of MRI on the need for unplanned mastectomy

Author	Number of Patients	% Mastectomy		P-value
		No MRI	MRI	
Bleicher et al[36]	290	5.9	9.8	NS
Pengel et al[37]	355	5.1	2.5	NS
Drew et al[38]	1623	7.6	5.9	NS

Abbreviation: NS, not significant.

involving 107 participating surgeons in the United Kingdom that was designed to address the question of the role of MRI in improving outcomes in patients undergoing BCT.[38] The sample included 1623 women believed to be candidates for BCT who were stratified on the basis of age, breast density, and treating surgeon, and randomized to receive MRI or not. In the MRI group, 58 patients (7.1%) underwent an immediate mastectomy as a result of the MRI findings, and 10 patients in the no-MRI group (1.2%) changed their treatment decision after randomization and opted for a mastectomy. Of the remainder who attempted BCT, conversion to mastectomy was required in 5.9% of the MRI group and 7.6% of the no-MRI group (see P = NS, see **Table 3**).[38] The overall result was a 13% mastectomy rate in the MRI group, and an 8.8% rate in the no-MRI group. In the study by Pengel and colleagues,[37] the mastectomy rate was doubled in the MRI group (11.6% vs 5.1%), and in the report by Bleicher and colleagues,[36] the use of MRI increased the mastectomy rate from 25% to 38%, an odds ratio of 1.80 after adjustment for tumor size and patient age (P = .024). These studies provide no suggestion that MRI decreases the likelihood of unplanned mastectomy, but do show a consistent pattern of an increased mastectomy rate in patients undergoing MRI.

In contrast to patient selection for BCT, which is not a major clinical problem, the need for reexcision because of margins involved with tumor after the initial lumpectomy is a common clinical occurrence. Morrow and colleagues[35] observed that 22% of 800 women undergoing successful BCT in a population-based sample derived from the SEER registry required at least 1 reexcision to complete surgical therapy. **Table 4** summarizes 4 retrospective studies and 1 prospective study that have examined the effect of MRI on the need for reexcision.[36–40] In spite of the inclusion of almost 2500 patients, none of the individual studies show a significant reduction in the need for reexcision in patients undergoing MRI. One additional study, limited to patients with infiltrating lobular carcinoma, showed a benefit for MRI. Mann and colleagues[41]

Table 4
Effect of MRI on the likelihood of positive margins after initial surgical excision

Author	Number of Patients	% Positive Margins		P-value
		No MRI	MRI	
Bleicher et al[36]	290	14	22	NS
Pengel et al[37]	355	19	14	NS
Schiller et al[39]	730	18	14	NS
Hwang et al[40]	472	14	12	NS
Drew et al[38]	1623	11	10	NS

Abbreviation: NS, not significant.

studied 90 patients who did not have MRI, and 55 who did and in whom BCT was attempted, and reported a 27% rate of reexcision in the no-MRI group compared with 9% in the MRI group (P = .01), as well as a significantly higher mastectomy rate in the no-MRI group (23% vs 7%; P = .013). Patients included in this study were treated between 1993 and 2005. It is not clear whether those undergoing MRI were more commonly treated later in the study period and whether criteria for reexcision were uniform over time, and how MRI reduced the mastectomy rate is not stated. Other larger studies have not confirmed a difference in the need for reexcision in patients with infiltrating lobular and infiltrating ductal histology. In a study of 318 patients with infiltrating lobular cancer who were matched by stage, year of diagnosis, and menopausal status to 2 controls with infiltrating ductal cancer (n = 636), 25% of patients with lobular cancer required reexcision, compared with 21% of those with ductal cancer; a difference that was not statistically significant after adjusting for tumor size and patient age.[42] One potential explanation for the inability of MRI to reduce the need for reexcision concerns its accuracy in determining tumor size. Although multiple studies have shown that MRI is more accurate than mammography in determining tumor size,[43–45] the degree of precision of measurement, and the ability to relate the imaging findings to the amount of tissue removed in the operating room, may be insufficient to see a reduction in margin positivity.

The available data on the use of MRI in the setting of newly diagnosed breast cancer do not provide evidence of patient benefit in short-term surgical outcomes, and raise some concerns. In addition to the increased mastectomy rate seen in patients undergoing MRI (discussed earlier), there are concerns about false-positive findings and the need for additional radiologic workup to evaluate these findings, leading to increased health-care costs and delays in therapy. In the meta-analysis by Houssami and colleagues,[29] the false-positive rate of MRI was 5.5% (95% CI, 3.1%–9.5%), and it is likely that false-positive rates outside the centers of expertise included in this meta-analysis are higher. Pettit and colleagues[46] reported that 36 of 410 patients considered to be candidates for BCT were converted to mastectomy on the basis of additional MRI lesions. In 23 cases, biopsy confirmation of malignancy in the additional lesion was not performed, and no additional cancer was found in more than half of these patients. Although the problem of inappropriate surgery due to false-positive MRI results can be minimized with biopsy confirmation of malignancy, there are some practical difficulties associated with this approach.

The current algorithm for evaluating an MRI abnormality involves targeted ultrasound to try to identify the lesion to allow an ultrasound-guided biopsy. If the lesion cannot be visualized by ultrasound and the patient is seeking treatment at a different institution than the one in which the MRI was obtained, then the MRI is often repeated to verify the presence of a target before the time of biopsy. In the study by Bleicher and colleagues,[36] there was a 22.4-day delay in the time from histologic diagnosis to initial surgery in patients who had MRI compared with those who did not (P = .01). The need for additional biopsies, particularly at multiple sites, is traumatic for patients, and Berg and colleagues[31] found that 12% of patients underwent a medically unnecessary mastectomy rather than undergo further workup of abnormal MRI findings. The risk of unnecessary surgery is present in the ipsilateral and the contralateral breast. King and colleagues[47] compared presenting characteristics of 2558 women who underwent unilateral mastectomy and 407 who had a contralateral prophylactic mastectomy (CPM) between 1997 and 2005 at Memorial Sloan-Kettering Cancer Center. Patients having preoperative MRI were significantly more likely to undergo CPM (43% vs 16%; P = .0001), and this was particularly true if the unaffected breast required a biopsy for a benign finding.

An exception to the general lack of usefulness of MRI for surgical treatment selection is the 1% of breast cancer patients whose breast cancers present as axillary nodal metastases with an occult primary tumor that cannot be detected by physical examination, mammography, or ultrasound. These cases have traditionally been treated with mastectomy to ensure removal of the primary tumor, but, in approximately one-third of the breast specimens, cancer is not identified by pathologic evaluation.[48] Although mastectomy was a reasonable approach to this problem in earlier years when the tumor burden that was undetected clinically could be large, in more recent studies,[49,50] the identification of cancer in the breast specimen has been infrequent. Although breast conservation has been successfully performed in patients with occult tumors using whole-breast irradiation without surgical excision, this deprives the patient of the benefit of a boost dose of radiation to the primary tumor site. The use of MRI to identify the primary tumor, allowing surgical excision and the use of a radiation boost, is a clinically valuable tool in this uncommon circumstance.

Studies evaluating the use of MRI in cases of occult breast cancer have been small and retrospective, but typically show detection of tumor in more than two-thirds of these cases with low false-negative rates (as summarized in **Table 5**).[51–57] A meta-analysis by de Bresser and colleagues,[58] which included 220 patients in 8 studies, found that MRI identified a suspicious lesion in 72% of cases, with a sensitivity of 90% and a specificity of 31% (range, 22%–50%). The mean size of tumors identified on pathologic examination ranged from 5 mm to 16 mm, and more than 90% (pooled mean, 96%) were invasive carcinomas.

The largest study included in the meta-analysis, by Buchanan and colleagues,[51] examined 55 patients with axillary lymphadenopathy and occult primary without evidence of distant disease. MRI revealed suspicious lesions in 76%, of which 62% (26 of 42) were pathologically confirmed to be the primary tumor, resulting in 15 of these patients being considered candidates for BCT. Conversely, MRI failed to identify the primary tumor in 25 patients (12 false-positive MRI and 13 negative MRI). Twelve of these patients underwent mastectomy, yielding cancer in only 4 cases (33%).

In an earlier investigation from the same institution (and an overlapping study period), Olson and colleagues[53] looked at the effect of MRI on breast conservation in 40 women with occult breast cancer. Of the 28 patients whose primary tumors were identified by MRI, 11 elected lumpectomy/axillary lymph node dissection. Two of the lumpectomy patients ultimately required mastectomy because of positive margins. Of the 12 patients with negative MRI, 5 underwent mastectomy, yielding

Table 5
MRI in occult breast cancer presenting as axillary adenopathy: identification and false-negative rates

Study	No. of Patients	MRI-detected Cancer (%)	False-Negatives
Buchanan et al[51]	55	26/55 (47)	2/13
McMahon et al[52]	18	12/18 (67)	NA
Olson et al[53]	40	28/40 (70)	1/5
Orel et al[54]	22	17/20 (85)	2/3
Henry-Tillman et al[55]	10	8/8 (100)	0/2
Morris et al[56]	12	9/12 (75)	0/2
Ko et al[57]	12	10/12 (83)	NA

Abbreviation: NA, not applicable.

cancer in only 1 patient. Negative MRI in this group of patients was predictive of low tumor yield, and potentially identified a subset of patients that could be adequately treated with whole-breast irradiation instead of mastectomy. Overall, MRI identifies the primary tumor in approximately 60% of cases presenting as adenopathy. Patients found to have small unifocal tumors are candidates for conventional BCT, whereas negative MRI provides reassurance that a large tumor burden is unlikely and that the patient may be adequately treated locally with axillary dissection and whole-breast irradiation. Mastectomy remains the most common form of local therapy in this situation, even when MRI is used.

Effect of MRI on Long-Term Cancer Outcomes

Local recurrence

A potential major benefit to patients of preoperative MRI would be a reduction in the incidence of local recurrence after BCT. Since the publication of the initial trials that established the suitability of BCT as a breast cancer treatment modality, rates of local recurrence have steadily declined. Pass and colleagues[7] examined the effect of changes in the processes of care between 1981 and 1996 on local recurrence rates in a group of 607 patients treated at a single institution. Between 1981 and 1985, the 5-year rate of ipsilateral breast tumor recurrence (IBTR) was 8%, decreasing to 1% between 1991 and 1996. In a similar study, Ernst and colleagues[6] observed 8-year rates of locoregional recurrence after BCT to decrease from 20.1% between 1985 and 1992, to 5.4% from 1993 to 1999. In contrast, rates of locoregional recurrence after mastectomy did not change between the 2 time periods. In the National Surgical Adjuvant Breast and Bowel Project (NSABP) trials conducted since the 1990s, rates of IBTR at 10 years were less than 8% in women who were node positive and node negative receiving systemic therapy.[27,28] These findings emphasize that local recurrence may be due to 2 mechanisms. The first mechanism, an excessive tumor burden in the breast that cannot be controlled with x-ray therapy (XRT), is the type of local recurrence that is potentially amenable to reduction through the use of MRI for patient selection. The second mechanism, local recurrence that occurs due to biologically aggressive disease, is a first site of metastases and will only be affected by improvements in systemic therapy. The proportion of local recurrences due to each of these mechanisms is unknown; however, the observation from the Early Breast Cancer Trialists overview analysis[59] that local recurrence is seen on the chest wall after mastectomy and XRT in 3% of node-negative cases and 7% of node-positive cases (figures similar to current rates of IBTR after BCT) strongly suggests that most recurrences after BCT in the current era are due to aggressive biology, not a heavy residual disease burden in the breast.

Three studies have retrospectively examined the effect of patient selection with MRI on IBTR. Fischer and colleagues[60] retrospectively compared 121 patients who had a preoperative MRI with 225 who did not. After a mean follow-up of approximately 40 months, IBTR occurred in 1.2% of the MRI group and 6.8% of the no-MRI group ($P<.001$). The 6.8% incidence of IBTR at less than 5 years follow-up is unusually high by current standards, making the outcome of this study difficult to interpret. In addition, although patients in the MRI group were more likely to have T1 tumors (64% vs 48%), more likely to be node negative (61% vs 54%), and less likely to have high-grade lesions (13% vs 28%), no adjustments for differences in tumor characteristics between the groups were made. Despite the more favorable profile of the MRI patients, chemotherapy was administered to 95% of patients in this group with indications for treatment, compared with 82% in the no-MRI group, and no adjustment was made for this difference. The combination of an unusually high rate of IBTR in the no-MRI group in comparison with other reports of patients treated without MRI in the same time period,[27,28] and the lack of adjustment for major differences in tumor and treatment variables which affect the incidence of IBTR, prevent reliable conclusions from being drawn from this study. Solin and colleagues[61] also examined the effect of MRI on IBTR in 215 patients who had the examination, and 541 who did not. Appropriate statistical adjustments were made for differences between patient groups. At 8 years, the rate of IBTR in the MRI group was 3%; it was 4% in the non-IBTR group. Hwang and colleagues[40] also examined the effect of MRI on IBTR with adjustment for differences between groups. After a median follow-up of 54 months, the 8-year actuarial rates of local recurrence were 1.8% in the MRI group and 2.5% in the no-MRI group: a nonsignificant difference. Based on the results of the Houssami and colleagues[29] meta-analysis showing a 6% to 11% conversion rate from BCT to mastectomy based on the findings of MRI, between 21 and 38 of the patients in the Hwang and colleagues[40] study and between 32 and 60 patients in the Solin and colleagues[61] study who were treated without MRI had inappropriate BCT; however, the number of patients who recurred was 9 and 13, respectively. The COMICE trial will provide additional data on MRI and IBTR when further follow-up is available, but it is evident from the information available now that the use of MRI will not have an effect on breast cancer–specific survival. The Early Breast Cancer Trialists overview[59] showed that, to observe a survival difference at 15 years, differences in local failure rates of 10% or greater between treatments must be present at 5 years of follow-up. The rate of IBTR after BCT in patients selected for the procedure without MRI is less than 10% at 10 years, so a difference of the magnitude needed to show a survival gain cannot be anticipated with the addition of MRI. Even if the group that seems to be at the highest risk for IBTR after BCT (ie, women with ER, PR, and HER2 negative disease[62]) were to be studied, it is unlikely that MRI would result in a survival benefit because these patients also have the highest risk for local recurrence after mastectomy,[63] strongly suggesting that these recurrences are a reflection of aggressive tumor biology rather than a heavy tumor burden in the breast.

Contralateral cancer

The other long-term outcome with the potential to be affected by MRI is the synchronous versus metachronous diagnosis of contralateral breast cancer. Women with unilateral breast carcinoma are at increased risk for the development of second cancers, but the absolute magnitude of this risk is low in women who do not have BRCA gene mutations. In 134,501 women diagnosed with unilateral DCIS, stage 1, and stage 2 breast carcinoma between 1973 and 1996 and reported to SEER, the 10-year actuarial risk of a contralateral cancer was 6.1%, and the 20-year risk was 12%.[64] For those less than 45 years of age at initial diagnosis, these figures were 3.1% and 6.2%, respectively. A diagnosis of DCIS was associated with a 6.0% risk of a second cancer at 10 years, and a diagnosis of infiltrating lobular carcinoma was associated with a 6.4% risk at 10 years. Based on these low incidence rates, it is difficult to argue that more intensive surveillance of the contralateral breast added to an annual mammogram is a cost-effective strategy for the general population of women with breast cancer. However, Lehman and colleagues[65] examined the role of MRI for evaluation of the contralateral breast in 969 women with unilateral breast cancer. Cancer was detected by MRI in 30 women (3.1%) with clinically and mammographically normal breasts within 12 months of the initial breast cancer diagnosis. The mean patient age was 53.3 years, and only 19.6% had 1 or more first-degree relatives with breast cancer. Of the cancers detected, 18 were invasive carcinoma and 12 were DCIS. An additional 3 cases of DCIS not detected by MRI were identified in prophylactic mastectomy specimens. The investigators concluded that MRI of the contralateral breast at the time of a unilateral breast cancer diagnosis was useful to allow the detection of early-stage carcinoma and synchronous rather than metachronous treatment of second primary tumors. The same arguments have been used to support the use of mirror image, contralateral breast biopsy, a procedure with similar results. Cody[66] identified contralateral cancer with mirror image biopsy in 3% of 871 women with unilateral cancer and a normal examination and mammogram treated between 1979 and 1993, and half of the cancers were invasive, whereas Pressman[67] reported a 6.2% identification rate with contralateral biopsy in an earlier time period. To reconcile the findings of Lehman and colleagues[65] and the contralateral biopsy studies[66,67] with the low rates of cancer observed at 5 and 10 years in the SEER study by Gao and colleagues,[64] one must make the assumption that virtually all contralateral cancer that occurs in the first 5 years after diagnosis is present at the time of diagnosis, and that it is all detectable by MRI. This seems unlikely and ignores clinical data which indicate that the use of endocrine therapy reduces the clinical incidence of contralateral breast cancer by 50%.[68] Even the use of conventional chemotherapy reduces contralateral cancer by 20%,[68] raising the distinct possibility that MRI of the contralateral breast identifies some cancers that would never become clinically evident, resulting in unnecessary treatment. In a meta-analysis of MRI of the contralateral breast, Brennan and colleagues[69] reported a 9.3% incidence of MRI-detected abnormalities in the contralateral breast (true-positive plus false-positive), with a positive predictive value (PPV) of 47.9%. In the already-anxious woman with a new diagnosis of breast cancer, this low PPV may have significant clinical consequences. In a large study examining factors associated with CPM, King and colleagues[47] found that undergoing a preoperative MRI increased the risk of CPM by a factor of 3.2 in multivariate analysis. Similarly, Sorbero and colleagues[70] examined the use of CPM in 3606 stage 1 to 3 breast cancer patients between 1998 and 2005 and found that, in multivariate analysis, the use of preoperative MRI was associated with an increased use of CPM (odds ratio, 2.04; $P = .001$) in women with stage 1 and 2 disease, although the overall rates of CPM were significantly lower than those reported by King and colleagues.[47]

In addition, the 1-year follow-up in the study of Lehman and colleagues[65] is insufficient to judge the effect of MRI on the incidence of contralateral cancer, and there are limited clinical data that address this question. Solin and colleagues[61] reported a 6% incidence of cancer at 8 years of follow-up in women who did and did not have preoperative MRI, indicating that more data are needed before concluding that MRI is routinely indicated in women with unilateral cancer for the purpose of screening the contralateral breast.

MRI FOR DETECTION OF LOCAL RECURRENCE

The current recommendations for detection of local recurrence after BCT are monthly breast self-examination; physician examination every 3 to 6 months for 5 years, then annually; and a mammogram 6 to 12 months after the completion of RT, then yearly.[5] With this approach, one-half to one-third of recurrences are identified as nonpalpable lesions detected by mammography alone, and 85% to 90% of patients have operable disease when a local recurrence is detected.[71,72] Evidence suggests that current methods of surveillance are highly successful; the inoperable recurrences are primarily inflammatory type skin recurrences (an aggressive subtype of recurrence the biology of which is unlikely to be affected by detection method[73]) and the average size of recurrent tumors is 1 to 2 cm.[74,75] It is not clear whether there is any benefit to detecting local recurrence at a smaller size. Mastectomy is the standard treatment of local recurrence, regardless of size, in patients who have received prior whole-breast irradiation, so the choice of therapy is not related to tumor size. Attempts to reconserve the breast with wide excision alone, even for small tumors with favorable histologic characteristics, have resulted in further local recurrence in 19% to 48% of cases,[72,74,76–78] an unacceptable rate given what is understood about the effect of failure to maintain local control on long-term survival.[59] Perhaps most importantly, there is no evidence that earlier identification of local recurrence improves patient outcomes. Most studies indicate that tumors with aggressive biology recur locally and distantly in a shorter time interval. In a study by Millar and colleagues,[79] the 10-year rate of IBTR for luminal A cancers (ER or PR positive, HER2 negative) was 3.6%, and the median time to recurrence was 80.5 months. For basal cancers (ER, PR, HER2 negative) there was a 9.6% incidence of IBTR at 10 years, with a median time to recurrence of 20 months. Despite the shorter time to the detection of IBTR in the basal group, the incidence of breast cancer death at a median follow-up of 96 months was 13.5% compared with 7.4% in the luminal A group. Veronesi and colleagues[75] reported that the risk of distant metastases after a local recurrence detected within 1 year of initial treatment was 6.6 times the risk seen in patients with local recurrence detected more than 3 years after surgery ($P = .004$). Other studies have confirmed the association between a short interval to the detection of local recurrence and poor survival.[76,80,81] Thus, the extrapolation from trials of screening mammography in which detection of a tumor at a smaller size, and presumably earlier in its natural history, results in a survival advantage does not seem relevant to the problem of local recurrence. In addition, given current rates of local recurrence of less than 1% per year,[27,28] and the prolonged period of risk for local recurrence that occurs at a median interval of 5 to 6 years posttreatment,[75,76,79] it is difficult to argue that 10 years of follow-up with MRI is cost-effective.

SUMMARY

MRI is able to visualize small tumor deposits that previously could only be identified on pathologic examination. Although this presents new opportunities, it also results in problems when this information results in more aggressive therapy in clinical situations in which outcomes are well documented and known to be good. At present, the clinical value of MRI is most evident in areas in which patient management has been problematic. These include screening women with known or suspected BRCA 1 and 2 mutations, a group for whom mammographic screening is associated with a high rate of interval cancers, and identification of the primary tumor site in patients presenting with axillary adenopathy. The role of MRI for treatment selection in the patient with newly diagnosed breast cancer remains controversial. Success rates for patients selected for BCT without MRI are high, and rates of IBTR are low. An expanding body of evidence indicates that tumor biology, as well as tumor burden, is a major determinant of the outcome of local and systemic therapy. Future efforts to improve the local therapy for breast cancer must acknowledge the heterogeneity of the disease and tailor approaches to the biology of individual subsets, as has been done in newer trials of systemic therapy. This goal can only be accomplished through a multidisciplinary approach to studies that examine the applications of newer diagnostic modalities such as MRI.

REFERENCES

1. Berry DA, Cronin KA, Plevritis SK, et al. Effect of screening and adjuvant therapy on mortality from breast cancer. N Engl J Med 2005;353(17):1784–92.

2. Poggi MM, Danforth DN, Sciuto LC, et al. Eighteen-year results in the treatment of early breast carcinoma with mastectomy versus breast conservation therapy: the National Cancer Institute Randomized Trial. Cancer 2003;98(4):697–702.

3. van Dongen JA, Voogd AC, Fentiman IS, et al. Long-term results of a randomized trial comparing breast-conserving therapy with mastectomy: European Organization for Research and Treatment of Cancer 10801 trial. J Natl Cancer Inst 2000; 92(14):1143–50.

4. Kaufmann M, Morrow M, von Minckwitz G, et al. Locoregional treatment of primary breast cancer: consensus recommendations from an International Expert Panel. Cancer 2010;116(5):1184–91.

5. Morrow M, Harris JR. Practice guideline for breast conservation therapy in the management of invasive breast cancer. J Am Coll Surg 2007;205:362–76.

6. Ernst MF, Voogd AC, Coebergh JW, et al. Using loco-regional recurrence as an indicator of the quality of breast cancer treatment. Eur J Cancer 2004;40(4):487–93.

7. Pass H, Vicini FA, Kestin LL, et al. Changes in management techniques and patterns of disease recurrence over time in patients with breast carcinoma treated with breast-conserving therapy at a single institution. Cancer 2004; 101(4):713–20.

8. Otto SJ, Fracheboud J, Looman CW, et al. Initiation of population-based mammography screening in Dutch municipalities and effect on breast-cancer mortality: a systematic review. Lancet 2003;361(9367):1411–7.

9. Pisano ED, Gatsonis C, Hendrick E, et al. Diagnostic performance of digital versus film mammography for breast-cancer screening. N Engl J Med 2005; 353(17):1773–83.

10. Kerlikowske K. Efficacy of screening mammography among women aged 40 to 49 years and 50 to 69 years: comparison of relative and absolute benefit. J Natl Cancer Inst Monogr 1997;22:79–86.

11. Brekelmans CT, Seynaeve C, Bartels CC, et al. Effectiveness of breast cancer surveillance in BRCA1/2 gene mutation carriers and women with high familial risk. J Clin Oncol 2001;19(4):924–30.

12. Kuhl CK, Schrading S, Leutner CC, et al. Mammography, breast ultrasound, and magnetic resonance imaging for surveillance of women at high familial risk for breast cancer. J Clin Oncol 2005;23(33):8469–76.

13. Lakhani SR, Jacquemier J, Sloane JP, et al. Multifactorial analysis of differences between sporadic breast cancers and cancers involving BRCA1 and BRCA2 mutations. J Natl Cancer Inst 1998;90(15):1138–45.

14. Sardanelli F, Giuseppetti GM, Panizza P, et al. Sensitivity of MRI versus mammography for detecting foci of multifocal, multicentric breast cancer in Fatty and dense breasts using the whole-breast pathologic examination as a gold standard. AJR Am J Roentgenol 2004;183(4):1149–57.

15. Warner E, Messersmith H, Causer P, et al. Systematic review: using magnetic resonance imaging to screen women at high risk for breast cancer. Ann Intern Med 2008;148(9):671–9.

16. Warner E, Plewes DB, Hill KA, et al. Surveillance of BRCA1 and BRCA2 mutation carriers with magnetic resonance imaging, ultrasound, mammography, and clinical breast examination. JAMA 2004;292(11):1317–25.

17. Kriege M, Brekelmans CT, Boetes C, et al. Efficacy of MRI and mammography for breast-cancer screening in women with a familial or genetic predisposition. N Engl J Med 2004;351(5):427–37.

18. Leach MO, Boggis CR, Dixon AK, et al. Screening with magnetic resonance imaging and mammography of a UK population at high familial risk of breast

cancer: a prospective multicentre cohort study (MARIBS). Lancet 2005; 365(9473):1769–78.

19. Hagen AI, Kvistad KA, Maehle L, et al. Sensitivity of MRI versus conventional screening in the diagnosis of BRCA-associated breast cancer in a national prospective series. Breast 2007;16(4):367–74.
20. Kuhl CK, Schrading S, Bieling HB, et al. MRI for diagnosis of pure ductal carcinoma in situ: a prospective observational study. Lancet 2007;370(9586):485–92.
21. Port ER, Park A, Borgen PI, et al. Results of MRI screening for breast cancer in high-risk patients with LCIS and atypical hyperplasia. Ann Surg Oncol 2007; 14(3):1051–7.
22. Saslow D, Boetes C, Burke W, et al. American Cancer Society guidelines for breast screening with MRI as an adjunct to mammography. CA Cancer J Clin 2007;57(2):75–89.
23. Morrow M, Bucci C, Rademaker A. Medical contraindications are not a major factor in the underutilization of breast conserving therapy. J Am Coll Surg 1998;186(3):269–74.
24. Holland R, Veling SH, Mravunac M, et al. Histologic multifocality of Tis, T1-2 breast carcinomas. Implications for clinical trials of breast-conserving surgery. Cancer 1985;56(5):979–90.
25. Lagios MD. Multicentricity of breast carcinoma demonstrated by routine correlated serial subgross and radiographic examination. Cancer 1977;40(4): 1726–34.
26. Schwartz GF, Patchesfsky AS, Feig SA, et al. Multicentricity of non-palpable breast cancer. Cancer 1980;45(12):2913–6.
27. Anderson SJ, Wapnir I, Dignam JJ, et al. Prognosis after ipsilateral breast tumor recurrence and locoregional recurrences in patients treated by breast-conserving therapy in five National Surgical Adjuvant Breast and Bowel Project protocols of node-negative breast cancer. J Clin Oncol 2009;27(15):2466–73.
28. Wapnir IL, Anderson SJ, Mamounas EP, et al. Prognosis after ipsilateral breast tumor recurrence and locoregional recurrences in five National Surgical Adjuvant Breast and Bowel Project node-positive adjuvant breast cancer trials. J Clin Oncol 2006;24(13):2028–37.
29. Houssami N, Ciatto S, Macaskill P, et al. Accuracy and surgical impact of magnetic resonance imaging in breast cancer staging: systematic review and meta-analysis in detection of multifocal and multicentric cancer. J Clin Oncol 2008;26(19):3248–58.
30. Mann RM, Hoogeveen YL, Blickman JG, et al. MRI compared to conventional diagnostic work-up in the detection and evaluation of invasive lobular carcinoma of the breast: a review of existing literature. Breast Cancer Res Treat 2008;107(1): 1–14.
31. Berg WA, Gutierrez L, NessAiver MS, et al. Diagnostic accuracy of mammography, clinical examination, US, and MR imaging in preoperative assessment of breast cancer. Radiology 2004;233(3):830–49.
32. Liberman L, Morris EA, Dershaw DD, et al. MR imaging of the ipsilateral breast in women with percutaneously proven breast cancer. AJR Am J Roentgenol 2003; 180(4):901–10.
33. Katipamula R, Degnim AC, Hoskin T, et al. Trends in mastectomy rates at the Mayo Clinic Rochester: effect of surgical year and preoperative magnetic resonance imaging. J Clin Oncol 2009;27(25):4082–8.
34. Morrow M, Schmidt R, Hassett C. Patient selection for breast conservation therapy with magnification mammography. Surgery 1995;118(4):621–6.

35. Morrow M, Jagsi R, Alderman AK, et al. Surgeon recommendations and receipt of mastectomy for treatment of breast cancer. JAMA 2009;302(14):1551–6.
36. Bleicher RJ, Ciocca RM, Egleston BL, et al. Association of routine pretreatment magnetic resonance imaging with time to surgery, mastectomy rate, and margin status. J Am Coll Surg 2009;209(2):180–7 [quiz: 294–5].
37. Pengel KE, Loo CE, Teertstra HJ, et al. The impact of preoperative MRI on breast-conserving surgery of invasive cancer: a comparative cohort study. Breast Cancer Res Treat 2009;116(1):161–9.
38. Drew PJ, Harvey I, Hanby A, et al. The UK NIHR multi-centre randomised COMICE trial of MRI planning for breast conserving treatment for breast cancer. Cancer Res 2009;69(Suppl 2) [abstract 51].
39. Schiller DE, Le LW, Cho BC, et al. Factors associated with negative margins of lumpectomy specimen: potential use in selecting patients for intraoperative radiotherapy. Ann Surg Oncol 2008;15(3):833–42.
40. Hwang N, Schiller DE, Crystal P, et al. Magnetic resonance imaging in the planning of initial lumpectomy for invasive breast carcinoma: its effect on ipsilateral breast tumor recurrence after breast-conservation therapy. Ann Surg Oncol 2009;16(11):3000–9.
41. Mann RM, Loo CE, Wobbes T, et al. The impact of preoperative breast MRI on the re-excision rate in invasive lobular carcinoma of the breast. Breast Cancer Res Treat 2010;119(2):415–22.
42. Morrow M, Keeney K, Scholtens D, et al. Selecting patients for breast-conserving therapy: the importance of lobular histology. Cancer 2006;106(12):2563–8.
43. Schouten van der Velden AP, Boetes C, Bult P, et al. Magnetic resonance imaging in size assessment of invasive breast carcinoma with an extensive intraductal component. BMC Med Imaging 2009;9:5.
44. Van Goethem M, Schelfout K, Kersschot E, et al. MR mammography is useful in the preoperative locoregional staging of breast carcinomas with extensive intraductal component. Eur J Radiol 2007;62(2):273–82.
45. Wasif N, Garreau J, Terando A, et al. MRI versus ultrasonography and mammography for preoperative assessment of breast cancer. Am Surg 2009;75(10):970–5.
46. Pettit K, Swatske ME, Gao F, et al. The impact of breast MRI on surgical decision-making: are patients at risk for mastectomy? J Surg Oncol 2009;100(7):553–8.
47. King TA, Sakr R, Gurevich I, et al. Clinical management factors contribute to the decision for contralateral prophylactic mastectomy. Cancer Res 2009;69(Suppl 24):494s [#438].
48. Fourquet A, Kirova YM, Campana F. Occult primary cancer with axillary metastases. In: Harris JR, Lippman ME, Morrow M, et al, editors. Diseases of the breast. 4th edition. Philadelphia: Lippincott Williams & Wilkins; 2010. p. 817–21.
49. Ellerbroek N, Holmes F, Singletary E, et al. Treatment of patients with isolated axillary nodal metastases from an occult primary carcinoma consistent with breast origin. Cancer 1990;66(7):1461–7.
50. Kemeny MM, Rivera DE, Terz JJ, et al. Occult primary adenocarcinoma with axillary metastases. Am J Surg 1986;152(1):43–7.
51. Buchanan CL, Morris EA, Dorn PL, et al. Utility of breast magnetic resonance imaging in patients with occult primary breast cancer. Ann Surg Oncol 2005;12(12):1045–53.
52. McMahon K, Medoro L, Kennedy D. Breast magnetic resonance imaging: an essential role in malignant axillary lymphadenopathy of unknown origin. Australas Radiol 2005;49(5):382–9.

53. Olson JA Jr, Morris EA, Van Zee KJ, et al. Magnetic resonance imaging facilitates breast conservation for occult breast cancer. Ann Surg Oncol 2000;7(6): 411–5.
54. Orel SG, Weinstein SP, Schnall MD, et al. Breast MR imaging in patients with axillary node metastases and unknown primary malignancy. Radiology 1999;212(2): 543–9.
55. Henry-Tillman RS, Harms SE, Westbrook KC, et al. Role of breast magnetic resonance imaging in determining breast as a source of unknown metastatic lymphadenopathy. Am J Surg 1999;178(6):496–500.
56. Morris EA, Schwartz LH, Dershaw DD, et al. MR imaging of the breast in patients with occult primary breast carcinoma. Radiology 1997;205(2):437–40.
57. Ko EY, Han BK, Shin JH, et al. Breast MRI for evaluating patients with metastatic axillary lymph node and initially negative mammography and sonography. Korean J Radiol 2007;8(5):382–9.
58. de Bresser J, de Vos B, van der Ent F, et al. Breast MRI in clinically and mammographically occult breast cancer presenting with an axillary metastasis: a systematic review. Eur J Surg Oncol 2010;36(2):114–9.
59. Clarke M, Collins R, Darby S, et al. Effects of radiotherapy and of differences in the extent of surgery for early breast cancer on local recurrence and 15-year survival: an overview of the randomised trials. Lancet 2005;366(9503):2087–106.
60. Fischer U, Zachariae O, Baum F, et al. The influence of preoperative MRI of the breasts on recurrence rate in patients with breast cancer. Eur Radiol 2004; 14(10):1725–31.
61. Solin LJ, Orel SG, Hwang WT, et al. Relationship of breast magnetic resonance imaging to outcome after breast-conservation treatment with radiation for women with early-stage invasive breast carcinoma or ductal carcinoma in situ. J Clin Oncol 2008;26(3):386–91.
62. Nguyen PL, Taghian AG, Katz MS, et al. Breast cancer subtype approximated by estrogen receptor, progesterone receptor, and HER-2 is associated with local and distant recurrence after breast-conserving therapy. J Clin Oncol 2008; 26(14):2373–8.
63. Kyndi M, Sorensen FB, Knudsen H, et al. Estrogen receptor, progesterone receptor, HER-2, and response to postmastectomy radiotherapy in high-risk breast cancer: the Danish Breast Cancer Cooperative Group. J Clin Oncol 2008;26(9):1419–26.
64. Gao X, Fisher SG, Emami B. Risk of second primary cancer in the contralateral breast in women treated for early-stage breast cancer: a population-based study. Int J Radiat Oncol Biol Phys 2003;56(4):1038–45.
65. Lehman CD, Gatsonis C, Kuhl CK, et al. MRI evaluation of the contralateral breast in women with recently diagnosed breast cancer. N Engl J Med 2007;356(13): 1295–303.
66. Cody HS 3rd. Routine contralateral breast biopsy: helpful or irrelevant? Experience in 871 patients, 1979–1993. Ann Surg 1997;225(4):370–6.
67. Pressman PI. Selective biopsy of the opposite breast. Cancer 1986;57(3):577–80.
68. Effects of chemotherapy and hormonal therapy for early breast cancer on recurrence and 15-year survival: an overview of the randomised trials. Lancet 2005; 365(9472):1687–717.
69. Brennan ME, Houssami N, Lord S, et al. Magnetic resonance imaging screening of the contralateral breast in women with newly diagnosed breast cancer: systematic review and meta-analysis of incremental cancer detection and impact on surgical management. J Clin Oncol 2009;27(33):5640–9.

70. Sorbero ME, Dick AW, Beckjord EB, et al. Diagnostic breast magnetic resonance imaging and contralateral prophylactic mastectomy. Ann Surg Oncol 2009;16(6): 1597–605.

71. van Tienhoven G, Voogd AC, Peterse JL, et al. Prognosis after treatment for loco-regional recurrence after mastectomy or breast conserving therapy in two randomised trials (EORTC 10801 and DBCG-82TM). EORTC Breast Cancer Cooperative Group and the Danish Breast Cancer Cooperative Group. Eur J Cancer 1999;35(1):32–8.

72. Voogd AC, van Tienhoven G, Peterse HL, et al. Local recurrence after breast conservation therapy for early stage breast carcinoma: detection, treatment, and outcome in 266 patients. Dutch Study Group on Local Recurrence after Breast Conservation (BORST). Cancer 1999;85(2):437–46.

73. Gage I, Schnitt SJ, Recht A, et al. Skin recurrences after breast-conserving therapy for early-stage breast cancer. J Clin Oncol 1998;16(2):480–6.

74. Fisher ER, Anderson S, Redmond C, et al. Ipsilateral breast tumor recurrence and survival following lumpectomy and irradiation: pathological findings from NSABP protocol B-06. Semin Surg Oncol 1992;8(3):161–6.

75. Veronesi U, Marubini E, Del Vecchio M, et al. Local recurrences and distant metastases after conservative breast cancer treatments: partly independent events. J Natl Cancer Inst 1995;87(1):19–27.

76. Galper S, Blood E, Gelman R, et al. Prognosis after local recurrence after conservative surgery and radiation for early-stage breast cancer. Int J Radiat Oncol Biol Phys 2005;61(2):348–57.

77. Kurtz JM, Jacquemier J, Amalric R, et al. Is breast conservation after local recurrence feasible? Eur J Cancer 1991;27(3):240–4.

78. Salvadori B, Veronesi U. Conservative methods for breast cancer of small size: the experience of the National Cancer Institute, Milan (1973–1998). Breast 1999;8(6):311–4.

79. Millar EK, Graham PH, O'Toole SA, et al. Prediction of local recurrence, distant metastases, and death after breast-conserving therapy in early-stage invasive breast cancer using a five-biomarker panel. J Clin Oncol 2009;27(28):4701–8.

80. Fortin A, Larochelle M, Laverdiere J, et al. Local failure is responsible for the decrease in survival for patients with breast cancer treated with conservative surgery and postoperative radiotherapy. J Clin Oncol 1999;17(1):101–9.

81. Fourquet A, Campana F, Zafrani B, et al. Prognostic factors of breast recurrence in the conservative management of early breast cancer: a 25-year follow-up. Int J Radiat Oncol Biol Phys 1989;17(4):719–25.

Clinical Significance of Minimal Sentinel Node Involvement and Management Options

Anees B. Chagpar, MD, MA, MSc, MPH, FRCSC[a,b,*]

KEYWORDS

- Sentinel node • Breast cancer • Axillary lymph node dissection
- Biopsy

Since its introduction in the mid-1990s,[1,2] sentinel lymph node (SLN) biopsy has revolutionized the management of breast cancer patients, allowing for a minimally invasive method to accurately stage the axilla without the need for axillary lymph node dissection (ALND) and its concomitant morbidity in node-negative patients. The ability to identify the lymph nodes most likely to harbor metastases has allowed for increased scrutiny of these lymph nodes, often finding minimal disease in the SLNs. The relevance of such minute disease has been controversial, and there has been considerable debate as to how best to manage such patients.

WHAT CONSTITUTES A POSITIVE SENTINEL LYMPH NODE?

SLNs are frequently subjected to increased pathologic scrutiny, often involving serial sectioning, the use of immunohistochemistry (IHC), and molecular techniques using polymerase chain reaction (PCR). Such careful evaluation has led to an upstaging of patients who may have been found to be node negative on routine histopathologic examination. Several studies have found that up to a third of patients may be found to have SLN metastases when their SLNs are subjected to more intensive examination (**Table 1**). When investigators re-examined ALND specimens of patients in older studies, such as the Ludwig Trial V, using serial sectioning and IHC, they found

This work was supported in part by NIH R21 CA 131688.

[a] Department of Surgery, University of Louisville, 315 East Broadway, Suite 312, Louisville, KY 40202, USA

[b] Multidisciplinary Breast Program, James Graham Brown Cancer Center, Louisville, KY 40202, USA

* Department of Surgery, University of Louisville, 315 East, Broadway, Suite 312, Louisville, KY 40202.

E-mail address: Anees.chagpar@nortonhealthcare.org

Surg Oncol Clin N Am 19 (2010) 493–505
doi:10.1016/j.soc.2010.03.002
1055-3207/10/$ – see front matter © 2010 Elsevier Inc. All rights reserved.

Table 1
Upstaging SLNs by immunohistochemistry, serial sectioning and molecular analysis

Study	No. of Patients	Technique	No. Upstaged (%)
Inokuchi (2003)[46]	342	IHC	5 (2)
Mullenix (2005)[47]	183	IHC	8 (4)
Wong (2001)[48]	869	IHC	58 (7)
Schreiber (1999)[49]	210	IHC	17 (9)
Pendas (1999)[50]	385	IHC	41 (11)
McIntosh (1999)[51]	52	IHC	8 (14)
Ryden (2007)[52]	132	IHC/SS	3 (2)
Weaver (2000)[53]	489	IHC/SS	20 (4)
Pargaonkar (2003)[54]	64	IHC/SS	5 (8)
Weaver (2009)[55]	54	IHC/SS	5 (9)
Stitzenberg (2002)[56]	55	IHC/SS	7 (13)
Yared (2002)[57]	96	IHC/SS	19 (20)
Inokuchi (2003)[46]	342	RT-PCR	31 (9)
Sakaguchi (2003)[58]	80	RT-PCR	13 (16)
Manzotti (2001)[59]	117	RT-PCR	23 (20)
Gillanders (2004)[60]	344	RT-PCR	112 (33)

micrometastases in 7% to 9% of patients who had previously been categorized as node negative. Further, these patients had a significantly worse overall and disease-free survival than those who were truly node negative.[3,4] Although hematoxylin-eosin (H&E) staining remains the gold standard for detecting metastases, many pathologists continue to use IHC in the evaluation of SLNs.[5] The Association of Directors of Anatomic and Surgical Pathology recommends that the results of IHC should be evaluated in the context of routine histopathology.[6]

Although the modality used to detect nodal metastases should be recorded, the seventh edition of the American Joint Committee on Cancer staging system uses the size of the tumor deposit to determine lymph node positivity.[7] Tumor deposits should be measured as the largest dimension of any group of contiguous cells, regardless of whether or not they are confined to the node.[7] Tumor deposits less than 0.2 mm are considered isolated tumor cells (ITCs) of unknown biologic significance (ie, node negative).[7] Tumor deposits measuring 0.2 to 2.0 mm or those containing more than 200 individual tumor cells in a single node section are considered micrometastases (N1[mic]) (ie, node positive).[7]

Although the prognostic impact of ITCs and micrometastasis is the subject of the American College of Surgeons Oncology Group (ACOSOG) Z-0010 trial and the National Surgical Adjuvant Breast and Bowel Project (NSABP) B-32 trial,[8] other studies have provided some insight into their relevance. For example, in a multicenter study of 1259 patients with a mean follow-up of 4.9 years, distant recurrence rates were significantly different between SLN-negative patients (6%) and those with ITCs (8%), micrometastases (14%), and macrometastases (21%).[9] Similarly, a study from Memorial Sloan-Kettering in which ALND specimens of 368 patients treated between 1976 and 1978 were evaluated with serial section and IHC found that 17 patients (5%) were found to have micrometastases and 5 patients (1%) were found to have macrometastases.[10] The finding of these deposits was associated with a significantly worse disease-free survival than those who were truly node negative.[10]

Several studies have assessed the incidence of finding non-SLN metastases in the setting of ITCs and micrometastases (**Table 2**). A meta-analysis demonstrated that in patients with SLN micrometastasis, approximately 20% would have nonsentinel metastasis.[11] Therefore, micrometastases constitute node-positive disease, and completion ALND is currently recommended. Patients with ITCs or clusters measuring less than 0.2 mm, however, are considered node negative and no further axillary surgery is required. In a recent survey of American Society of Clinical Oncology members, the finding of micrometastases were found to "always" or "sometimes"

Table 2
Incidence of non-SLN metastases with SLN ITCs/micrometastases

Study	No. of SLN + Patients	ITC/ Micrometastases	No. of NSLN Positive (%)
Cserni (2007)[61]	26	ITC	0 (0)
Calhoun (2005)[62]	61	ITC	3 (4.9)
Van Rijk (2006)	54	ITC	4 (7.4)
Schrenk (2005)[63]	44	ITC	4 (9.1)
Van Deurzen (2007)[64]	23	ITC	3 (13.0)
Viale (2005)[65]	116	ITC	17 (15.8)
Houvenaeghel (2006)[66]	187	ITC	30 (16.0)
Menes (2005)[67]	31	ITC	6 (19.4)
Fournier (2004)[68]	16	ITC/micrometastasis	1 (6.3)
Nos (2003)[69]	123	ITC/micrometastasis	8 (6.5)
Yu (2005)[70]	70	ITC/micrometastasis	5 (7.1)
van Iterson (2003)[71]	54	ITC/micrometastasis	6 (11.1)
Hung (2005)[72]	24	ITC/micrometastasis	4 (16.7)
Fleming (2004)[73]	16	ITC/micrometastasis	3 (18.8)
Mignotte (2002)[42]	68	ITC/micrometastasis	15 (22.1)
den Bakker (2002)[74]	32	ITC/micrometastasis	11 (34.4)
Rutledge (2005)[75]	29	Micrometastasis	1 (3.4)
Zgajnar (2005)[76]	36	Micrometastasis	4 (11.1)
Gipponi (2006)[77]	116	Micrometastasis	16 (13.8)
Houvenaeghel (2006)[66]	301	Micrometastasis	43 (14.3)
Fink (2008)[78]	12	Micrometastasis	2 (16.7)
Chagpar (2005)[79]	84	Micrometastasis	15 (17.9)
Van Deurzen (2007)[64]	101	Micrometastasis	20 (19.8)
Reynolds (1999)[80]	27	Micrometastasis	6 (22.2)
Schrenk (2005)[63]	78	Micrometastasis	78 (23.1)
Leidenius (2005)[37]	84	Micrometastasis	22 (26.2)
Li (2007)[81]	68	Micrometastasis	18 (26.4)
Menes (2005)[67]	30	Micrometastasis	6 (20.0)
Viale (2005)[65]	318	Micrometastasis	68 (21.3)
Cserni (2004)[82]	32	Micrometastasis	8 (33.3)

influence clinical decisions in 54.7% and 43.8% of respondents, respectively, whereas 52.9% stated that ITCs never had an impact.[12] Only 22.1% of respondents stated, however, they would "always" recommend an ALND for micrometastases, whereas 73% stated they would recommend it "sometimes."[12] Factors influencing this decision included primary tumor size, patient age, tumor grade, lymphovascular invasion, and size of the metastasis.[12]

TREATMENT OF SENTINEL NODE POSITIVE DISEASE: THE NEED FOR ALND?

Although controversial, there is little evidence that ALND improves survival. The 25-year follow-up from the landmark NSABP B-04 trial showed no difference in survival for patients who received elective ALND compared with those who did not.[13] Nonetheless, ALND provides excellent local control.[13] Many patients with SLN metastases have no further disease in the axilla (**Table 3**), thus raising the question of whether or not ALND is needed in all SLN-positive patients. The University of Louisville Breast Sentinel Node Study, a multicenter prospective trial of 4131 patients, found that 63.1% of SLN-positive patients had disease limited to the sentinel nodes. ALND is associated with significant morbidity, including numbness, swelling, and decreased range of motion of the shoulder. Therefore, there has been considerable interest in identifying a subset of SLN-positive patients in whom the risk of non-SLN metastases is so low that ALND may be avoided.

Another reason to advocate that all patients with a positive SLN should undergo completion ALND is to obtain accurate staging information that may affect adjuvant therapy decisions. Although it may be argued that contemporary use of systemic therapy is often guided by primary tumor information and that the absolute number of total lymph nodes involved may be of little consequence to therapy decisions, others may find information, in particular regarding lymph node ratio, to affect their decision making.[14,15] Furthermore, the number of positive nodes may affect decisions regarding postmastectomy radiation therapy (PMRT). Although the American Society of Clinical Oncology and the American Society of Therapeutic Radiology and

Table 3
Rate of Nonsentinel Node Metastases in SLN-Positive Patients

Study	No. of Patients	% Patients with No Non-SLN Metastases
Yu et al (2005)[70]	286	34.3
Viale (2005)[65]	794	49.7
van Deurzen (2007)[64]	193	51.8
Degnim et al (2005)[24]	574	58.3
Soni et al (2005)[26]	149	58.4
Cserni et al (2004)[82]	150	60.0
Kocsis et al (2004)[25]	140	61.0
Van Zee et al (2003)[21]	1075	61.1
Schrenk et al (2005)[63]	379	62.3
van Iterson et al (2003)[71]	135	66.0
Nos et al (2003)[69]	263	76.0
Houvenaeghel (2009)[83]	490	84.9
Houvenaeghel (2006)[66]	301	85.7

Oncology continue to recommend PMRT in the setting of 4 or more positive nodes,[16,17] more recent data suggest that PMRT may be of benefit even in the 1 to 3 node-positive group.[18] Proponents of treating all node-positive patients with PMRT on the basis of these data may argue, therefore, that information obtained from completion ALND will not affect their management.

Finally, accurate staging is dependent on the absolute number of positive nodes[7] and provides prognostic information. ALND has not been found to adversely affect long-term quality of life[19,20] and, therefore, remains standard of care after a positive SLN biopsy.

PREDICTIVE MODELS

If it were possible, however, to accurately define a subset of patients in whom no further non-SLNs would be positive, there would be the ability to have accurate staging and treatment information without the morbidity of an ALND. This quest has been the subject of inquiry for many investigators, and several models have been developed for this purpose.

Perhaps the best known of these is the Memorial Sloan-Kettering nomogram developed by Van Zee and colleagues.[21] This model predicts the probability of non-SLN status based on several factors, including pathologic tumor size, grade, lymphovascular invasion, multifocality, estrogen receptor status, the number of positive and negative SLNs, and the method used to identify SLN metastases (by IHC, routine H&E staining, serial sectioning with H&E, or frozen section). Although several investigators have validated this nomogram,[22,23] some have found that it could not predict nonsentinel node status, particularly in patients at low likelihood of having nonsentinel node disease.[24–26] Although the nomogram has been found to predict nonsentinel node metastasis better than clinicians' best guess, most surgeons would not change patient management based on the findings of the nomogram.[27] Perhaps this is because many surgeons opt to complete the ALND based on intraoperative examination of the SLN, and the nomogram requires final histopathology and, therefore, would mandate delaying the ALND to a separate operative setting. Given that the sensitivity of intraoperative evaluation of SLNs has been reported to be between 50% and 85% (depending on the technique used),[28] this nomogram (available online at http://www.mskcc.org/mskcc/html/15938.cfm;) is useful in discussing with patients the probability of non-SLN metastases and in deciding whether or not a return to the operating room for a completion ALND is worth the concomitant risk.

Others have created similar models to predict non-SLN metastases. Kohrt and colleagues[29] at Stanford used multivariate logistic regression informed by classification and regression trees to develop a model involving 3 variables to predict non-SLN status: tumor size, angiolymphatic invasion, and size of metastasis. Pal and colleagues[30] from Cambridge similarly developed a nomogram based on histologic grade, overall metastasis size from the SLN, and the proportion of positive SLNs. Despite the fact that these models only contained 3 variables each, they both found (in their populations) that their models were superior to the Memorial Sloan-Kettering nomogram.

The Tenon model, developed by Barranger and colleagues,[31] is a simple point system in which points are assigned on the basis of presence of macrometastases, histologic tumor size, and proportion of involved lymph nodes. In this simple model, 2 points are assigned if macrometastases are noted in the SLN, 1.5 points if the tumor size is 11 to 20 mm, and 3 points if the tumor size is greater than 2 cm; 1 point if 50% to 99% of the SLNs removed are positive; and 2 points if all of the SLNs removed were involved. Using this scoring system, patients with a score of 3.5 or less had a 97.3% chance of having no further non-SLNs involved.[31] This model has also been validated in a prospective multicenter trial.[32] Given the variety of prediction models available, several groups have compared these. Although each model has its strengths and weaknesses, the Memorial Sloan-Kettering nomogram seems to be the most robust of the models available.[33,34]

Although acknowledging the power the Memorial Sloan-Kettering nomogram obtains from postoperative pathologic information, the University of Louisville group sought to define a clinical prediction rule based on preoperative and intraoperative factors alone that might guide intraoperative decision-making. Their simple model, based on a multivariate analysis of a multi-institutional series of 1253 SLN-positive patients, assigns 1 point for more than 1 positive SLN, 1 point if more than 50% of the SLNs harvested were positive, and up to 4 points for increasing tumor size (T1a = 1, T1b or T1c = 2, T2 = 3, and T3 = 4).[35] In their series, patients with only 1 point had a 95% probability of having no further axillary disease. This model has been validated in other data sets.[36] Furthermore, although not truly evaluating this model, Leidenius and colleagues[37] found that the risk of non-SLN metastasis was negligible in patients with a single positive SLN who had more than 4 SLNs removed. Silverstein and colleagues[38] similarly argued that in patients with small tumors (T1a) with a positive SLN, non-SLN metastases are rare. Others, however, have criticized this model. Despite finding progressively increasing non-SLN metastases rates with higher point values, Scow and colleagues[39] argued that given that 1 of their 6 patients (17%) with 1 point had SLN metastases, this rate was too high to presume that this model was valid. Although their findings may have been related to the small sample size in which they tested the model, one of the legitimate criticisms of the University of Louisville model is that few patients are assigned 1 point.

Given the limitations of data available preoperatively and intraoperatively to inform the prediction of the likelihood of non-SLN metastases, efforts were made to refine the University of Louisville model using novel quantitative intraoperative reverse transcription (RT)-PCR–based assay data. A multicenter trial to evaluate an intraoperative molecular assay had found that assay data corresponded with the metastatic volume in the SLN.[40] Given that the burden of the disease in the SLN is often correlated with SLN metastases, Chagpar and colleagues[41] used the quantitative data to define a new score using the quantitative cycle time values for mammoglobin and cytokeratin-19. This score combined with tumor size and the proportion of SLNs harboring metastatic disease based on intraoperative histopathology was found to improve the prediction of non-SLN metastases, such that even in patients with tumors greater than 2 cm and those with more than 50% of their SLNs involved, a probability of non-SLN metastases of less than 8% could be achieved if their assay score was low (**Fig. 1**).

It remains difficult to define a highly selected group in whom the risk of non-SLN metastases is low,[42,43] and the probability of non-SLN metastasis at which ALND can be omitted is unclear. Until such time as nomograms or clinical prediction rules can be consistently validated, especially at low probabilities of non-SLN metastases, completion ALND will continue to be recommended in patients with a positive SLN.

Some investigators, however, have sought to define models to predict the likelihood of having 4 or more positive nodes—because this is a group in whom extensive disease is present and those who are unlikely to have significant disease may be treated by adjuvant radiation rather than ALND or because this is a population in whom PMRT is mandatory and prediction of which patients are at low likelihood of requiring PMRT may proceed with immediate reconstruction without significant fear

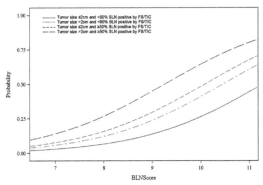

Fig. 1. Smoothed curves for prediction model including tumor size, proportion of positive lymph nodes, and breast lymph node (BLN) score. BLN score is defined as 10.2586–2.8053 × min (MG_CT/IC_CT, CK19_CT/IC_CT) + 1.7164 × BLN positive rate in SLNs, where MG_CT/ refers to the cycle time for mammoglobin divided by the cycle time for the internal control, CK19_CT/ IC_CT refers to the cycle time for cytokeratin-19 divided by the cycle time for the internal control, and the BLN positive rate in SLNs refers to the proportion of SLNs positive based on previously established cutoffs. FS, frozen section; TIC, touch imprint cytology. (*From* Chagpar AB, Blumencranz P, Whitworth PW, et al. Use pre- and intra-operative data to predict probability of positive non-sentinel lymph nodes. Cancer Res 2010;69(4):513 [abstract]; with permission.)

of compromising their outcomes. Currently, there are at least 2 prediction models that address this issue. The first was proposed by the University of Louisville group who, based on a multivariate analysis of 1132 patients, proposed a point system in which 1 point was given for each positive SLN,[1–3] 1 point was given for T2 (vs T1) disease, and 1 point was given for more than 50% of SLNs removed being positive for metastatic disease.[44] Patients with a single point had a less than 4% risk of having 4 or more positive lymph nodes.[44] Unlike this model, which used only preoperative and intraoperative data, Katz and colleagues proposed a more comprehensive nomogram including primary tumor size, number of positive SLNs, lymphovascular invasion, lobular histology, extranodal extension, micro- versus macrometastasis, and whether or not more than 1 SLN was positive. Both of these models have been validated in independent series.[36,45]

CLINICAL TRIALS

The ACOSOG Z-0010 and the NSABP B-32 trials will shed significant light on the biologic significance of SLN metastases found by IHC and the clinical management of patients with micrometastatic disease. The Z-011 trial, designed to evaluate the need for ALND in patients with a positive SLN undergoing partial mastectomy followed by whole breast irradiation, closed due to poor accrual. The International Breast Cancer Study Group (IBCSG) trial 23-01, however, currently evaluates the role of completion axillary dissection in patients who are found to have micrometastases on SLN biopsy (**Fig. 2**).

Furthermore, the European Organization for Research and Treatment of Cancer After Mapping of the Axilla: Radiotherapy or Surgery study compares completion axillary dissection with axillary radiotherapy in patients with positive SLN. Until these data are available, however, and with increasing use of accelerated partial breast irradiation, ALND remains standard for local control of the axilla in SLN positive patients.

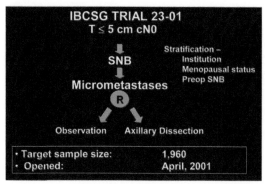

Fig. 2. IBCSG TRIAL on sentinel node micrometastases.

SUMMARY

The advent of SLN biopsy has obviated ALND for the majority of breast cancer patients who have node-negative disease. With increasing scrutiny of the SLNs, however, minimal disease is recognized. Such disease would have heretofore been missed, and therefore, there remains controversy as to the true significance of such minimal SLN involvement and the management of these patients. In particular, several prediction models have been introduced to identify a subset of SLN-positive patients who are unlikely to have further disease in the axilla. Although these models may help tailor therapy, no threshold of non-SLN metastases has been widely accepted. ALND remains relatively well tolerated and provides staging information that may affect prognosis and adjuvant treatment decisions. Therefore, current recommendations are for SLN metastases greater than 0.2 mm to be followed by completion ALND.

REFERENCES

1. Giuliano AE. Sentinel lymphadenectomy in primary breast carcinoma: an alternative to routine axillary dissection. J Surg Oncol 1996;62(2):75–7.
2. Albertini JJ, Lyman GH, Cox C, et al. Lymphatic mapping and sentinel node biopsy in the patient with breast cancer. JAMA 1996;276(22):1818–22.
3. Neville AM, Price KN, Gelber RD, et al. Axillary node micrometastases and breast cancer. Lancet 1991;337(8749):1110.
4. Cote RJ, Peterson HF, Chaiwun B, et al. Role of immunohistochemical detection of lymph-node metastases in management of breast cancer. International Breast Cancer Study Group. Lancet 1999;354(9182):896–900.
5. Cserni G, Amendoeira I, Apostolikas N, et al. Discrepancies in current practice of pathological evaluation of sentinel lymph nodes in breast cancer. Results of a questionnaire based survey by the European Working Group for Breast Screening Pathology. J Clin Pathol 2004;57(7):695–701.
6. Association of Directors of Anatomic and Surgical Pathology. ADASP recommendations for processing and reporting lymph node specimens submitted for evaluation of metastatic disease. Am J Surg Pathol 2001;25(7):961–3.
7. American Joint Committee on Cancer. Breast. In: Edge SB, Byrd DR, Compton CC, et al, editors. AJCC cancer staging handbook. New York: Springer-Verlag; 2010. p. 417–60.

8. White RL Jr, Wilke LG. Update on the NSABP and ACOSOG breast cancer sentinel node trials. Am Surg 2004;70(5):420–4.

9. Reed J, Rosman M, Verbanac KM, et al. Prognostic implications of isolated tumor cells and micrometastases in sentinel nodes of patients with invasive breast cancer: 10-year analysis of patients enrolled in the prospective East Carolina University/Anne Arundel Medical Center Sentinel Node Multicenter Study. J Am Coll Surg 2009;208(3):333–40.

10. Tan LK, Giri D, Hummer AJ, et al. Occult axillary node metastases in breast cancer are prognostically significant: results in 368 node-negative patients with 20-year follow-up. J Clin Oncol 2008;26(11):1803–9.

11. Cserni G, Gregori D, Merletti F, et al. Meta-analysis of non-sentinel node metastases associated with micrometastatic sentinel nodes in breast cancer. Br J Surg 2004;91(10):1245–52.

12. Wasif N, Ye X, Giuliano AE. Survey of ASCO members on management of sentinel node micrometastases in breast cancer: variation in treatment recommendations according to specialty. Ann Surg Oncol 2009;16(9):2442–9.

13. Fisher B, Jeong JH, Anderson S, et al. Twenty-five-year follow-up of a randomized trial comparing radical mastectomy, total mastectomy, and total mastectomy followed by irradiation. N Engl J Med 2002;347(8):567–75.

14. Vinh-Hung V, Verkooijen HM, Fioretta G, et al. Lymph node ratio as an alternative to pN staging in node-positive breast cancer. J Clin Oncol 2009;27(7):1062–8.

15. Truong PT, Vinh-Hung V, Cserni G, et al. The number of positive nodes and the ratio of positive to excised nodes are significant predictors of survival in women with micrometastatic node-positive breast cancer. Eur J Cancer 2008;44(12):1670–7.

16. Recht A, Edge SB, Solin LJ, et al. Postmastectomy radiotherapy: clinical practice guidelines of the American Society of Clinical Oncology. J Clin Oncol 2001;19(5):1539–69.

17. Harris JR, Halpin-Murphy P, McNeese M, et al. Consensus Statement on postmastectomy radiation therapy. Int J Radiat Oncol Biol Phys 1999;44(5):989–90.

18. Truong PT, Jones SO, Kader HA, et al. Patients with t1 to t2 breast cancer with one to three positive nodes have higher local and regional recurrence risks compared with node-negative patients after breast-conserving surgery and whole-breast radiotherapy. Int J Radiat Oncol Biol Phys 2009;73(2):357–64.

19. Barranger E, Dubernard G, Fleurence J, et al. Subjective morbidity and quality of life after sentinel node biopsy and axillary lymph node dissection for breast cancer. J Surg Oncol 2005;92(1):17–22.

20. Peintinger F, Reitsamer R, Stranzl H, et al. Comparison of quality of life and arm complaints after axillary lymph node dissection vs sentinel lymph node biopsy in breast cancer patients. Br J Cancer 2003;89(4):648–52.

21. Van Zee KJ, Manasseh DM, Bevilacqua JL, et al. A nomogram for predicting the likelihood of additional nodal metastases in breast cancer patients with a positive sentinel node biopsy. Ann Surg Oncol 2003;10(10):1140–51.

22. Lambert LA, Ayers GD, Hwang RF, et al. Validation of a breast cancer nomogram for predicting nonsentinel lymph node metastases after a positive sentinel node biopsy. Ann Surg Oncol 2006;13(3):310–20.

23. Smidt ML, Kuster DM, van der Wilt GJ, et al. Can the Memorial Sloan-Kettering Cancer Center nomogram predict the likelihood of nonsentinel lymph node metastases in breast cancer patients in the Netherlands? Ann Surg Oncol 2005;12(12):1066–72.

24. Degnim AC, Reynolds C, Pantvaidya G, et al. Nonsentinel node metastasis in breast cancer patients: assessment of an existing and a new predictive nomogram. Am J Surg 2005;190(4):543–50.
25. Kocsis L, Svebis M, Boross G, et al. Use and limitations of a nomogram predicting the likelihood of non-sentinel node involvement after a positive sentinel node biopsy in breast cancer patients. Am Surg 2004;70(11):1019–24.
26. Soni NK, Carmalt HL, Gillett DJ, et al. Evaluation of a breast cancer nomogram for prediction of non-sentinel lymph node positivity. Eur J Surg Oncol 2005;31(9):958–64.
27. Specht MC, Kattan MW, Gonen M, et al. Predicting nonsentinel node status after positive sentinel lymph biopsy for breast cancer: clinicians versus nomogram. Ann Surg Oncol 2005;12(8):654–9.
28. Krishnamurthy S, Meric-Bernstam F, Lucci A, et al. A prospective study comparing touch imprint cytology, frozen section analysis, and rapid cytokeratin immunostain for intraoperative evaluation of axillary sentinel lymph nodes in breast cancer. Cancer 2009;115(7):1555–62.
29. Kohrt HE, Olshen RA, Bermas HR, et al. New models and online calculator for predicting non-sentinel lymph node status in sentinel lymph node positive breast cancer patients. BMC Cancer 2008;8:66.
30. Pal A, Provenzano E, Duffy SW, et al. A model for predicting non-sentinel lymph node metastatic disease when the sentinel lymph node is positive. Br J Surg 2008;95(3):302–9.
31. Barranger E, Coutant C, Flahault A, et al. An axilla scoring system to predict non-sentinel lymph node status in breast cancer patients with sentinel lymph node involvement. Breast Cancer Res Treat 2005;91(2):113–9.
32. Coutant C, Rouzier R, Fondrinier E, et al. Validation of the Tenon breast cancer score for predicting non-sentinel lymph node status in breast cancer patients with sentinel lymph node metastasis: a prospective multicenter study. Breast Cancer Res Treat 2009;113(3):537–43.
33. Coutant C, Olivier C, Lambaudie E, et al. Comparison of models to predict non-sentinel lymph node status in breast cancer patients with metastatic sentinel lymph nodes: a prospective multicenter study. J Clin Oncol 2009;27(17):2800–8.
34. Gur AS, Unal B, Johnson R, et al. Predictive probability of four different breast cancer nomograms for nonsentinel axillary lymph node metastasis in positive sentinel node biopsy. J Am Coll Surg 2009;208(2):229–35.
35. Chagpar AB, Scoggins CR, Martin RC, et al. Prediction of sentinel lymph node-only disease in women with invasive breast cancer. Am J Surg 2006;192(6):882–7.
36. Cserni G, Bianchi S, Vezzosi V, et al. Validation of clinical prediction rules for a low probability of nonsentinel and extensive lymph node involvement in breast cancer patients. Am J Surg 2007;194(3):288–93.
37. Leidenius MH, Vironen JH, Riihela MS, et al. The prevalence of non-sentinel node metastases in breast cancer patients with sentinel node micrometastases. Eur J Surg Oncol 2005;31(1):13–8.
38. Silverstein MJ, Gierson ED, Waisman JR, et al. Axillary lymph node dissection for T1a breast carcinoma. Is it indicated? Cancer 1994;73(3):664–7.
39. Scow JS, Degnim AC, Hoskin TL, et al. Simple prediction models for breast cancer patients with solitary positive sentinel nodes–are they valid? Breast J 2009;15(6):610–4.
40. Julian TB, Blumencranz P, Deck K, et al. Novel intraoperative molecular test for sentinel lymph node metastases in patients with early-stage breast cancer. J Clin Oncol 2008;26(20):3338–45.

41. Chagpar AB, Blumencranz P, Whitworth PW, et al. Use pre- and intra-operative data to predict probability of positive non-sentinel lymph nodes [abstract]. Cancer Res 2010;69(4):513.

42. Mignotte H, Treilleux I, Faure C, et al. Axillary lymph-node dissection for positive sentinel nodes in breast cancer patients. Eur J Surg Oncol 2002;28(6): 623–6.

43. Travagli JP, Atallah D, Mathieu MC, et al. Sentinel lymphadenectomy without systematic axillary dissection in breast cancer patients: predictors of non-sentinel lymph node metastasis. Eur J Surg Oncol 2003;29(4):403–6.

44. Chagpar AB, Scoggins CR, Martin RC, et al. Predicting patients at low probability of requiring post-mastectomy radiation therapy. Ann Surg Oncol 2006;14(2):670–7.

45. Unal B, Gur AS, Beriwal S, et al. Predicting likelihood of having four or more positive nodes in patient with sentinel lymph node-positive breast cancer: a nomogram validation study. Int J Radiat Oncol Biol Phys 2009;75(4):1035–40.

46. Inokuchi M, Ninomiya I, Tsugawa K, et al. Quantitative evaluation of metastases in axillary lymph nodes of breast cancer. Br J Cancer 2003;89(9):1750–6.

47. Mullenix PS, Brown TA, Meyers MO, et al. The association of cytokeratin-only-positive sentinel lymph nodes and subsequent metastases in breast cancer. Am J Surg 2005;189(5):606–9.

48. Wong SL, Chao C, Edwards MJ, et al. The use of cytokeratin staining in sentinel lymph node biopsy for breast cancer. Am J Surg 2001;182(4):330–4.

49. Schreiber RH, Pendas S, Ku NN, et al. Microstaging of breast cancer patients using cytokeratin staining of the sentinel lymph node. Ann Surg Oncol 1999; 6(1):95–101.

50. Pendas S, Dauway E, Cox CE, et al. Sentinel node biopsy and cytokeratin staining for the accurate staging of 478 breast cancer patients. Am Surg 1999;65(6): 500–5.

51. McIntosh SA, Going JJ, Soukop M, et al. Therapeutic implications of the sentinel lymph node in breast cancer. Lancet 1999;354(9178):570.

52. Ryden L, Chebil G, Sjostrom L, et al. Determination of sentinel lymph node (SLN) status in primary breast cancer by prospective use of immunohistochemistry increases the rate of micrometastases and isolated tumour cells: analysis of 174 patients after SLN biopsy. Eur J Surg Oncol 2007;33(1):33–8.

53. Weaver DL, Krag DN, Ashikaga T, et al. Pathologic analysis of sentinel and non-sentinel lymph nodes in breast carcinoma: a multicenter study. Cancer 2000; 88(5):1099–107.

54. Pargaonkar AS, Beissner RS, Snyder S, et al. Evaluation of immunohistochemistry and multiple-level sectioning in sentinel lymph nodes from patients with breast cancer. Arch Pathol Lab Med 2003;127(6):701–5.

55. Weaver DL, Le UP, Dupuis SL, et al. Metastasis detection in sentinel lymph nodes: comparison of a limited widely spaced (NSABP protocol B-32) and a comprehensive narrowly spaced paraffin block sectioning strategy. Am J Surg Pathol 2009;33(11):1583–9.

56. Stitzenberg KB, Calvo BF, Iacocca MV, et al. Cytokeratin immunohistochemical validation of the sentinel node hypothesis in patients with breast cancer. Am J Clin Pathol 2002;117(5):729–37.

57. Yared MA, Middleton LP, Smith TL, et al. Recommendations for sentinel lymph node processing in breast cancer. Am J Surg Pathol 2002;26(3):377–82.

58. Sakaguchi M, Virmani A, Dudak MW, et al. Clinical relevance of reverse transcriptase-polymerase chain reaction for the detection of axillary lymph node metastases in breast cancer. Ann Surg Oncol 2003;10(2):117–25.

59. Manzotti M, Dell'Orto P, Maisonneuve P, et al. Reverse transcription-polymerase chain reaction assay for multiple mRNA markers in the detection of breast cancer metastases in sentinel lymph nodes. Int J Cancer 2001;95(5):307–12.

60. Gillanders WE, Mikhitarian K, Hebert R, et al. Molecular detection of micrometa-static breast cancer in histopathology-negative axillary lymph nodes correlates with traditional predictors of prognosis: an interim analysis of a prospective multi-institutional cohort study. Ann Surg 2004;239(6):828–37.

61. Cserni G, Bianchi S, Vezzosi V, et al. Sentinel lymph node biopsy in staging small (up to 15 mm) breast carcinomas. Results from a European multi-institutional study. Pathol Oncol Res 2007;13(1):5–14.

62. Calhoun KE, Hansen NM, Turner RR, et al. Nonsentinel node metastases in breast cancer patients with isolated tumor cells in the sentinel node: implications for completion axillary node dissection. Am J Surg 2005;190(4):588–91.

63. Schrenk P, Konstantiniuk P, Wolfl S, et al. Prediction of non-sentinel lymph node status in breast cancer with a micrometastatic sentinel node. Br J Surg 2005; 92(6):707–13.

64. van Deurzen CH, van HR, Hobbelink MG, et al. Predictive value of tumor load in breast cancer sentinel lymph nodes for second echelon lymph node metastases. Cell Oncol 2007;29(6):497–505.

65. Viale G, Maiorano E, Pruneri G, et al. Predicting the risk for additional axillary metastases in patients with breast carcinoma and positive sentinel lymph node biopsy. Ann Surg 2005;241(2):319–25.

66. Houvenaeghel G, Nos C, Mignotte H, et al. Micrometastases in sentinel lymph node in a multicentric study: predictive factors of nonsentinel lymph node involve-ment–Groupe des Chirurgiens de la Federation des Centres de Lutte Contre le Cancer. J Clin Oncol 2006;24(12):1814–22.

67. Menes TS, Tartter PI, Mizrachi H, et al. Breast cancer patients with pN0(i+) and pN1(mi) sentinel nodes have high rate of nonsentinel node metastases. J Am Coll Surg 2005;200(3):323–7.

68. Fournier K, Schiller A, Perry RR, et al. Micrometastasis in the sentinel lymph node of breast cancer does not mandate completion axillary dissection. Ann Surg 2004;239(6):859–63.

69. Nos C, Harding-MacKean C, Freneaux P, et al. Prediction of tumour involvement in remaining axillary lymph nodes when the sentinel node in a woman with breast cancer contains metastases. Br J Surg 2003;90(11):1354–60.

70. Yu JC, Hsu GC, Hsieh CB, et al. Prediction of metastasis to non-sentinel nodes by sentinel node status and primary tumor characteristics in primary breast cancer in Taiwan. World J Surg 2005;29(7):813–8.

71. van Iterson V, Leidenius M, Krogerus L, et al. Predictive factors for the status of non-sentinel nodes in breast cancer patients with tumor positive sentinel nodes. Breast Cancer Res Treat 2003;82(1):39–45.

72. Hung WK, Chan MC, Mak KL, et al. Non-sentinel lymph node metastases in breast cancer patients with metastatic sentinel nodes. ANZ J Surg 2005;75(1-2):27–31.

73. Fleming FJ, Kavanagh D, Crotty TB, et al. Factors affecting metastases to non-sentinel lymph nodes in breast cancer. J Clin Pathol 2004;57(1):73–6.

74. den Bakker MA, van Weeszenberg A, de Kanter AY, et al. Non-sentinel lymph node involvement in patients with breast cancer and sentinel node micrometasta-sis; too early to abandon axillary clearance. J Clin Pathol 2002;55(12):932–5.

75. Rutledge H, Davis J, Chiu R, et al. Sentinel node micrometastasis in breast carci-noma may not be an indication for complete axillary dissection. Mod Pathol 2005; 18(6):762–8.

76. Zgajnar J, Besic N, Podkrajsek M, et al. Minimal risk of macrometastases in the non-sentinel axillary lymph nodes in breast cancer patients with micrometastatic sentinel lymph nodes and preoperatively ultrasonically uninvolved axillary lymph nodes. Eur J Cancer 2005;41(2):244–8.

77. Gipponi M, Canavese G, Lionetto R, et al. The role of axillary lymph node dissection in breast cancer patients with sentinel lymph node micrometastases. Eur J Surg Oncol 2006;32(2):143–7.

78. Fink AM, Lass H, Hartleb H, et al. S-classification of sentinel lymph node predicts axillary nonsentinel lymph node status in patients with breast cancer. Ann Surg Oncol 2008;15(3):848–53.

79. Chagpar A, Middleton LP, Sahin AA, et al. Clinical outcome of patients with lymph node-negative breast carcinoma who have sentinel lymph node micrometastases detected by immunohistochemistry. Cancer 2005;103(8):1581–6.

80. Reynolds C, Mick R, Donohue JH, et al. Sentinel lymph node biopsy with metastasis: can axillary dissection be avoided in some patients with breast cancer? J Clin Oncol 1999;17(6):1720–6.

81. Li J, Rudas M, Kemmner W, et al. The location of small tumor deposits in the SLN predicts non-SLN macrometastases in breast cancer patients. Eur J Surg Oncol 2008;34(8):857–62.

82. Cserni G, Burzykowski T, Vinh-Hung V, et al. Axillary sentinel node and tumour-related factors associated with non-sentinel node involvement in breast cancer. Jpn J Clin Oncol 2004;34(9):519–24.

83. Houvenaeghel G, Nos C, Giard S, et al. A nomogram predictive of non-sentinel lymph node involvement in breast cancer patients with a sentinel lymph node micrometastasis. Eur J Surg Oncol 2009;35(7):690–5.

Clinical Significance and Management of Extra-Axillary Sentinel Lymph Nodes: Worthwhile or Irrelevant?

Hiram S. Cody III, MD

KEYWORDS

- Sentinel lymph node • Mastectomy • Lymphoscintigraphy
- Internal mammary nodes

Sentinel lymph node (SLN) biopsy is well established as standard care for axillary lymph node staging in breast cancer, based on the results of at least 69 observational studies[1] and 5 randomized trials.[2–6] SLN biopsy works well using a variety of techniques, but it seems in general that the overall success of lymphatic mapping is maximized, and the false-negative rate is minimized, by the combination of blue dye and radioisotope.[3,7,8] Radioisotope mapping in turn has validated the long-standing observation that the predominant lymphatic drainage of the breast is to the axilla[9–12] and has revived debate over the significance of lymphatic drainage to nonaxillary sites. This article addresses the clinical implications and management of nonaxillary SLNs, including the internal mammary (IM), intramammary, Rotter, supraclavicular, and contralateral axillary sites.

INTERNAL MAMMARY SLNs
Extended Radical Mastectomy

The guiding premise in Halsted's[13] 1894 report of his technique for radical mastectomy (RM) was that local control and survival were related and that an operation that minimized local recurrence would maximize survival. This concept was extended to its limit by Wangensteen's[14] "super-radical mastectomy" (a staged operation, which included resection of the breast, IM, mediastinal, and supraclavicular nodes), first described in 1949 and eventually abandoned because of high operative mortality

Breast Service, Department of Surgery, Memorial Sloan-Kettering Cancer Center, 300 East 66th Street, #831, New York, NY 10065, USA
E-mail address: codyh@mskcc.org

Surg Oncol Clin N Am 19 (2010) 507–517
doi:10.1016/j.soc.2010.04.002
1055-3207/10/$ – see front matter © 2010 Elsevier Inc. All rights reserved.

(12.5%) and few survivors.[15] In 1951, Urban[16] observed a high rate of parasternal chest wall recurrence (18%–28%) after RM in patients with inner-quadrant breast cancers. He logically hypothesized that extended RM (ERM), an operation that combined RM with a full-thickness resection of the parasternal chest wall and IM nodes, might offer a survival advantage for a subset of patients at increased risk for IM node involvement, specifically those with central or inner quadrant tumors. In his initial series of ERM, done for patients with stage I-II disease, he reported good results and no operative mortality.[17]

The goal of improved survival with more radical versions of mastectomy was never met: Veronesi and Valagussa's[18] randomized trial comparing ERM with RM demonstrates a 1.1% to 3.5% reduction in the 10-year rate of parasternal chest wall recurrence but no difference in any other outcomes or in survival at 30 years' follow-up.[19] These studies clearly establish the prognostic significance of IM node metastases: Veronesi and colleagues[20] trial, the final 10-year report from Cody and Urban,[21] and the overall literature on ERM[22] collectively show that the prognostic significance of axillary and IM node metastases is comparable. The prognosis of patients with disease limited to axillary or IM nodes is intermediate between that of patients with negative nodes and those with IM and axillary metastases. These results would seem to confirm the Fisher hypothesis[23] that lymph node metastases have prognostic value but that occult systemic disease governs survival and that variations in local control are therefore unlikely to affect survival. More recently, the 2005 Early Breast Cancer Trialists' Collaborative Group[24] meta-analysis has made the historic observation that local control and survival are related but that survival is improved only when local relapse is reduced by more than 10%.

IM Nodes: Implications for the SLN Era

Three studies have reviewed the collective literature on IM nodes[22,25,26] and are relevant and instructive for the SLN era. Klauber-DeMore and colleagues[22] examined the results of ERM, comprising 4172 patients in 7 studies. IM node metastases were present in 19% to 33% of all cases, were more frequent in axillary node–positive (29%–52%) than node–negative (4%–18%) patients, were equally frequent for central/medial versus lateral tumors if the axillary nodes were negative (8%–10% vs 3%–13%), and were more frequent for medial/central tumors if the axillary nodes were positive (36%–49% vs 22%–26%). An exhaustive overview by Bevilacqua and colleagues[25] (summarized in **Table 1** and comprising 9 series of unselected patients and 16 series of patients selected for an increased risk of IM node involvement) and a more recent review by Chen and colleagues[26] are substantially similar.

Current treatment protocols for stage I-II breast cancer do not include any IMN treatment, yet local recurrence in the IMN or parasternal area is rare, occurring in less than 1% of patients treated by mastectomy[27] or breast conservation.[28] If local recurrence must be reduced by more than 10% to improve survival[24] and is already rare in untreated IM nodes, then it is inconceivable that any further reduction in local recurrence could improve survival. The identification of IM node metastases would, therefore, seem to be of importance mainly for the identification of increased systemic risk in patients who would not otherwise be candidates for systemic adjuvant chemo- or hormonal therapy by current National Comprehensive Cancer Network guidelines (ie, those with negative axillary nodes, negative hormone receptors, and tumors less than 0.5 cm).[29] Within this small subset, perhaps 5% of all patients, only 10% would have positive IM nodes, changing their treatment, and only a minority of these would experience a survival benefit.

Table 1
Patterns of IMN positivity by tumor location and axillary node status in unselected versus selected patient populations

	Axillary Node–Negative Patients—IMN Positive % (#) by Tumor Location				Axillary Node–Positive Patients—IMN Positive % (#) by Tumor Location				Total IMN Positive % (#)
	Medial	Central	Lateral	All Sites	Medial	Central	Lateral	All Sites	Total
9 studies of unselected patients	10 (49/478)	7 (16/242)	4 (29/677)	67 (121/1802)	38 (153/401)	40 (90/226)	23 (177/776)	31 (530/1706)	19 (663/3533)
16 studies of selected patients	14 (102/716)	8 (12/147)	5 (19/408)	11 (267/2478)	52 (275/534)	41 (120/290)	22 (123/534)	37 (923/2508)	24 (1329/5575)
TOTAL	13 (143/1090)	7 (24/345)	4 (40/937)	9 (317/3421)	46 (370/808)	43 (185/433)	23 (263/1130)	36 (117/3244)	23 (1639/7279)

Adapted from Bevilacqua J, Gucciardo G, Cody HS, et al. Proposed patient selection algorithm for internal mammary sentinel lymph node biopsy in breast cancer. Eur J Surg Oncol 2002;28:603–14.

IM-SLN Biopsy

Lymphoscintigraphy (LSG) done routinely as part of lymphatic mapping identifies IM-SLN in a minority of all patients; high-resolution LSG done by a dedicated team has found IM-SLN in as many as 34% of cases,[30] but most investigators have reported a lower yield. It is worth noting that intradermal isotope injection maximizes the success of SLN identification in the axilla[31,32] but rarely drains to the IM nodes; intra-tumoral, peritumoral, or intraparenchymal injections are required to access the deeper lymphatics leading to the IM nodes.[33] In a remarkable series of 700 SLN biopsy procedures (done with meticulous lymphatic mapping by intratumoral injection), Estourgie and colleagues[34] report results that largely recapitulate those from the era of ERM: by preoperative LSG, 95% of patients drained to the axilla and 22% to the IM nodes. IM nodes were seen most frequently in the third (36%), second (27%), and fourth (24%) interspaces.

Six series[35–40] using comparable methods have reported strikingly similar results for IM-SLN biopsy and are summarized in **Table 2**. The routine pursuit of IM-SLN biopsy in these series identified metastasis limited to the IM nodes in only 1% of all patients, a small incremental benefit. Beyond a potential change in systemic therapy, the investigators argue other benefits for this approach, including the addition or avoidance of IM RT and the avoidance of axillary dissection in patients draining only to the IM nodes. Nevertheless, in an era when virtually all patients receive some form of systemic therapy and in which local recurrence in untreated IM nodes is rare, the rationale for routine IM-SLN biopsy remains unclear.

IM-SLN Biopsy: Is It Ever Indicated?

These data suggest that the benefit of routine IM-SLN biopsy accrue to few patients. Nevertheless, there are several clear indications for the procedure.

- A preoperative LSG showing drainage only to the IM nodes. IM node drainage on LSG is almost always accompanied by axillary drainage and isolated IM drainage is infrequent; in a recent series, LSG showed drainage only to the IMN in 4% of patients but in 75% of these axillary SLNs were found at surgery.[41] For those few patients with exclusive IM drainage and with axillary SLNs, negative or absent,

Table 2
Comparable series of IM-SLN biopsy

Author/Year	IMN Imaged[a]	IMN Found[a]	IMN Positive[a]	IMN-Only Positive[a]
Estourgie/2003[35]	22%	19%	3%	1.3%
n = 691		(86%)	(16%)	(43%)
Farrus/2004[36]	17%	12%	1.6%	0
n = 120		(71%)	(13%)	(0)
Paredes/2005[37]	14%	8%	2.8%	0.3%
n = 391		(57%)	(35%)	(11%)
Leidenius/2006[38]	14%	11%	1.8%	0.8%
n = 984		(79%)	(16%)	(44%)
Madsen/2007[39]	22%	17%	4%	1%
n = 505		(77%)	(24%)	(25%)
Heuts/2007[40]	20%	14%	3%	0.9%
n = 1008		(70%)	(21%)	(30%)

[a] Bold percents represent the proportion of the total number of patients mapped; percentagess in parentheses represent the proportion of the preceding column.

IM-SLN biopsy makes sense and allows the surgeon to avoid unnecessary axillary dissection.

- A preoperative LSG showing drainage to IM and axillary nodes and when (1) the axillary SLN is benign on intraoperative examination and (2) the patient is not already a candidate for adjuvant chemotherapy based on other criteria. Although IM-SLN biopsy makes sense for any patient in whom a positive result would alter the plan for systemic therapy, this decision is increasingly based on factors other than lymph node status, among them estrogen receptor/progesterone receptor/her2 status, lymphovascular invasion, and (increasingly) gene expression profiles.
- Evidence of IM node involvement on preoperative imaging (CT, MRI, positron emission tomography). Grossly enlarged IMN are usually amenable to CT-guided core biopsy and are thus a debatable indication for IM-SLN biopsy. As discussed previously, most patients with visible IMN metastases are candidates for chemotherapy on the basis of other criteria and there are no data to suggest that surgical excision of grossly involved IM nodes (and specifically IM-SLN) will improve local control beyond that achieved by chemotherapy and radiotherapy (RT).
- Reoperative SLN biopsy with drainage to IM nodes. SLN biopsy is feasible in patients who have had prior axillary surgery (SLN biopsy or axillary dissection) for breast cancer and present with local recurrence.[42] LSG in the reoperative setting is particularly useful because the prior surgery may have altered the lymphatic drainage of the breast unpredictably. The author has observed non-axillary drainage (most often to the IM nodes) in 30% of reoperative SLN biopsies versus 6% of first-time procedures.[43] Ipsilateral recurrence in the conserved breast occurs in approximately 5% to 10% of all patients,[44,45] and these are the patients for whom LSG and IM-SLN biopsy may ultimately prove most useful.

IM-SLN Biopsy: Technical Considerations

The author's technique of axillary SLN biopsy has previously been described in detail.[46] Preoperative LSG, which the author does routinely, is of limited benefit if the goal at surgery is to identify axillary SLNs (a handheld gamma probe is more sensitive that a full field-of-view gamma camera) but is essential to identify nonaxillary patterns of lymphatic drainage, in particular IM-SLN. All of the isotope injections are given intradermally, because this maximizes identification of axillary SLNs,[31] a result confirmed in a randomized trial by Povoski and colleagues.[32] When the author has a specific aim to identify IM-SLN, then the isotope is injected peritumorally.

In the operating room, a subdermal injection is given next (1 to 5 mL of isosulfan blue dye) in 1 of 3 ways: directly over the tumor, just cephalad to the prior excision scar, or in the subareolar location. As the dye fills the dermal lymphatics, particularly in reoperative SLN biopsy, lymphatic flow as a blush extending laterally toward the axilla or medially toward the IM nodes if often seen. Using a handheld gamma probe, the breast is scanned, identifying and marking the site of isotope injection, any hot spots in the axillary or parasternal areas, and any hot spots in between (suggesting the presence of intramammary SLN).

For patients having mastectomy, the skin incisions are marked out appropriately for conventional, skin-sparing, or skin and nipple–sparing mastectomy. If immediate reconstruction is planned, the incision is designed in collaboration with a plastic surgeon. For patients having breast conservation therapy (BCT), a circumareolar or transverse skin-line incision is made close to the tumor site but placed in such a way that if a completion mastectomy is required, the excision scar could be encompassed with minimal skin sacrifice.

The breast incision should be of adequate length to allow good exposure for the tumor excision and the IM-SLN biopsy. For mastectomy, the IM-SLN biopsy is easily done through the mastectomy incision after removal of the breast. For breast conservation therapy, the IM-SLN biopsy is done through the breast incision by dissecting in the retromammary fascial plane and retracting the breast medially as needed to expose the parasternal area. This is easily done even through lateral excision cavities. Some report using a separate parasternal breast incision for IM-SLN biopsy[35,47] but the author has never found this necessary.

After identification of one or more a hot spots parasternally (most commonly in the second, third or fourth interspaces), the pectoralis major is split in the direction of its fibers, exposing the intercostal muscles. These are carefully divided from the sternal border laterally for approximately 3 to 4 cm. Lateral to this, the parietal pleural forms a single layer. Medially the pleura splits into an anterior and posterior portion, with the IM nodes, IM artery, and IM veins lying between the anterior and posterior pleural leaflets.

After division of the intercostal muscles parasternally, the fatty tissue containing the IM nodes and IM vessels is seen directly beneath the thin anterior layer of the pleura. The lung may be seen moving beneath the pleura more laterally where the anterior and posterior pleural layers have fused. The anterior layer of pleura is carefully divided proceeding from the sternal border laterally. The goal is to expose the IM nodes and vessels but not to divide the pleura so far laterally that the pleural cavity is entered.

The IM area is carefully inspected and scanned to identify any blue or hot nodes, which in general are much smaller than axillary nodes and can be found medial or lateral to the IM artery and (usually) paired IM veins. The IM nodes are dissected free with gentle sharp and blunt dissection, taking care not to injure the vessels, removing if necessary the adjacent fatty tissue, and submitting each node as a separate specimen labeled by interspace of origin and position relative to the vessels (medial or lateral). The IM nodes are submitted for permanent pathology, not frozen section. Processing, as for axillary SLN, includes serial sections and staining with hematoxylin-eosin and anticytokeratins.

IM-SLN biopsy is usually simple and straightforward, taking 5 to 10 minutes, but this is not always the case and surgeons must carefully weigh the small benefit of IM-SLN biopsy against the added morbidity of a more extended procedure. IM-SLNs that are inaccessible beneath the sternum or manubrium should be left in place. IM-SLNs that are inaccessible within a tight interspace (usually the fourth or fifth) or behind the costal cartilages should in general also be left, although the removal of a small segment of costal cartilage for exposure is usually safe. IM-SLNs, which are adherent to deeper structures or part of a large underlying tumor mass, should be biopsied but not excised; more radical chest wall resections are reserved for patients who have failed chemotherapy and RT and should not in general be done de novo.

Bleeding from small vessels is easily controlled with cautery, but significant bleeding from inadvertent injury to the IM artery or veins may require ligation/clipping of the vessels (through the adjacent interspaces or by resection of a costal cartilage for exposure). Inadvertent entry into the pleural cavity is easily recognized and treated. Some recommend suturing the pleural defect, but because the pleura is stretched tightly between the ribs this is easier said than done. For patients under positive pressure ventilation, the author prefers to hyperinflate the lungs and cover the pleural defect with a plug of moistened Surgicel, held in place by the overlying muscle layers.

For patients breathing on their own under sedation, the pneumothorax is simply evacuated with a red rubber catheter, the pleural defect plugged, and the catheter pulled.

The intercostal muscles cannot be closed, but the pectoralis major is reapproximated over the IM-SLN biopsy site and the operative incisions are closed conventionally, with drains as needed. After IM-SLN biopsy, all patients have a chest radiograph in the recovery room; stable patients with pneumothorax are monitored with serial chest radiographs, and chest tubes are almost never required.

IM-SLN biopsy has little morbidity. In the 6 comparable series of IM-SLN biopsy (see **Table 2**),[35–40] entry into the pleural cavity occurred in approximately 1% of patients, most of whom did not develop pneumothorax, and significant hemorrhage from the IM artery or veins occurred in less than 1%. The author and colleagues have previously reported a similar rate of complications in 142 IM-SLN biopsy procedures done at their institution and the European Institute of Oncology,[48] which recently updated its own experience in 663 patients, with similar results.[49]

OTHER SITES OF NONAXILLARY SLN
Intramammary SLN

Estourgie and colleagues,[34] using meticulous LSG to study the breast lymphatics, have identified intramammary SLNs in 7.4% of 700 SLN biopsy procedures, two-thirds lying laterally and one-third medially within the breast. In practice, intramammary SLNs are found much less often. In the authors' experience,[50] intramammary SLNs were found in 151 of 7140 patients (2%), but most of these were found by a pathologist and only 15 (0.2%) were actually identified at surgery. For patients with positive intramammary SLNs, (1) axillary metastases were found in 61% and (2) a negative axillary SLN reliably predicted a negative axilla. Intra and colleagues[51] have reported a similar result, finding intramammary SLNs in 15 of 9632 SLN biopsy procedures (0.2%). Both studies suggest that management of the axilla should depend on the status of the axillary, not the intramammary, SLN.

Rotter (Interpectoral) SLN

Estourgie and colleagues[34] identified infraclavicular lymph node drainage in 2.7% of their patients, some of which may have been Rotter nodes. Cody and colleagues[52] have examined the pattern of metastasis to Rotter nodes, removing them as a separate specimen in 500 consecutive modified radical mastectomies; Rotter nodes were positive in 14 cases (2.8%) but were the sole site of nodal metastasis in only 2 patients (0.4%), both of whom were long-term survivors. Although it is absolutely reasonable to remove Rotter nodes when they map as SLN or when they are palpated in the setting of gross axillary disease, the effect of Rotter node status on clinical management in early-stage breast cancer is debatable.

Supraclavicular SLNs

Estourgie and colleagues[34] identified supraclavicular drainage in 0.5% of their patients. Brito and colleagues[53] have shown that the prognosis of patients with supraclavicular and without distant metastases was comparable to that of stage IIIB disease and more than that of patients with distant metastases, suggesting that they should be treated with curative intent. Accordingly, supraclavicular node metastases were recategorized in the American Joint Committee on Cancer *Cancer Staging Manual* (6th edition) from M1 to N3 disease.[54] Supraclavicular SLNs are rarely identified in practice, and the incidence of subclinical supraclavicular node metastases is unknown. It is reasonable to remove supraclavicular SLNs when they are present and to treat patients with positive supraclavicular nodes by conventional criteria.

Contralateral Axillary SLNs

Contralateral axillary metastasis (CAM) in patients previously treated for breast cancer is the subject of an extensive and largely anecdotal literature but is not rare. CAM developed in 3.6% of 1440 patients reported by Devitt and Michalchuk[55] and in 5% of 123 patients reported by Daoud and colleagues.[56] For patients without evidence of distant metastases, the first clinical dilemma in CAM is to distinguish between a CAM from the previous cancer versus an occult primary in the contralateral breast; virtually all CAM represent contralateral spread.[57] The second clinical dilemma is one of definition: should CAM be treated as distant metastasis or locoregional recurrence? In the absence of other disease sites, most oncologists give the benefit of the doubt and treat with curative intent.

In the author's experience with reoperative SLN biopsy[42,43] there has been an increased incidence of nonaxillary drainage. Preoperative LSG was positive in 55% of cases and 30% of these drained to nonaxillary sites. In order of frequency, the nonaxillary sites were IM (68%), contralateral axilla (26%), intramammary (11%), supraclavicular (5%), and infraclavicular (5%). Proper management of a contralateral axillary SLN remains undefined. Because all patients with CAM receive some form of systemic adjuvant therapy, surgical management of CAM should focus on local control. At present, it seems reasonable to perform SLN biopsy for cN0 patients who map to the contralateral axilla and to perform axillary dissection for patients with CAM.

SUMMARY

Nonaxillary drainage is demonstrable by LSG in up to one-third of breast cancer patients, and nonaxillary SLN biopsy (most frequently of the IM nodes) is the subject of a growing body of literature. It is not yet clear that the identification of nonaxillary SLNs significantly affects treatment or outcome in patients with primary operable disease. The greatest future potential for nonaxillary SLN biopsy is in the management of patients with ipsilateral breast tumor recurrence, where prior axillary surgery may have unpredictably altered the lymphatic drainage of the breast.

REFERENCES

1. Kim T, Giuliano AE, Lyman GH. Lymphatic mapping and sentinel lymph node biopsy in early-stage breast carcinoma. Cancer 2006;106:4–16.
2. Veronesi U, Paganelli G, Viale G, et al. A randomized comparison of sentinel-node biopsy with routine axillary dissection in breast cancer. N Engl J Med 2003;349:546–53.
3. Krag DN, Anderson SJ, Julian TB, et al. Technical outcomes of sentinel-lymph-node resection and conventional axillary-lymph-node dissection in patients with clinically node-negative breast cancer: results from the NSABP B-32 randomised phase III trial. Lancet Oncol 2007;8:881–8.
4. Mansel RE, Fallowfield L, Kissin M, et al. Randomized multicenter trial of sentinel node biopsy versus standard axillary treatment in operable breast cancer: the ALMANAC Trial. J Natl Cancer Inst 2006;98:599–609.
5. Zavagno G, De Salvo GL, Scalco G, et al. A randomized clinical trial on sentinel lymph node biopsy versus axillary lymph node dissection in breast cancer: results of the Sentinella/GIVOM trial. Ann Surg 2008;247:207–13.

6. Gill G. Sentinel-lymph-node-based management or routine axillary clearance? One-year outcomes of sentinel node biopsy versus axillary clearance (SNAC): a randomized controlled surgical trial. Ann Surg Oncol 2009;16:266–75.
7. Cody HS, Fey J, Akhurst T, et al. Complementarity of blue dye and isotope in sentinel node localization for breast cancer: univariate and multivariate analysis of 966 procedures. Ann Surg Oncol 2001;8:13–9.
8. McMasters KM, Tuttle TM, Carlson DJ, et al. Sentinel lymph node biopsy for breast cancer: a suitable alternative to routine axillary dissection in multi-institutional practice when optimal technique is used. J Clin Oncol 2000;18:2560–6.
9. Stibbe EP. The internal mammary lymphatic glands. J Anat 1918;52:258–64.
10. Handley RS, Thackray AC. Invasion of the internal mammary lymph glands in carcinoma of the breast. Br J Surg 1947;1:15–20 (The Bradshaw Lecture).
11. Turner-Warwick RT. The lymphatics of the breast. Br J Surg 1959;46:574–82.
12. Haagensen CD. The ILymphatics of the breast. In: Haagensen CD, Feind CR, Herter FP, editors. The lymphatics in cancer. Philadelphia: WB Saunders; 1972. p. 340–4.
13. Halsted WS. The results of operations for the cure of cancer of the breast performed at the Johns Hopkins Hospital from June 1889 to January 1894. Johns Hopkins Hosp Rep 1894;4:297–350.
14. Wangensteen OH. Remarks on extension of the Halsted operation for cancer of the breast. Ann Surg 1949;130:315–6.
15. Wangensteen OH, Lewis FJ, Athelger SW. The extended or super-radical operation for carcinoma of the breast. Surg Clin North Am 1956;36:1051–63.
16. Urban JA. Radical excision of the chest wall for mammary cancer. Cancer 1951;4:1263–85.
17. Urban JA. Radical mastectomy in continuity with en bloc resection of internal mammary lymph node chain: new procedure for primary operable cancer of breast. Cancer 1952;5:992–1008.
18. Veronesi U, Valagussa P. Inefficacy of internal mammary nodes dissection in breast cancer surgery. Cancer 1981;47:170–5.
19. Veronesi U, Marubini E, Mariani L, et al. The dissection of internal mammary nodes does not improve the survival of breast cancer patients. 30-year results of a randomised trial. Eur J Cancer 1999;35:1320–5.
20. Veronesi U, Cascinelli N, Bufalino R. Risk of internal mammary lymph node metastases and its relevance on prognosis of breast cancer patients. Ann Surg 1983;198:681–4.
21. Cody HS, Urban JA. Internal mammary node status: a major prognosticator in axillary node-negative breast cancer. Ann Surg Oncol 1995;2:32–7.
22. Klauber-DeMore N, Bevilacqua JB, VanZee KJ, et al. Comprehensive review of the management of internal mammary metastases in breast cancer. J Am Coll Surg 2001;193:547–55.
23. Fisher B. Laboratory and clinical research in breast cancer: a personal adventure: the David A. Karnofsky memorial lecture. Cancer Res 1980;40:3863–74.
24. Early Breast Cancer Trialists' Collaborative Group. Effects of radiotherapy and of differences in the extent of surgery for early breast cancer on local recurrence and 15-year survival: an overview of the randomised trials. Lancet 2005;366:2087–106.
25. Bevilacqua J, Gucciardo G, Cody HS, et al. Proposed patient selection algorithm for internal mammary sentinel lymph node biopsy in breast cancer. Eur J Surg Oncol 2002;28:603–14.

26. Chen RC, Lin NU, Golshan M, et al. Internal mammary nodes in breast cancer: diagnosis and implications for patient management – a systematic review. J Clin Oncol 2008;26:4981–9.

27. Fisher B, Redmond C, Fisher E. Ten-year results of a randomized clinical trial comparing radical mastectomy and total mastectomy with or without radiation. N Engl J Med 1985;312:674–81.

28. Harris EE, Hwang WT, Seyednejad F, et al. Prognosis after regional lymph node recurrence in patients with stage I-II breast carcinoma treated with breast conservation therapy. Cancer 2003;98:2144–51.

29. Nccn. NCCN clinical practice guidelines in oncology: breast cancer v.1. 2010. Available at: http://www.nccn.org/professionals/physician_gls/PDF/breast.pdf. Accessed March 1, 2010

30. Spillane AJ, Noushi F, Cooper RA, et al. High-resolution lymphoscintigraphy is essential for recognition of the significance of internal mammary nodes in breast cancer. Ann Oncol 2009;20:977–84.

31. Linehan DC, Hill ADK, Akhurst T, et al. Intradermal radiocolloid and intraparenchymal blue dye injection optimize sentinel node identification in breast cancer patients. Ann Surg Oncol 1999;6:450–4.

32. Povoski SP, Olsen JO, Young DC, et al. Prospective randomized clinical trial comparing intradermal, intraparenchymal, and subareolar injection routes for sentinel lymph node mapping and biopsy in breast cancer. Ann Surg Oncol 2006;13:1412–21.

33. Tanis PJ, Nieweg OE, Valdes Olmos RA, et al. Anatomy and physiology of lymphatic drainage of the breast from the perspective of sentinel node biopsy. J Am Coll Surg 2001;192:399–409.

34. Estourgie SH, Nieweg OE, Olmos RA, et al. Lymphatic drainage patterns from the breast. Ann Surg 2004;239:232–7.

35. Estourgie SH, Tanis PJ, Nieweg OE, et al. Should the hunt for internal mammary chain sentinel nodes begin? An evaluation of 150 breast cancer patients. Ann Surg Oncol 2003;10:935–41.

36. Farrus B, Vidal-Sicart S, Velasco M, et al. Incidence of internal mammary node metastases after a sentinel lymph node technique in breast cancer and its implication in the radiotherapy plan. Int J Radiat Oncol Biol Phys 2004;60: 715–21.

37. Paredes P, Vidal-Sicart S, Zanon G, et al. Clinical relevance of sentinel lymph nodes in the internal mammary chain in breast cancer patients. Eur J Nucl Med Mol Imaging 2005;32:1283–7.

38. Leidenius MH, Krogerus LA, Toivonen TS, et al. The clinical value of parasternal sentinel node biopsy in breast cancer. Ann Surg Oncol 2006;13:321–6.

39. Madsen E, Gobardhan P, Bongers V, et al. The impact on post-surgical treatment of sentinel lymph node biopsy of internal mammary lymph nodes in patients with breast cancer. Ann Surg Oncol 2007;14:1486–92.

40. Heuts EM, Van der Ent FWC, von Meyenfeldt MF, et al. Internal mammary lymph drainage and sentinel node biopsy in breast cancer - A study on 1008 patients. Eur J Surg Oncol 2009;35:252–7.

41. van der Ploeg IM, Tanis PJ, Valdes Olmos RA, et al. Breast cancer patients with extra-axillary sentinel nodes only may be spared axillary lymph node dissection. Ann Surg Oncol 2008;15:3239–43.

42. Port ER, Fey J, Gemignani ML, et al. Reoperative sentinel lymph node biopsy: a new option for patients with primary or locally recurrent breast carcinoma. J Am Coll Surg 2002;195:167–72.

43. Port ER, Garcia-Etienne CA, Park J, et al. Reoperative sentinel lymph node biopsy: a new frontier in the management of ipsilateral breast tumor recurrence. Ann Surg Oncol 2007;14:2209–14.

44. Anderson SJ, Wapnir I, Dignam JJ, et al. Prognosis after ipsilateral breast tumor recurrence and locoregional recurrences in patients treated by breast-conserving therapy in five National Surgical Adjuvant Breast and Bowel Project protocols of node-negative breast cancer. J Clin Oncol 2009;27:2466–73.

45. Wapnir IL, Anderson SJ, Mamounas EP, et al. Prognosis after ipsilateral breast tumor recurrence and locoregional recurrences in five National Surgical Adjuvant Breast and Bowel Project node-positive adjuvant breast cancer trials. J Clin Oncol 2006;24:2028–37.

46. Cody HS, Borgen PI. State-of-the-art approaches to sentinel node biopsy for breast cancer: study design, patient selection, technique, and quality control at Memorial Sloan-Kettering Cancer Center. Surg Oncol 1999;8:85–91.

47. van der Ent FW, Kengen RA, van der Pol HA, et al. Halsted revisited: internal mammary sentinel lymph node biopsy in breast cancer. Ann Surg 2001;234:79–84.

48. Sacchini G, Borgen PI, Galimberti V, et al. Surgical approach to internal mammary lymph node biopsy. J Am Coll Surg 2001;193:709–13.

49. Veronesi U, Arnone P, Veronesi P, et al. The value of radiotherapy on metastatic internal mammary nodes in breast cancer. Results on a large series. Ann Oncol 2008;19:1553–60.

50. Pugliese MS, Stempel MM, Cody HS III, et al. Surgical management of the axilla: do intramammary nodes matter? Am J Surg 2009;198:532–7.

51. Intra M, Garcia-Etienne CA, Renne G, et al. When sentinel lymph node is intra-mammary. Ann Surg Oncol 2008;15:1304–8.

52. Cody HS, Egeli RA, Urban JA. Rotter's node metastases: therapuetic and prognostic considerations in early breast carcinoma. Ann Surg 1984;199:266–70.

53. Brito RA, Valero V, Buzdar AU, et al. Long-term results of combined-modality therapy for locally advanced breast cancer with ipsilateral supraclavicular metastases: the University of Texas M.D. Anderson Cancer Center experience. J Clin Oncol 2001;19:628–33.

54. Singletary SE, Allred C, Ashley P, et al. Staging system for breast cancer: revisions for the 6th edition of the AJCC Cancer Staging Manual. Surg Clin North Am 2003;83:803–19.

55. Devitt JE, Michalchuk AW. Significance of contralateral axillary metastases in carcinoma of the breast. Can J Surg 1969;12:178–80.

56. Daoud J, Meziou M, Kharrat M, et al. [Contralateral axillary lymph node metastasis of cancer of the breast]. Bull Cancer 1998;85:713–5 [in French].

57. Huston TL, Pressman PI, Moore A, et al. The presentation of contralateral axillary lymph node metastases from breast carcinoma: a clinical management dilemma. Breast J 2007;13:158–64.

Sentinel Lymph Node Biopsy Before or After Neoadjuvant Chemotherapy: Pros and Cons

Michael S. Sabel, MD

KEYWORDS

- Sentinel lymph node biopsy • Breast cancer
- Neoadjuvant chemotherapy

There are few innovations in surgery that have so rapidly and drastically changed the management of a disease as the introduction of sentinel lymph node (SLN) biopsy has changed breast surgery. Beyond the obvious of greatly minimizing the morbidity associated with the surgical staging of breast cancer, our knowledge of the anatomy of the breast and axilla and the biology of breast cancer metastasis has improved. However, no great advance comes without great controversy, and it is almost stunning how a procedure so beautifully simple in concept has led to such vigorous debate. Among several areas of debate, perhaps the most controversial is that of the timing of SLN biopsy in the patient receiving neoadjuvant therapy.

Before the introduction of sentinel lymph node biopsy as a method of staging the axilla, there was little consequence surgically on whether patients received neoadjuvant chemotherapy or not, as either way they would be receiving an axillary lymph node dissection. The most significant impact of preoperative therapy on axillary staging was that there were going to be patients who may have been node positive initially but were node negative after chemotherapy and so their true pretreatment nodal status was never known. At the time, however, this would not alter their surgery and the associated risks, nor did it significantly impact therapy decisions.

This changed dramatically as lymphatic mapping and SLN biopsy assumed greater prominence in the surgical therapy of breast cancer. Now patients who opted for neoadjuvant chemotherapy to shrink their primary tumor and potentially avoid mastectomy were obligated to undergo axillary lymph node dissection (ALND) as part of their surgery, whereas if they had a mastectomy, they would be candidates for SLN

Department of Surgery, University of Michigan Comprehensive Cancer Center, 3304 Cancer Center, 1500 East Medical Center Drive, Ann Arbor, MI 48109, USA
E-mail address: msabel@umich.edu

Surg Oncol Clin N Am 19 (2010) 519–538
doi:10.1016/j.soc.2010.03.004
1055-3207/10/$ – see front matter © 2010 Elsevier Inc. All rights reserved.

surgonc.theclinics.com

biopsy and potentially avoid ALND. This put patients in the awkward position of having to decide which was the lesser of 2 evils: losing the breast or the increased risk of lymphedema.

In addition to the surgical dilemma, the controversy was further fueled by the increasing desire, and ability, to tailor care to the individual patient. The nodal status of the patient took on increased importance in deciding whether adjuvant chemotherapy was indicated, what regimen, and whether radiation therapy would be recommended after mastectomy. As the question of how to best incorporate SLN biopsy into the neoadjuvant paradigm became more critical, 2 approaches emerged. Several institutions initiated prospective trials of SLN biopsy performed after neoadjuvant chemotherapy in conjunction with a completion ALND, with the goal of ultimately showing that SLN biopsy could be safely and accurately performed after the patient completed systemic therapy. Other institutions adopted a policy of performing SLN biopsy before initiation of chemotherapy. This avoided the issue surrounding the accuracy of SLN biopsy after chemotherapy and potentially provided information that might influence adjuvant therapy decisions.

This article summarizes the relative pros and cons surrounding the timing of SLN biopsy in patients undergoing neoadjuvant chemotherapy (**Table 1**), as well as addresses the clinical questions regarding the 2 approaches including the accuracy of the procedure and the prognostic information gleaned.

POTENTIAL ADVANTAGES TO SLN BIOPSY BEFORE NEOADJUVANT CHEMOTHERAPY

The first approach is to perform the SLN biopsy before beginning chemotherapy. Although this requires an additional surgery, and could potentially delay the initiation of chemotherapy, the strongest argument for this approach is the perceived accuracy of the procedure. When SLN biopsy was first introduced there was some concern as to the accuracy of the procedure in the presence of a large primary tumor, which constituted most patients being considered for neoadjuvant therapy. However, 2 series looking specifically at SLN biopsy in this patient population demonstrated that this was not a concern.[1,2] Several institutions that adopted pretreatment SLN biopsy subsequently reported their results with this specific approach (**Table 2**). Given the documented safety of avoiding ALND for a negative SLN biopsy, patients who are found to be SLN negative before treatment can safely avoid ALND at the time of their surgical therapy. This is in contrast with concerns raised regarding the accuracy of SLN biopsy after chemotherapy, as is discussed in more detail later in this article. With very little data on regional recurrence rates among patients who have a negative SLN biopsy after neoadjuvant chemotherapy, without completion ALND, the risks of this approach remain unclear. Performing SLN biopsy before chemotherapy avoids these concerns.

The other primary advantage of performing SLN biopsy is that the true pretreatment nodal status of the patient is known. This is important if the nodal status might affect the decision to give chemotherapy at all, the regimen used, or the decision to give chest wall radiation if the patient ultimately requires mastectomy or include the regional nodes in the radiation fields. Whether this is a true advantage or not is controversial, as this represents a moving target. The optimal agents and regimens used for systemic therapy are constantly evolving. For example, several years ago when this controversy was first emerging, the addition of a taxane to an anthracycline-based regimen, or the use of trastuzumab (Herceptin) in the face of Her-2/neu overexpression, was limited to node-positive patients as there were few data in the node-negative population. Thus there was a greater importance of the pretreatment nodal status in

Table 1
Arguments for and against performing SLN biopsy before or after neoadjuvant chemotherapy

	SLN Biopsy Before Chemotherapy	SLN Biopsy After Chemotherapy
Accuracy	PRO Most accurate regional staging of patients before starting therapy. Low regional recurrence rates documented.	PRO Large series and meta-analyses suggest false negative rates similar to SLN in general. CON High false negative rates reported in rare studies or when nodes are clinically involved before chemotherapy.
Convenience	PRO More surgical experience with SLN biopsy in this setting. CON Requires at least 2 operations. Delays onset of chemotherapy.	PRO Surgical sequence more in line with conventional neoadjuvant approach. May begin chemotherapy quickly and limit number of operations. CON May be a learning curve associated with SLN biopsy after chemotherapy.
Prognosis	PRO Knowing nodal status may guide whether neoadjuvant therapy is appropriate. Prechemotherapy nodal status may guide choice of chemotherapy or adjuvant postmastectomy radiation. CON Nodal status becoming less important for many adjuvant therapy decisions. Nodal status after chemotherapy may be more predictive.	PRO Incorporating response to chemotherapy may better predict risk of recurrence and need for radiation therapy. Newer approaches may guide adjuvant decisions without need for pretreatment nodal status. CON Presently, data suggest that both pre-and posttreatment nodal status is important.
Outcome	PRO Low axillary recurrence rate documented. CON Unnecessary ALNDs in women with nodal disease eradicated by chemotherapy.	PRO Decreased morbidity by decreasing need for ALND. CON Limited data regarding axillary recurrence in this setting.

deciding what regimen to use. As more data emerged regarding the benefits in the node-negative population, the pretreatment nodal status became less important. For most patients being considered for neoadjuvant therapy, the clinical tumor size and information from the core biopsy became sufficient to select therapy, and the importance of the SLN status before chemotherapy diminished.

The pendulum began to swing back when Oncotype DX (Genomic Health, Redwood City, CA, USA) was introduced.[3,4] Now genomic profiling could be used to identify hormone-receptor–positive, node-negative patients who, despite a large-sized tumor, received very little benefit from adjuvant chemotherapy, and may ultimately be better

Table 2
Published reports of sentinel lymph node biopsy before neoadjuvant chemotherapy

First Author	Year	N	ID Rate	SLN Positive	Patients With Positive NSLN After Chemotherapy
Zirngibl[50]	2002	15	93%	43%	0%
Schrenk[51]	2003	21	100%	43%	66%
Sabel[52]	2003	26	100%	52%	70%
Ollila[53]	2003	22	100%	45%	40%
Jones[54]	2005	52	100%	58%	NR
Van Rijk[55]	2006	25	100%	44%	40%
Cox[56]	2006	47	98%	83%	65%
Grube[57]	2008	55	100%	55%	45%
Papa[58]	2008	86	99%	67%	NR
Straver[7]	2009	75	100%	29%	32%

served with neoadjuvant hormonal therapy. Therefore, in some patients, knowing the nodal status might be crucial to neoadjuvant therapy decisions. The ground may shift again as new data emerge suggesting that Oncotype DX may still be useful in identifying patients who can avoid chemotherapy even if they are node positive,[5,6] or as new agents are introduced into the adjuvant/neoadjuvant setting. The increasing use of immunohistochemical staining, genomics, and possibly proteomics in the selection of targeted therapies may continue to reduce the importance of SLN status.

POTENTIAL ADVANTAGES TO SLN BIOPSY AFTER NEOADJUVANT CHEMOTHERAPY

If patients have an SLN biopsy before neoadjuvant chemotherapy, they are committing themselves to at least 2 operations: 1 before chemotherapy and at least 1 after chemotherapy. This deviates from the current convention of neoadjuvant treatment where all of the chemotherapy is completed, followed by all of the surgery. If SLN biopsy can be safely performed after neoadjuvant chemotherapy, a greater percentage of patients can complete their surgical therapy in 1 trip to the operating room. And, whereas breast cancer patients are regularly asked to commit to more than 1 operation (patients undergoing SLN biopsy know they may need to return to the operating room [OR] for an ALND, patients undergoing breast-conserving therapy [BCT] know they may need to return to the OR for a reexcision lumpectomy or mastectomy), in today's health care economic climate, the need to conserve costs is becoming increasingly important. In addition, depending on the surgeon's schedule, the time required to schedule and perform the SLN biopsy may delay the onset of chemotherapy.

A more significant criticism of performing SLN biopsy before neoadjuvant therapy is that it commits more patients to an ALND even though the chemotherapy may have eradicated any remaining disease from the axilla. Performing the SLN biopsy after chemotherapy takes advantage of the potential downstaging effect of chemotherapy on axillary nodes. In the reported series of SLN biopsy before chemotherapy, the SLN was positive in between 30% and 80% of patients, all of whom then had completion ALND in addition to either lumpectomy or mastectomy at the completion of systemic therapy (**Table 3**). Some patients who would have a positive SLN biopsy before neoadjuvant therapy and thus require ALND may have a negative SLN biopsy following

Table 3
Published reports of SLN biopsy followed by ALND after neoadjuvant chemotherapy

First Author	Year	N	ID Rate	SLN Positive	FN Rate
Cohen[59]	2000	38	82%	52%	17%
Breslin[60]	2000	51	84%	51%	12%
Nason[61]	2000	15	87%	69%	33%
Fernandez[62]	2001	40	90%	59%	20%
Tafra[63]	2001	29	93%	52%	0%
Stearns[64]	2002	34	85%	45%	14%
Brady[65]	2002	14	93%	77%	0%
Julian[66]	2002	34	91%	39%	0%
Miller[67]	2002	35	86%	30%	0%
Vigario[68]	2003	37	97%	50%	28%
Balch[69]	2003	32	97%	58%	5%
Reitsamer[70]	2003	30	87%	54%	7%
Schwartz[71]	2003	21	100%	48%	9%
Piato[72]	2003	42	98%	56%	17%
Haid[73]	2003	45	93%	45%	5%
Kang[74]	2004	54	72%	62%	11%
Shimazu[75]	2004	47	94%	66%	12%
Lang[76]	2004	53	94%	47%	4%
Patel[77]	2004	42	95%	42%	0%
Aihara[78]	2004	20	85%	35%	17%
Kinoshita[79]	2005	77	93.5%	33%	18%
Mamounas[29]	2005	428	85%	36%	11%
Jones[54]	2005	36	80.6%	55%	11%
Tanaka[80]	2006	70	90%	90%	5%
Lee[26]	2007	219	78%	69%	5.6%
Papa[58]	2008	31	87%	59%	16%
Tausch[81]	2008	167	85%	42%	8%
Gimbergues[82]	2008	129	93.8%	46%	14.3%
Hino[83]	2008	55	71%	46%	0%
Classe[84]	2008	195	90%	23.5%	11.5%
Hunt[42]	2009	84	NR	NR	5.9%
Shwartz[85]	2010	79	98.7%	29%	4.1%

therapy and not require a complete node dissection, further minimizing the morbidity of treatment. Studies of patients with cytologically confirmed axillary metastases before neoadjuvant chemotherapy have reported pathologic complete response (pCR) in the axillary nodes in 20% to 36% of patients,[7-11] and it is feasible that patients with micrometastases in the SLN may have a higher rate of pCR.

A third potential advantage to SLN biopsy after chemotherapy is that the information may be more useful to the practitioner than the pretreatment nodal status. Proponents of pretreatment SLN biopsy argue that knowing the SLN status may help guide treatment and having a negative SLN biopsy after chemotherapy does not allow you to know whether the patient was node positive to begin with. However, knowing the response of the disease in the axilla may be more important in determining risk of recurrence, and the decision to proceed with postmastectomy radiation, than knowing the nodal status before treatment. If a patient has a positive SLN biopsy before chemotherapy, and a negative ALND afterward, it is often unclear whether there was additional disease that responded or whether all nodal disease was removed with the first operation. Proponents of SLN biopsy after chemotherapy would argue that the presence or absence of disease in the nodes *after* chemotherapy may be a better criterion by which to choose which patients should receive postmastectomy radiation than the nodal status before chemotherapy.

MUST A POSITIVE PRETREATMENT SLN BIOPSY COMMIT A PATIENT TO AN ALND AFTER CHEMOTHERAPY?

The strongest argument for performing SLN biopsy after neoadjuvant chemotherapy is that a positive node before chemotherapy commits the patient to an ALND and the associated morbidity. Thus, the patient does not realize the potential benefit of the chemotherapy downstaging the nodal status to N0. Presently, patients in whom the prechemotherapy SLN was positive are recommended to undergo complete ALND at the time of either lumpectomy or mastectomy. This approach is open to question, just as we are now questioning whether non-neoadjuvant patients with a positive SLN biopsy require an ALND. Several nomograms and statistical models predicting the likelihood of residual disease after a positive SLN biopsy have been reported, guiding patients and surgeons in the decision to perform a completion ALND.[12,13] Data from the National Cancer database suggest that today over 20% of patients with a positive SLN biopsy are not having the completion node dissection.[14] Forthcoming data from the American College of Surgeons Oncology Group Z0011 trial, which randomized patients with a positive SLN biopsy to ALND versus observation, as well as institutional series of SLN-positive patients who did not undergo ALND, may further support a selective use of ALND. Although these nomograms have less utility in predicting nonsentinel lymph node (NSLN) involvement after neoadjuvant chemotherapy,[15] new models could be applied to completing the ALND after neoadjuvant chemotherapy, incorporating additional factors unique to the neoadjuvant approach. Straver and colleagues[7] found several factors that may predict an axillary pCR, including Her-2 overexpression, triple negative subtype, pCR in the primary tumor, initial clinical, and histology. Jeruss and colleagues[16] examined 18 factors among patients treated with neoadjuvant chemotherapy at the M. D. Anderson Cancer Center for their ability to predict positive NSLNs, and then tested the resulting nomogram on patients from the University of Michigan who had either prechemotherapy fine needle aspiration (FNA) or SLN biopsy to assess nodal status. This nomogram incorporated 5 variables: lymphovascular invasion, initial lymph node status, method to detect the nodal disease, multicentricity, and the pathologic tumor size. When applied to the University of Michigan cohort, the area under the curve (AUC) was 0.78 (95% CI, 0.62–0.92). Predictive models such as these might be used to help determine the potential benefit of a completion ALND after neoadjuvant chemotherapy in patients who had a positive SLN biopsy before therapy.

IS SLN BIOPSY ACCURATE AFTER NEOADJUVANT CHEMOTHERAPY?

In weighing the relative advantages and disadvantages, the first question one must address is whether the SLN status is a reliable and accurate procedure in the patient who has had systemic therapy. When first introduced, the most significant concern regarding the performance of SLN biopsy after chemotherapy was the accuracy of the procedure. There were 2 theoretical concerns. The first was the effect of the chemotherapy on the lymphatic pathways and the lymph nodes themselves. This could impact the identification rate, increasing the number of cases where a complete ALND needed to be performed for staging purposes.

The second area of concern was whether or not the status of the SLN truly reflected the status of the axillary nodes. As the first node that receives drainage from the site of the cancer (or the breast), the SLN is the most likely to contain malignant cells if metastases have occurred. False negative findings could either be biologic (cells passed through the SLN to the NSLN) or technical, representing either the surgeon's removal and labeling of an NSLN as an SLN, or the pathologist missing disease that was present in the SLN. When SLN biopsy is performed after chemotherapy, another form of biologic false negative is introduced. For the concept of the SLN to be true after chemotherapy, 1 of 2 assumptions must be made. The first is that the response in the nodes is "all or none," meaning any disease in the lymph nodes will be either completely eradicated or remain present, but not disappear from some nodes and not others. The alternate possibility is "front to back, back to front," meaning that if at the start of therapy disease was present in the SLN and NSLN, then it is eradicated in the NSLN before disappearing from the SLN. This is not an unreasonable assumption, as the volume of disease within the SLN is typically greater than that in the NSLN. However, in cases where disease is eradicated from the SLN but not the NSLN, false negative findings would occur. This latter possibility is not unreasonable to believe either, as there may be a biologic difference between spread from the primary to the SLN and spread beyond the SLN to the NSLN.[17]

Of course all patients with newly diagnosed breast cancer need a careful workup and clinical staging before proceeding with therapy. This includes at least a detailed history, a thorough physical examination, and a bilateral mammogram. However, clinical examination alone is notoriously inaccurate in determining the nodal status, with both a significant false negative rate and a false positive rate.[18] A recent addition to the staging workup of the breast cancer patient is ultrasound of the axilla. In combination with physical examination and FNA biopsy of any abnormal nodes, this approach can identify a significant percentage of patients with regional metastases, avoiding the need for SLN biopsy to document nodal status.[19–24] For patients not being considered for neoadjuvant therapy, or for whom nodal staging is to be performed before neoadjuvant chemotherapy, these patients avoid SLN biopsy and proceed directly to ALND. In the context of regional staging after neoadjuvant chemotherapy, this divides the patients into 2 groups: those with clinically involved nodes before chemotherapy, and those with clinically negative nodes, for whom the nodal status before chemotherapy is unknown.

ACCURACY IN THE FACE OF CLINICALLY INVOLVED NODES BEFORE CHEMOTHERAPY

Most of the studies described of SLN biopsy after chemotherapy were limited to, or contained a majority of, patients who had no clinical evidence of disease within their lymph nodes before the initiation of systemic therapy; therefore, many of the patients were node negative at the onset of chemotherapy. Three studies have specifically examined the accuracy of SLN biopsy in patients who were documented to have regional metastases at the onset of neoadjuvant therapy (**Table 4**). Shen and colleagues,[25] from the University of Texas M. D. Anderson Cancer Center, looked at SLN biopsy in 69 patients who had FNA-documented disease in the regional nodes before chemotherapy. Sixty-one ultimately underwent a completion ALND, and in 5 the SLN was not identified (identification rate of 92.8%), leaving 56 patients for evaluation. The SLN identification rate was 92.8% and the false negative rate was 25%,

Table 4
Studies of SLN biopsy after neoadjuvant chemotherapy in the face of clinically involved nodes before the onset of chemotherapy

First Author	Year	N	Definition of Node Positive	Identification Rate	False Negative Rate
Shen[25]	2007	69	FNA +	92.8%	25%
Lee[26]	2007	238	FNA + or + by ultrasound and PET criteria	77.6%	5.6%
Newman[9]	2007	54	FNA or SLN +	98%	10.7%

leading the investigators to conclude that SLN biopsy cannot be considered a reliable indicator of the presence or absence of disease in the axilla after chemotherapy in this patient population. Lee and colleagues[26] looked at 219 node-positive patients undergoing neoadjuvant chemotherapy. In this case, the definition of positive could be either FNA-positive or greater than 1-cm thick with loss of fat hilum on ultrasound and uptake on positron emission tomography (PET) scan of greater than 2.5. The investigators report a false negative rate of only 5.6%, which was not significantly different from the false negative rate at their institution for SLN biopsy in general. Finally, Newman and colleagues[9] reported a false negative rate of 10.7% among 28 patients who underwent neoadjuvant chemotherapy. In this study, pretreatment nodal status was determined either by FNA or by SLN biopsy.

ACCURACY IN THE FACE OF CLINICALLY NEGATIVE NODES

As stated, most of the patients enrolled in prospective trials of SLN biopsy and ALND after neoadjuvant chemotherapy were clinically node negative, although the use of axillary ultrasound in addition to physical examination was rare. In addition, the method of lymphatic mapping, whether blue dye alone, radiocolloid alone, or the combination, also varied. A summary of these published reports is presented in **Table 2**. The identification rate in these publications ranged from 72% to 100% and the false negative rate ranged from 0% to 39%. It should be pointed out that in some of these studies the false negative rate was inappropriately reported as the percentage of false negative SLN among all the negative results (which is actually the negative predictive value), as opposed to the proportion of positive instances that were erroneously reported as negative (number of false negatives/total number of positives), an error that has occurred in other series of SLN biopsy in both breast cancer and melanoma.

Some authors of these single-institution series concluded that SLN biopsy was inaccurate following neoadjuvant chemotherapy, whereas most felt the data supported its accuracy. Many of these studies involved relatively small numbers of patients, particularly node-positive patients, varied greatly in technique, and possibly involved a learning curve. A more accurate picture of the safety of SLN biopsy after systemic therapy may come from looking at a meta-analysis of the single-institution reports and the use of postchemotherapy SLN biopsy in prospective multicenter trials.

For the meta-analysis, 21 studies incorporating more than 1200 patients were analyzed.[27] For inclusion, each patient had to have operable breast cancer and had to have a subsequent ALND. In this study, the pooled identification rate was 90%. The sensitivity of SLN biopsy ranged from 67% to 100%, with a pooled estimate of 88% (95% confidence interval 85 to 90). Meta-analyses performed using Bayesian modeling resulted in (posterior) estimates for identification rate and sensitivity of 91% (95% confidence interval 88 to 94) and 88% (95% confidence interval 84 to 91) respectively. Even this false negative rate of 12% may slightly overestimate the true false negative (FN) rate, as this meta-analysis included studies from 1993 to 2004. Studies conducted since 2004 continue to have wide variability in the false negative rate (5% to 25%) but collectively have a false negative rate of 9%.[28]

Additional data come from the National Surgical Adjuvant Breast and Bowel Project (NSABP) B-27, a study of 4 cycles of neoadjuvant doxorubicin/cyclophosphamide (AC) chemotherapy versus neoadjuvant or adjuvant docetaxel following 4 cycles of AC.[29] Although level I and II axillary dissection was mandated as part of the study, surgeons had the option of performing an SLN biopsy before the planned ALND. Of the 2365 patients analyzed at the completion of the study, 428 (18%) had lymphatic mapping and SLN biopsy performed at the time of ALND. The overall false negative rate was 11%. The data also suggested that the use of radiocolloid (with or without blue dye) was more accurate than blue dye alone, with false negative rates of 8% and 14% respectively.

How does this compare with SLN biopsy in general? It is important to keep in mind that when SLN biopsy is performed before any systemic therapy, the false negative rate is not zero. The first multicenter trial of SLN for breast cancer, reported by Krag and colleagues,[30] reported a false negative rate of 11%; this article paved the way for SLN biopsy without completion ALND if the SLN biopsy is negative to become standard practice in the surgical management of breast cancer. In 2002, Lyman and colleagues[31] reported the results of a meta-analysis of 69 trials involving more than 10,000 patients where SLN biopsy was performed before a completion ALND. The false negative rate in that study was 8.4% and it was 5.1% and 9.0% in 2 other meta-analyses of SLN biopsy.[32,33] The NSAPB B-32 study was a randomized trial comparing SLN biopsy alone versus SLN biopsy plus ALND. In this trial, the false negative rate among patients having SLN biopsy followed by immediate ALND was 9.7%.[34] All of these numbers are very close to the 11% false negative rate reported in NSABP B-27.

IS IT SAFE TO AVOID ALND AFTER A NEGATIVE SLN BIOPSY FOLLOWING NEOADJUVANT CHEMOTHERAPY?

For patients who have clinically documented nodal metastases before the initiation of systemic therapy, there are only 3 studies, with false negative rates ranging from 5% to 25%. Given the paucity of data and the concerning possibility of leaving behind disease, it is probably premature to abandon ALND in this setting. More data are needed, and are presently being collected in a prospective, multicenter trial through the American College of Surgeons Oncology Group (ACOSOG).

What of clinically node-negative patients? Proponents of SLN biopsy after neoadjuvant chemotherapy argue that a false negative rate of 11% or 12%, based on the meta-analyses and multicenter studies, is not much higher than the false negative rate of SLN biopsy in general, reported between 5% to 10% in meta-analyses and multicenter trials. The argument may also be made that in women undergoing neoadjuvant chemotherapy, the impact of understaging the axilla is less significant, as the decision to proceed with systemic therapy has already been made. There are, however, some outstanding questions as to whether we are comparing apples and oranges.

In NSABP B-32, SLN biopsy and ALND were performed by all participating surgeons, whereas in NSABP B-27, performing SLN biopsy after chemotherapy was elective, and represented only a subset of patients. Therefore, there may be some bias involving patient selection and surgeon experience in performing SLN biopsy after chemotherapy in NSABP B-27. The false negative rate might have been higher had all participating surgeons performed an SLN biopsy. The impact of surgeon experience on the false negative rate is demonstrated in the meta-analysis by Lyman and colleagues,[31] who showed that in studies of 100 or more patients, the false negative rate was only 6.7% compared with 9.0% for studies of fewer than 100 patients.

A second question is whether the routine pathologic examination of the NSLN accurately reflects the false negative rate. This question arose in the early days of routine SLN biopsy. The SLN is typically subjected to thin sectioning and in some cases immunohistochemical (IHC) staining to identify micrometastases, and this has been shown to increase the detection rate. The NSLN are typically bivalved only. When SLN biopsy was first introduced, there was concern that the false negative rate might be higher than reported because of micrometastases in the NSLN missed by routine bivalving. To address this issue, several studies performed thin sectioning and IHC staining of the NSLN in cases where the SLN was negative.[35,36] Sabel and colleagues[35] performed this detailed histologic examination of 775 NSLNs among 42 consecutive SLN cases and found no cases where micrometastases were present in the NSLN when the SLN biopsy was negative. These studies provided support for both the SLN concept and the accuracy of the procedure. In the multiple reported series of SLN biopsy and ALND performed after neoadjuvant chemotherapy, this detailed analysis of the NSLN is absent.

The most important outstanding question is that of the impact on regional recurrence. Even if one accepts that the FN rate after neoadjuvant chemotherapy is similar to that of SLN biopsy in general, is the regional control rate the same? For patients having SLN biopsy before adjuvant therapy, although some may not receive adjuvant chemotherapy based on a false negative SLN result, most patients will have some form of systemic therapy based on tumor size, grade, and other factors. Thus, the clinical impact of leaving behind microscopic disease in the regional nodes may be relatively small, as this disease may likely be eradicated by chemotherapy or hormonal therapy. In fact, this appears to be the case, as the regional recurrence rate among patients who had a negative SLN biopsy and did not undergo ALND is extremely small, ranging from 0% to 3% (**Table 5**), much lower than the false negative rates of SLN biopsy followed by ALND might predict. Even among patients with a positive SLN biopsy who did not undergo ALND, although a more selected and biased population, the regional recurrence rate appears low.[37–40] However, patients with a false negative SLN biopsy after neoadjuvant chemotherapy have residual micrometastases left behind after having completed systemic chemotherapy. Radiation therapy or hormonal therapy in hormone-receptor–positive patients may help control regional metastases, but it is reasonable to believe the likelihood of recurrence of disease remaining after chemotherapy is greater than that remaining before chemotherapy. Although these patients are likely at a higher risk of systemic disease, the importance of locoregional control on overall survival cannot be underestimated.[41] Unfortunately, the one piece of information missing from this debate is the regional recurrence rate among patients who had a negative SLN biopsy after neoadjuvant chemotherapy and did not undergo completion ALND. Promising data have been reported by Hunt and colleagues.[42] Among 575 patients who had SLN biopsy after neoadjuvant chemotherapy, with a median follow-up of 55 months, the regional recurrence rate was 1.2%. However, 30% of these patients had a complete node dissection (either planned or because of a positive SLN biopsy), so it remains unclear what the follow-up and recurrence rate is among the subset who were SLN negative and did not have a complete node dissection. In addition, this series has a much lower SLN positivity rate (20.7%)

Table 5
Regional recurrence after a negative SLN biopsy without ALND

First Author	Year	N	Regional Recurrence Rate	Median Follow-up, Mo
Guiliano[86]	2000	67	0%	39
Schrenk[87]	2001	83	0%	22
Roumen[88]	2001	100	1%	24
Veronesi[89]	2001	280	0%	15
Chung[90]	2002	206	1.5%	26
Badgwell[91]	2003	159	0%	32
Blanchard[92]	2003	685	0.15%	29
Veronesi[93]	2003	167	0%	46
Reitsamer[94]	2004	200	0%	36
Naik[95]	2004	2340	0.1%	31
Imoto[96]	2004	112	3.6%	52
Torrenga[97]	2004	104	1.0%	57
Zavagno[98]	2005	479	0%	36
Langer[99]	2005	222	0.7%	42
Snoj[100]	2005	50	2%	32
Jeruss[39]	2005	633	0.3%	27
Swenson[101]	2005	580	0.5%	33
Smidt[102]	2005	439	0.5%	26
Sanjuan[103]	2005	163	0.6%	21
Palesty[104]	2006	320	0.6%	33
Rosing[105]	2006	89	1%	26
Domenech[106]	2007	95	2.1%	49
Takei[107]	2007	1062	1.0%	34
Bergkvist[108]	2008	2246	0.6%	37
Poletti[109]	2008	804	0.5%	39

than most of the series of SLN after neoadjuvant chemotherapy, which range from 24% to 77% (see **Table 2**). This may represent differences in patient selection or response to chemotherapy, but it makes it difficult to extrapolate these results. Further information regarding the recurrence rate among SLN-negative patients who do not have completion ALND is critical.

WHICH APPROACH PROVIDES THE MOST RELEVANT PROGNOSTIC/PREDICTIVE INFORMATION?

One significant argument for performing the SLN biopsy before chemotherapy is the impact that the information might have on the decision to include the regional lymph nodes in the fields or to recommend postmastectomy radiation should the patient not be eligible for breast-conserving surgery at the completion of therapy. This argument is based on the assumption that pretreatment nodal status is the most important prognostic information regarding locoregional recurrence, and this information is lost in patients who have a complete response. However, that assumption might not be correct. Response to systemic therapy, particularly a complete pathologic response, has clearly been shown to be strongly prognostic in regard to the development of distant metastases and overall survival. The postchemotherapy nodal status and the response to chemotherapy in the axilla may likewise provide additional, and perhaps more prognostic information than the prechemotherapy nodal status.[43]

The benefits of postmastectomy radiation on locoregional recurrence have been demonstrated in large randomized trials involving both pre- and postmenopausal women.[44–46] Not only did radiation decrease the risk of recurrence, but also improved overall survival. The data clearly suggest a benefit in women with 4 or more involved lymph nodes, although controversy still remains among women with 1 to 3 involved nodes. The magnitude of the survival benefit is correlated with the reduction in local-regional recurrence (LRR), which is clearly going to be related to the risk of developing LRR in the absence of radiation.

So which is a better predictor of chest wall recurrence: the pretreatment nodal stage or the posttreatment nodal stage and response to chemotherapy? The data are mixed. In a retrospective analysis, Bucholz and colleagues[47] compared 150 patients who underwent neoadjuvant chemotherapy followed by mastectomy without postmastectomy radiation therapy (RT) to more than 1000 patients treated by mastectomy and adjuvant chemotherapy. Despite a lower pathologic stage after treatment, the neoadjuvant group had a higher 5-year LRR rate compared with the adjuvant group (27% vs 15%). The data imply that the LRR rate based on pathologic staging after neoadjuvant chemotherapy may be underestimated by ignoring (or not knowing) the pretreatment clinical staging. Further data from the M. D. Anderson Cancer Center suggest the importance of pretreatment clinical staging for using postmastectomy RT despite a good response to neoadjuvant chemotherapy.[48] Although one might be tempted to use these findings as an argument for the importance of SLN biopsy before treatment, interpretation is limited by small numbers, limited follow-up for the neoadjuvant group, the retrospective nature of the data, and the inaccuracy of clinically staging the axilla. One must be careful in extrapolating the results from pretreatment clinically node-positive patients with 1 to 3 nodes identified by pretreatment axillary ultrasound and FNA biopsy to pretreatment clinically node-negative patients with nodes containing micrometastatic disease that would be detected only by pretreatment SLN biopsy. This latter group has a different tumor burden, and likely a lower locoregional recurrence risk.

Support of the posttreatment nodal status and response to chemotherapy on predicting LRR comes from the NSABP neoadjuvant chemotherapy trials B-18 and B-27. Preliminary analysis of more than 2000 patients, none of whom had postmastectomy RT, suggest that rates of LRR can be defined based on pretherapy clinical factors (such as clinical tumor size and clinical nodal status) and post-therapy factors without knowing the pretreatment histologic nodal status. Patients with negative nodes after therapy had an extremely low risk of chest wall recurrence (1.5% if they had a pCR, 5.0% if they did not) compared with patients who were node positive after therapy (11.2%), and are unlikely to benefit from postmastectomy radiation. Again, however, data must be interpreted carefully, as it is unknown how many patients who were node negative after therapy had microscopic disease in their nodes at the onset of therapy, and what the LRR rate was in this subset. In the NSABP data, 14 (5%) of 270 patients who were node negative and did not have a complete response had a chest wall recurrence. As an example, if we assume that 50% of the patients were node negative before treatment, and most of the chest wall recurrences (13 of 14) were among the initially node-positive patients, then the LRR among patients node positive before chemotherapy but node negative afterward would be 10%, a recurrence rate for whom we might recommend postmastectomy RT. There are data to suggest that patients who are node positive before chemotherapy but node negative afterward have a worse outcome. Kilbride and colleagues[49] examined 114 patients who were node positive before neoadjuvant chemotherapy, determined either by FNA or prechemotherapy SLN biopsy. Patients were stratified as node negative before treatment, downstaged (node positive before treatment but node negative afterward), and node positive after treatment. The strongest predictor of treatment failure was the pretreatment nodal status, with a distant relapse rate of 8.1% in node-negative patients, 13.9% in the downstaged group, and 22.0% in the persistently positive group ($P = .047$). In addition, the use of RT was associated with a decreased local recurrence rate among the downstaged group (12.5% vs 3.7%), although these were small numbers and not statistically significant. It cannot be known whether patients SLN positive before chemotherapy and SLN negative afterward are negative because of response in NSLN, or negative because the disease was restricted to the SLN and surgically eradicated before therapy.

It is clear that we need to optimize our selection of patients for postmastectomy radiation to realize the full benefits on LRR, and possibly overall survival, while minimizing the morbidity. Additional research is necessary but this presents several challenges. After a prospective, randomized trial of postmastectomy radiation for patients with 1 to 3 positive nodes was closed secondary to poor accrual, the enthusiasm for future similar trials is diminished. As for using retrospective data, the NSABP and M. D. Anderson data come from clinical trial data before the use of postmastectomy radiation, giving a clearer picture of recurrence risk without treatment. More modern data series include many patients who received postmastectomy radiation, diluting numbers and introducing selection bias. When specifically examining the pre- or post-chemotherapy SLN biopsy, we face a surgical version of Heisenberg's Uncertainty Principle. If we perform the SLN biopsy after chemotherapy, we never truly know which patients were initially node positive, and if we examine the sentinel node before chemotherapy, we never really know which patients had a true regional response. Finally, like adjuvant chemotherapy, this is a moving target, with potential changes in recommendations for postmastectomy radiation as more information regarding the present trials, including subset analyses emerges, as well as the influx of genomic or proteomic approaches that may better identify patients at risk of locoregional recurrence than tumor size, nodal status, or response to systemic therapy.

MUST ONE APPROACH BE UNIVERSALLY APPLIED?

The reader may walk away from this article choosing one side or the other: that SLN biopsy should be performed either before or after neoadjuvant chemotherapy. However, the take-home message should be that as is true for many of these controversies, there is no right answer; no single approach or technique that should be universally applied. The management of breast cancer is multidisciplinary, and surgical staging and locoregional control will greatly impact medical and radiation oncologists in addition to the surgeon. It is therefore naïve to believe that there is one approach that should be used universally; whose advantages always trump its disadvantages. On the contrary, the timing of SLN biopsy in patients being considered for neoadjuvant chemotherapy should be discussed in a multidisciplinary setting, determining how the results may affect the choice of systemic agents, the fields for RT, or even the most appropriate surveillance. **Fig. 1** presents a reasonable approach to this debate. Any patient being considered for neoadjuvant chemotherapy should ideally have a thorough evaluation of the regional lymph nodes, including physical examination, axillary ultrasound, and FNA biopsy of any

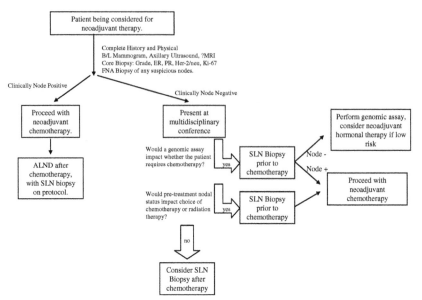

Fig. 1. Incorporation of SLN biopsy in patients being considered for neoadjuvant chemotherapy.

suspicious lymph nodes. Until additional information is available regarding false negative and regional recurrence rates, patients documented to be clinically node positive by FNA should proceed with systemic therapy and undergo ALND at the time of their surgery, hopefully with SLN biopsy performed at the time on protocol. Patients who are clinically node negative should ideally have their case presented at a tumor board, or discussed with medical oncology and radiation oncology, before a surgical decision is made. If the pretreatment nodal status would influence the decision to use neoadjuvant therapy, the type of neoadjuvant therapy, the use of postmastectomy radiation (should the patient not become eligible for BCT), or the radiation fields, then SLN biopsy should be performed before the initiation of chemotherapy. At this time, ALND in concert with either lumpectomy or mastectomy is recommended at the completion of the neoadjuvant therapy, although the use of predictive models or nomograms may be considered in having a balanced discussion with patients regarding the risks and benefits of completion ALND. For those patients for whom adjuvant therapy decisions can be made independent of the nodal status, a balanced discussion can be had with the patient regarding the relative pros and cons of the timing of SLN biopsy, with SLN biopsy after neoadjuvant chemotherapy being a reasonable option.

REFERENCES

1. Chung MH, Ye W, Giuliano AE. Role for sentinel lymph node dissection in the management of large (>5cm) invasive breast cancer. Ann Surg Oncol 2001; 8(9):688–92.
2. Bedrosian I, Reynolds C, Mick R, et al. Accuracy of sentinel lymph node biopsy in patients with large primary breast tumors. Cancer 2000;88:2540–5.
3. Paik S, Shak S, Tang G, et al. Multi-gene RT-PCR assay for predicting recurrence in node negative breast cancer patients- NSABP studies B20 and B14. 26th

Annual San Antonio Breast Cancer Symposium. Vol. Abstract #16. San Antonio (TX), December 3–6, 2003.

4. Paik S, Shak S, Tang G, et al. A multigene assay to predict recurrence of tamoxifen-treated, node-negative breast cancer. N Engl J Med 2004;351:2817–26.

5. Hayes DF, Thor AD, Dressler LG, et al. HER2 and response to paclitaxel in node-positive breast cancer. N Engl J Med 2007;357:1496–506.

6. Albain KS, Barlow W, Shak S, et al. Prognostic and predictive value of the 21-gene recurrence score assay in postmenopausal, node-positive, ER-positive breast cancer (S8814, INT0100) [abstract 10]. Breast Cancer Res Treat 2007; 106(Suppl 1).

7. Straver ME, Rutgers EJT, Russel NS, et al. Towards rational axillary treatment in relation to neoadjuvant therapy in breast cancer. Eur J Cancer 2009;45:2284–92.

8. Rouzier R, Extra J-M, Klijanienko J, et al. Incidence and prognostic significance of complete axillary downstaging after primary chemotherapy in breast cancer patients with T1 to T3 tumors and cytologically proven axillary metastatic lymph nodes. J Clin Oncol 2002;20(5):1304–10.

9. Newman EA, Sabel MS, Nees AV, et al. Sentinel lymph node biopsy performed after neoadjuvant chemotherapy is accurate in patients with documented node-positive breast cancer at presentation. Ann Surg Oncol 2007;14(10):2946–52.

10. Hennessy BT, Hortobagyi GN, Rouzier R, et al. Outcome after pathologic complete eradication of cytologically proven breast cancer axillary node metastases following primary chemotherapy. J Clin Oncol 2005;23(36):9304–11.

11. Beatty JD, Precht LM, Lowe K, et al. Axillary-conserving surgery is facilitated by neoadjuvant chemotherapy of breast cancer. Am J Surg 2009;197:637–42.

12. Van Zee KJ, Manasseh DM, Bevilacqua JL, et al. A nomogram for predicting the likelihood of additional nodal metastases in breast cancer patients with a positive sentinel node biopsy. Ann Surg Oncol 2003;10:1140–51.

13. Degnim AC, Reynolds C, Pantvaidya G, et al. Nonsentinel node metastasis in breast cancer patients: assessment of an existing and a new predictive nomogram. Am J Surg 2005;190(4):543–50.

14. Bilimoria KY, Bentrem DJ, Hansen NM, et al. Comparison of sentinel lymph node biopsy alone and completion axillary lymph node dissection for node-positive breast cancer. J Clin Oncol 2009;27(18):2946–53.

15. Evrensel T, Johnson R, Ahrendt G, et al. The predicted probability of having positive non-sentinel lymph nodes in patients who received neoadjuvant chemotherapy for large operable breast cancer. Int J Clin Pract 2007;62(9):1379–82.

16. Jeruss JS, Newman LA, Ayers GD, et al. Factors predicting additional disease in the axilla in patients with positive sentinel lymph nodes after neoadjuvant chemotherapy. Cancer 2008;112:2646–54.

17. Torisu-Itakura H, Lee JH, Scheri RP, et al. Molecular characterization of inflammatory genes in sentinel and nonsentinel nodes in melanoma. Clin Cancer Res 2007;13(11):3125–32.

18. Specht MC, Fey JV, Borgen PI, et al. Is the clinically positive axilla in breast cancer really a contraindication to sentinel lymph node biopsy? J Am Coll Surg 2005;200(1):10–4.

19. Oruwari JU, Chung MA, Koelliker S, et al. Axillary staging using ultrasound-guided fine needle aspiration biopsy in locally advanced breast cancer. Am J Surg 2002;184:307–9.

20. Krishnamurthy S, Sneige N, Bedi DG, et al. Role of ultrasound-guided fine-needle aspiration of indeterminate and suspicious axillary lymph nodes in the initial staging of breast carcinoma. Cancer 2002;95:982–8.

21. de Kanter AY, van Eijck CHJ, van Geel AN, et al. Multicentre study of ultrasonographically guided axillary node biopsy in patients with breast cancer. Br J Surg 1999;86(11):1459–62.

22. Lam WW, Yang WT, Chan YT, et al. Detection of axillary lymph node metastases in breast carcinoma by technetium-99m sestamibi breast scintigraphy, ultrasound, and conventional mammography. Eur J Nucl Med 1996;23(5):498–503.

23. Bonnema J, van Geel AN, van Ooijen B, et al. Ultrasound-guided aspiration biopsy for detection of nonpalpable axillary node metastases in breast cancer patients: new diagnostic method. World J Surg 1997;21(3):270–4.

24. Ciatto S, Brancato B, Risso G, et al. Accuracy of fine needle aspiration cytology (FNAC) of axillary lymph nodes as a triage test in breast cancer staging. Breast Cancer Res Treat 2007;103:85–91.

25. Shen J, Gilcrease MZ, Babiera GV, et al. Feasibility and accuracy of sentinel lymph node biopsy after preoperative chemotherapy in breast cancer patients with documented axillary metastases. Cancer 2007;109:1255–63.

26. Lee S, Kim EY, Kang SH, et al. Sentinel node identification rate, but not accuracy, is significantly decreased after pre-operative chemotherapy in axillary node-positive breast cancer patients. Breast Cancer Res Treat 2007;102: 283–8.

27. Xing Y, Foy M, Cox DD, et al. Meta-analysis of sentinel lymph node biopsy after preoperative chemotherapy in patients with breast cancer. Br J Surg 2006;93: 539–46.

28. Mamounas EP, Bellon JR. Local-regional therapy considerations in patients receiving preoperative chemotherapy. In: Harris JR, Lippman ME, Morrow M, et al, editors. Diseases of the breast. 4th edition. Philadelphia: Lippincott Williams & Wilkins; 2010. p. 730–44.

29. Mamounas EP, Brown A, Anderson S, et al. Sentinel node biopsy after neoadjuvant chemotherapy in breast cancer: results from National Surgical Adjuvant Breast and Bowel Project Protocol B-27. J Clin Oncol 2005;23(12):2694–702.

30. Krag D, Weaver D, Ashikaga T, et al. The sentinel node in breast cancer—a multicenter validation study. N Engl J Med 1998;339(14):941–6.

31. Lyman GH, Kim TY, Giuliano AE. A systematic review and meta-analysis of lymphatic mapping and sentinel node biopsy (SNB) in early stage breast cancer [abstract 2001]. San Antonio Breast Conference. San Antonio (TX), December 2–11, 2004.

32. Fraile M, Rull M, Julian FJ, et al. Sentinel node biopsy as a practical alternative to axillary lymph node dissection in breast cancer patients: an approach to its validity. Ann Oncol 2000;11:701–5.

33. Miltenburg DM, Miller C, Karamlou TB, et al. Meta-analysis of sentinel lymph node biopsy in breast cancer. J Surg Res 1999;84:138–42.

34. Julian TB, Krag DN, Brown A, et al. Preliminary technical results of NSABP B-32, a randomized phase III clinical trial to compare sentinel node resection to conventional axillary dissection in clinically node-negative breast cancer patients [abstract 14]. San Antonio Breast Cancer Symposium. San Antonio (TX), December 2–11, 2004.

35. Sabel MS, Zhang P, Barnwell JM, et al. Accuracy of sentinel node biopsy in predicting nodal status in patients with breast carcinoma. J Surg Oncol 2001;77(4): 243–6.

36. Chu KU, Turner RR, Hansen NM, et al. Sentinel node metastasis in patients with breast carcinoma accurately predicts immunohistochemically detectable nonsentinel node metastasis. Ann Surg Oncol 1999;6(8):756–61.

37. Fant JS, Grant MD, Knox SM, et al. Preliminary outcome in patients with breast cancer and a positive sentinel lymph node who declined axillary dissection. Ann Surg Oncol 2003;10:126–30.

38. Zakaria S, Pantivaidya G, Reynolds CA, et al. Sentinel node positive breast cancer patients who do not undergo axillary dissection: are they different? Surgery 2007;143(5):641–7.

39. Jeruss JS, Winchester DJ, Sener SF, et al. Axillary recurrence after sentinel node biopsy. Ann Surg Oncol 2005;12:34–40.

40. Guenther JM, Hansen NM, DiFronzo LA, et al. Axillary dissection is not required for all patients with breast cancer and positive sentinel nodes. Arch Surg 2003; 138:52–6.

41. Sabel MS. Locoregional therapy of breast cancer: maximizing control, minimizing morbidity. Expert Rev Anticancer Ther 2007;6(9):1261–79.

42. Hunt KK, Yi M, Mittendorf EA, et al. Sentinel lymph node surgery after neoadjuvant chemotherapy is accurate and reduces the need for axillary dissection in breast cancer patients. Ann Surg 2009;250(4):558–66.

43. Klauber-Demore N, Ollila DW, Moore DT, et al. Size of residual lymph node metastasis after neoadjuvant chemotherapy in locally advanced breast cancer patients is prognostic. Ann Surg Oncol 2006;13(5):685–91.

44. Overgaard M, Hansen PS, Overgaard J, et al. Postoperative radiotherapy in high-risk premenopausal women with breast cancer who receive adjuvant chemotherapy. Danish Breast Cancer Cooperative Group 82b Trial. N Engl J Med 1997;337(14):949–55.

45. Overgaard M, Jensen MB, Overgaard J, et al. Postoperative radiotherapy in high-risk postmenopausal breast-cancer patients given adjuvant tamoxifen: Danish Breast Cancer Cooperative Group DBCG 82c randomised trial. Lancet 1999;353:1641–8.

46. Ragaz J, Jackson SM, Le N, et al. Adjuvant radiotherapy and chemotherapy in node-positive premenopausal women with breast cancer. N Engl J Med 1997; 337:956–62.

47. Buchholz TA, Tucker SL, Masullo L, et al. Predictors of local-regional recurrence after neoadjuvant chemotherapy and mastectomy without radiation. J Clin Oncol 2002;20(1):17–23.

48. McGuire SE, Gonzalez-Angulo AM, Huang EH, et al. Postmastectomy radiation improves the outcome of patients with locally advanced breast cancer who achieve a pathologic complete response to neoadjuvant chemotherapy. Int J Radiat Oncol Biol Phys 2007;68:1004–9.

49. Kilbride KE, Lee MC, Nees AV, et al. Axillary staging prior to neoadjuvant chemotherapy for breast cancer: predictors of recurrence. Ann Surg Oncol 2008;15(11):3252–8.

50. Zirngibl C, Steinfeld-Birg D, Vogt H, et al. Sentinel lymph node biopsy before neoadjuvant chemotherapy—conservation of breast and axilla [abstract]. Breast Cancer Res Treat 2002;76(Suppl 1):S129.

51. Schrenk P, Hochreiner G, Fridrik M, et al. Sentinel node biopsy performed before preoperative chemotherapy for axillary lymph node staging in breast cancer. Breast J 2003;9(4):282–7.

52. Sabel MS, Schott AF, Kleer CG, et al. Sentinel node biopsy prior to neoadjuvant chemotherapy. Am J Surg 2003;186(2):102–5.

53. Ollila DW, Neuman HB, Sartor C, et al. Lymphatic mapping and sentinel lymphadenectomy prior to neoadjuvant chemotherapy in patients with large breast cancers. Am J Surg 2005;190:371–5.

54. Jones JL, Zabicki K, Christian RL, et al. A comparison of sentinel node biopsy before and after neoadjuvant chemotherapy: timing is important. Am J Surg 2005;190(4):517–20.

55. van Rijk MC, Nieweg OE, Rutgers EJT, et al. Sentinel node biopsy before neoadjuvant chemotherapy spares breast cancer patients axillary lymph node dissection. Ann Surg Oncol 2006;13(4):475–9.

56. Cox CE, Cox JM, White LB, et al. Sentinel node biopsy before neoadjuvant chemotherapy for determining axillary status and treatment prognosis in locally advanced breast cancer. Ann Surg Oncol 2006;13(4):483–90.

57. Grube BJ, Christy CJ, Black D, et al. Breast sentinel lymph node dissection before preoperative chemotherapy. Arch Surg 2008;143(7):692–700.

58. Papa MZ, Zippel D, Kaufman B, et al. Timing of sentinel lymph node biopsy in patients receiving neoadjuvant chemotherapy for breast cancer. J Surg Oncol 2008;98:403–6.

59. Cohen LF, Breslin TM, Keurer HM, et al. Identification and evaluation of axillary sentinel lymph nodes in patients with breast carcinoma treated with neoadjuvant chemotherapy. Am J Surg Pathol 2000;24(9):1266–72.

60. Breslin TM, Cohen LF, Sahin AA, et al. Sentinel lymph node biopsy is accurate after neoadjuvant chemotherapy for breast cancer. J Clin Oncol 2000;18(20): 3480–6.

61. Nason KS, Anderson BO, Byrd DR, et al. Increased false negative sentinel node biopsy rates after preoperative chemotherapy for invasive breast carcinoma. Cancer 2000;89(11):2187–94.

62. Fernandez A, Cortes M, Benito E, et al. Gamma probe sentinel node localization and biopsy in breast cancer patients treated with a neoadjuvant chemotherapy scheme. Nucl Med Commun 2001;22:361–6.

63. Tafra L, Verbanac KM, Lannin DR. Preoperative chemotherapy and sentinel lymphadenectomy for breast cancer. Am J Surg 2001;182:312–5.

64. Stearns V, Ewing CA, Slack R, et al. Sentinel lymphadenectomy after neoadjuvant chemotherapy for breast cancer may reliably represent the axilla except for inflammatory breast cancer. Ann Surg Oncol 2002;9(3):235–42.

65. Brady EW. Sentinel lymph node mapping following neoadjuvant chemotherapy for breast cancer. Breast J 2002;8(2):97–100.

66. Julian TB, Dusi D, Wolmark N. Sentinel node biopsy after neoadjuvant chemotherapy for breast cancer. Am J Surg 2002;184(4):315–7.

67. Miller AR, Thomason VE, Yeh I-T, et al. Analysis of sentinel lymph node mapping with immediate pathologic review in patients receiving preoperative chemotherapy for breast carcinoma. Ann Surg Oncol 2002;9(3):243–7.

68. Vigario A, Sapienza MT, Sampaio AP, et al. Primary chemotherapy effect in sentinel node detection in breast cancer. Clin Nucl Med 2003;28(7):553–7.

69. Balch GC, Mithani SK, Richards KR, et al. Lymphatic mapping and sentinel lymphadenectomy after preoperative therapy for stage II and III breast cancer. Ann Surg Oncol 2003;10:616–21.

70. Reitsamer R, Peintiger F, Rettenbacher L, et al. Sentinel lymph node biopsy in breast cancer patients after neoadjuvant chemotherapy. J Surg Oncol 2003; 84:63–7.

71. Schwartz GF, Meltzer AJ. Accuracy of axillary sentinel lymph node biopsy following neoadjuvant (induction) chemotherapy for carcinoma of the breast. Breast J 2003;9:374–9.

72. Piato JR, Barros AC, Pincerato KM, et al. Sentinel lymph node biopsy in breast cancer after neoadjuvant chemotherapy. Eur J Surg Oncol 2003;29:118–20.

73. Haid A, Koeberle-Wuehrer R, Offner F, et al. Clinical usefulness and perspectives of sentinel node biopsy in the management of breast cancer. Chirurg 2003;74:657–64.
74. Kang SH, Kim SK, Kwon Y, et al. Decreased identification rate of sentinel lymph node after neoadjuvant chemotherapy. World J Surg 2004;28:1019–24.
75. Shimazu K, Tamaki Y, Taguchi T, et al. Sentinel lymph node biopsy using periareolar injection of radiocolloid for patients with neoadjuvant chemotherapy-treated breast carcinoma. Cancer 2004;100:2555–61.
76. Lang JE, Esserman LJ, Ewing CA, et al. Accuracy of selective sentinel lymphadenectomy after neoadjuvant chemotherapy: effect of clinical node status at presentation. J Am Coll Surg 2004;199:856–62.
77. Patel NA, Piper G, Patel JA, et al. Accurate axillary nodal staging can be achieved after neoadjuvant therapy for locally advanced breast cancer. Am Surg 2004;70(8):696–9.
78. Aihara T, Munakata S, Morino H, et al. Feasibility of sentinel node biopsy for breast cancer after neoadjuvant endocrine therapy. A pilot study. J Surg Oncol 2004;85:77–81.
79. Kinoshita T, Takasugi M, Iwamoto E, et al. Sentinel lymph node biopsy examination for breast cancer patients with clinically negative axillary lymph nodes after neoadjuvant chemotherapy. Am J Surg 2005;194(1):135–6.
80. Tanaka Y, Maeda H, Ogawa Y, et al. Sentinel node biopsy in breast cancer patients treated with neoadjuvant chemotherapy. Oncol Rep 2006;15:927–31.
81. Tausch C, Konstantiniuk P, Kugler F, et al. Sentinel lymph node biopsy after preoperative chemotherapy for breast cancer: findings from the Austrian Sentinel Node Group. Ann Surg Oncol 2008;15(12):3378–83.
82. Gimbergues P, Abrial C, Durando X, et al. Sentinel lymph node biopsy after neoadjuvant chemotherapy is accurate in breast cancer patients with a clinically negative axillary nodal status at presentation. Ann Surg Oncol 2008;15(5):1316–21.
83. Hino M, Sano M, Sato N, et al. Sentinel lymph node biopsy after neoadjuvant chemotherapy in a patient with operable breast cancer. Surg Today 2008;38:585–91.
84. Classe J-M, Bordes V, Campion L, et al. Sentinel lymph node biopsy after neoadjuvant chemotherapy for advanced breast cancer: results of Ganglion Sentinelle et Chimotherapie Neoadjuvante, a French prospective multicentric study. J Clin Oncol 2008;27(5):726–32.
85. Schwartz GF, Tannelbaum JE, Jernigan AM, et al. Axillary sentinel lymph node biopsy after neoadjuvant chemotherapy for carcinoma of the breast. Cancer 2010;116(5):1243–51.
86. Guiliano AE, Haigh PI, Brennan MB, et al. Prospective observational study of sentinel lymphadenectomy without further axillary dissection in patients with sentinel node-negative breast cancer. J Clin Oncol 2000;18:2553–9.
87. Schrenk P, Hatzl-Griesenhofer M, Shamiyeh A, et al. Follow-up of sentinel node negative breast cancer patients without axillary lymph node dissection. J Surg Oncol 2001;77:165–70.
88. Roumen RM, Kujit GP, Liem IH, et al. Treatment of 100 patients with sentinel node negative breast cancer without further axillary dissection. Br J Surg 2001;88:1639–43.
89. Veronesi U, Galimberti V, Zurrida S, et al. Sentinel lymph node biopsy as an indicator for axillary dissection in early breast cancer. Eur J Cancer 2001;37:454–8.
90. Chung MA, Steinhoff MM, Cady B. Clinical axillary recurrence after a negative sentinel node biopsy. Am J Surg 2002;184:310–4.

91. Badgwell BD, Povoski SP, Abdessalam SF, et al. Patterns of recurrence after sentinel lymph node biopsy for breast cancer. Ann Surg Oncol 2003;10:376–80.

92. Blanchard DK, Donohue JH, Reynolds C, et al. Relapse and morbidity in patients undergoing sentinel lymph node biopsy alone or with axillary dissection for breast cancer. Arch Surg 2003;138:482–7.

93. Veronesi U, Paganelli G, Viale G, et al. A randomized comparison of sentinel-node biopsy with routine axillary dissection in breast cancer. N Engl J Med 2003;349(6):546–53.

94. Reitsamer R, Peintiger F, Prokop E, et al. 200 sentinel lymph node biopsies without axillary lymph node dissection. No axillary recurrences after a 3-year follow-up. Br J Cancer 2004;90:1551–4.

95. Naik AM, Fey JV, Gemignani M, et al. The risk of axillary relapse after sentinel lymph node biopsy for breast cancer is comparable with that of axillary lymph node dissection. Ann Surg 2004;240:462–8.

96. Imoto S, Wada N, Murakami K, et al. Prognosis of breast cancer patients treated with sentinel node biopsy in Japan. Jpn J Clin Oncol 2004;34:452–6.

97. Torrenga H, Fabry H, van der Sijp JR, et al. Omitting axillary lymph node dissection in sentinel node negative breast cancer patients is safe: a long term follow-up analysis. J Surg Oncol 2004;88:4–7.

98. Zavagno G, Carcoforo P, Franchini Z, et al. Axillary recurrence after negative sentinel lymph node biopsy without axillary dissection: a study on 479 breast cancer patients. Eur J Surg Oncol 2005;31(7):715–20.

99. Langer I, Marti WR, Guller U, et al. Axillary recurrence rate in breast cancer patients with negative sentinel lymph node (SLN) or SLN micrometastases. Ann Surg 2005;241(1):152–8.

100. Snoj M, Bracko M, Zagar I. Axillary recurrence rate in breast cancer patients with negative sentinel lymph node. Croat Med J 2005;46(3):377–81.

101. Swenson KK, Mahipal A, Nissen MJ, et al. Axillary disease recurrence after sentinel lymph node dissection for breast carcinoma. Cancer 2005;104:1834–9.

102. Smidt ML, Janssen CM, Kuster DM, et al. Axillary recurrence after a negative sentinel node biopsy for breast cancer: incidence and clinical significance. Ann Surg Oncol 2001;12:29–33.

103. Sanjuan A, Vidal-Sicart S, Zanon g, et al. Clinical axillary recurrence after sentinel node biopsy in breast cancer: a follow-up study of 200 patients. Eur J Nucl Med Mol Imaging 2005;32(8):932–6.

104. Palesty JA, Foster JM, Hurd TC, et al. Axillary recurrence in women with a negative sentinel lymph node and no axillary dissection in breast cancer. J Surg Oncol 2006;93(2):129–32.

105. Rosing DK, Dauphine CE, Perla VM, et al. Axillary regional recurrence after sentinel lymph node biopsy for breast cancer. Am Surg 2006;72:939–42.

106. Domenech A, Benitez A, Bajen MT, et al. Patients with breast cancer and negative sentinel lymph node biopsy without additional axillary lymph node dissection: a follow-up study of up to 5 years. Oncology 2007;72(1–2):27–32.

107. Takei H, Suemasu K, Kurosumi M, et al. Recurrence after sentinel lymph node biopsy with or without axillary lymph node dissection in patients with breast cancer. Breast Cancer 2007;14(1):16–24.

108. Bergkvist L, de Boniface J, Jonsson P-E, et al. Axillary recurrence rate after negative sentinel node biopsy in breast cancer: three-year follow-up of the Swedish multicenter cohort study. Ann Surg 2008;247(1):150–6.

109. Poletti P, Fenaroli P, Milesi A, et al. Axillary recurrence in sentinel lymph node negative breast cancer patients. Ann Oncol 2008;19(11):1842–6.

Sentinel Lymph Node Surgery in Uncommon Clinical Circumstances

Bijan Ansari, MD, Judy C. Boughey, MD*

KEYWORDS

- Sentinel lymph node • Neoadjuvant chemotherapy
- Breast cancer in men • Multifocal breast cancer
- Internal mammary lymph node • Breast reduction
- Breast augmentation • Prophylactic mastectomy

Surgical staging of the axillary lymph nodes in patients with breast cancer has evolved from axillary lymph node dissection (ALND) to sentinel lymph node (SLN) surgery. Although SLN surgery has become the standard of care for clinically node-negative early-stage breast cancer, controversies exist regarding its applications in some special circumstances. American Society of Clinical Oncology (ASCO) published guideline recommendations for use of SLN surgery in 2005 with a section devoted to SLN in special circumstances.[1] The literature was more limited at that time, and additional data have since been published in these areas. In this article, an update of the information on the role of SLN surgery in uncommon circumstances is provided.

BREAST CANCER IN MEN

In general, men with breast cancer have larger tumors than women have and are more likely than women to have positive nodes.[2] At the time of issuance of the ASCO panel recommendations, data on the use of SLN surgery in men with early-stage breast cancer were limited.[3–10] Therefore, no categorical recommendations about the use of SLN surgery for men with breast cancer were made, despite it being unlikely that SLN surgery would be any less accurate in men than it was in women.[1]

There have been several additional studies with larger numbers of patients showing technical feasibility and accuracy of SLN surgery in men similar to that in women. Boughey and colleagues[2] compared 30 men and 2784 women with breast cancer who underwent SLN surgery. The SLN was identified in 100% of men and in 98.3% of women. The incidence of positive SLNs was higher in men than women (37.0%

Department of Surgery, Mayo Clinic, 200 First Street SW, Rochester, MN 55905, USA
* Corresponding author.
E-mail address: boughey.judy@mayo.edu

Surg Oncol Clin N Am 19 (2010) 539–553
doi:10.1016/j.soc.2010.03.001   surgonc.theclinics.com
1055-3207/10/$ – see front matter © 2010 Elsevier Inc. All rights reserved.

vs 22.3%), although this did not reach statistical significance. In cases with positive SLNs, male patients had increased risk of additional disease in nonsentinel axillary lymph nodes compared with women (62.5% vs 20.7%). Additional data and review of literature by Rusby and colleagues[11] reported combined data from 110 men who had undergone SLN surgery and showed a 96% SLN identification rate. There were no false negatives in the 13 patients with negative SLNs who had undergone concomitant ALND. Gentilini and colleagues[12] reported an identification rate of 100% in 32 men with early breast cancer who underwent SLN surgery. No backup axillary dissection was performed in 26 patients with negative SLNs; however, after a median follow-up of 30 months no axillary recurrence occurred. SLN surgery in 78 men at Memorial Sloan-Kettering Cancer Center reported an SLN identification rate of 97%. Negative SLNs were found in 39 of 76 (51%) patients. In 3 (8%) patients with negative SLNs, a positive non-SLN was identified by intraoperative palpation. At a median follow-up of 28 months, there were no axillary recurrences.[13]

As a result of data comparable to breast cancer in women, although not formally validated, SLN surgery is now advocated as the procedure of choice in men with clinically node-negative breast cancer.[11,12,14] Given the higher rate of SLN positivity in men and higher rate of non-SLN involvement in patients with a positive SLN, intraoperative evaluation of the SLN should be considered in the surgical management of male patients with breast cancer and completion ALND recommended in cases with positive SLN.[2]

PREGNANT PATIENTS WITH BREAST CANCER

Significant fetal radiation exposure may result in malformations, mental retardation, and childhood cancer. The ASCO 2005 guidelines on use of SLN surgery, while acknowledging that the dose of radiation to the fetus was minimal, nevertheless concluded that there were insufficient data to recommend the use of SLN surgery in pregnant women.[1] Understandably, the radiation effects are most harmful during early fetal life at the time of organogenesis. The use of phantom models, based on radiation-absorbed dose calculations in nonpregnant women who have undergone SLN surgery, estimated the fetal absorbed dose to be 0.014 mGy or less, using 0.5 mCi activity (18.5 MBq).[15] In another study, Keleher and colleagues[16] estimated the maximum absorbed dose to the fetus in 2 nonpregnant women using 92.5 MBq tracer activity to be 4.3 mGy. These absorbed doses are well below the acceptable radiation dose to the pregnant woman.[15–18]

More recent guidelines, however, including those on breast and head and neck cancers and melanoma, do not consider pregnancy a contraindication for SLN surgery, especially beyond the first trimester.[19–21] Despite theoretical safety, surgeons are reluctant, and currently studies of the use of SLN surgery in pregnancy are limited to a few case reports and series with few patients.[22–25] At the European Institute of Oncology in Milan, SLN surgery is offered to women with breast cancer diagnosed during pregnancy, and Gentilini and colleagues[25] recently reported on 12 pregnant patients who underwent SLN surgery. The SLN was identified in all patients. Of the 12 patients, 10 had pathologically negative SLNs. One patient had micrometastasis in 1 of 4 SLNs. One patient had metastasis in the SLN and underwent axillary clearance. No detrimental effect on the fetus was observed. There was no overt axillary recurrence in the patients with negative SLNs after a median follow-up of 32 months. Similar results have been reported from the Moffitt Cancer Center where 10 patients with an average gestation of 15.8 weeks underwent SLN surgery. In all cases the SLN was identified and the sentinel node was positive in 50%. Nine patients delivered healthy children and 1 patient elected to terminate her pregnancy.[23] Due to lack of data on the safety of blue dye in pregnancy, most surgeons performing SLN surgery in pregnant women use radioactive tracer only.[26]

SLN surgery in pregnant women must be considered on an individual basis, with thorough counseling regarding level of the risk of fetal damage and benefits. When SLN surgery is used, efforts should be made to reduce fetal radiation exposure including the use of same-day surgery following injection of the radiolabeled colloid, which allows reduction of injected activity down to 10 to 15 MBq and reduction of exposure time.[25]

DUCTAL CARCINOMA IN SITU

The management of the axilla for ductal carcinoma in situ (DCIS) has changed dramatically over the years. In the past, DCIS accounted for a small proportion of all breast cancer cases and was diagnosed after presentation with a palpable mass, nipple discharge, or Paget disease. DCIS now accounts for approximately 20% of all new breast cancers diagnosed in the United States, more than 90% of which are asymptomatic and detected on screening studies, most commonly by the presence of microcalcifications on mammography.[27–29] By definition DCIS is preinvasive, and should not have the potential to invade beyond the basement membrane and spread to the regional lymph nodes.

However, the need for SLN surgery in patients with a preoperative diagnosis of DCIS is debated. Some 10% to 30% of patients with a preoperative percutaneous biopsy diagnosis of DCIS will be found to have invasive disease in their final surgical pathology specimen. Such a finding results from sampling error as well as limitations of sampling techniques that may miss a small cancer within a large area of DCIS. These patients are thus upstaged to invasive cancer at final pathology and therefore need nodal evaluation.

Some investigators argue that performing SLN surgery in patients with a preoperative biopsy diagnosis of pure DCIS allows those found subsequently to have invasive disease to avoid further surgery.[30] There are several observational studies that report results of SLN surgery in patients with DCIS. In a meta-analysis of observational studies, Ansari and colleagues[31] reported that the frequency of a positive SLN in patients with a preoperative diagnosis of DCIS ranged from 0% to 16.7%, with an overall incidence of SLN positivity of 7.4%. This result contrasted with an overall SLN positivity rate of 3.7% in patients with a definitive (postoperative) diagnosis of DCIS.

Therefore, it is desirable to predict the subset of patients with a biopsy diagnosis of DCIS who are at higher risk of harboring invasive disease. For these patients, performing SLN surgery at the time of their tumor surgery would be advantageous. In most studies a palpable mass, a mammographic mass, a large-size lesion, and a high-grade lesion were associated with a significant risk of invasive disease in the final resection specimen.[31]

Current recommendations for SLN surgery in patients with biopsy revealing DCIS include those patients who are at high risk of occult invasive disease, in an attempt to prevent a second operation. This group may include patients with a palpable tumor, an extensive area of DCIS, high-grade DCIS, or microinvasion on preoperative biopsy. In addition, patients with DCIS who are undergoing mastectomy or breast reduction or reconstruction should also be considered for SLN surgery because should they be found to have invasive disease, SLN surgery is not usually possible after such procedures.[32,33] When immediate autologous tissue reconstruction is being performed in patients with DCIS (or invasive cancer), it may be appropriate to carry out SLN surgery as an initial separate procedure to avoid tissue reconstruction in node-positive patients in whom postmastectomy radiation may be recommended.[26,34–36]

MULTICENTRIC/MULTIFOCAL BREAST CANCER

Patients with multicentric and/or multifocal breast cancer were initially considered not to be candidates for SLN surgery because of concerns of higher false-negative rates and technical feasibility. The dominant view regarding the flow of the lymph in the breast considers the entire breast tissue as a single lymphatic unit that drains to specific primary SLNs. In other words, no matter where the sites of the tumors within the breast or what the methods of the injections are, the primary lymphatic drainage seems to be the same, although some controversy continues.[37–40] The implication of this concept has prompted the use of SLN surgery in multicentric/multifocal disease.

To date, numerous small and larger series have reported on the feasibility and accuracy of performing SLN surgery in multifocal/multicentric breast cancer. Identification rates and false-negative rates, from most series, have ranged from 90% to 100% and 0% to 15%, respectively. Various injection methods have been used, in particular subareolar or intradermal, with or without preoperative lymphoscintigraphy, with acceptable identification and false-negative rates.[41–49] Earlier smaller studies reported higher false-negative rates. One study of 21 patients using intratumoral blue dye only reported a 33% false-negative rate with a 85.7% identification rate,[50] and another study reported 21% (8 of 38 patients) false-negative rate in patients with multicentric/multifocal disease.[51] In one of the largest prospective series, out of 3730 patients in the Austrian Sentinel Node Study Group, a multi-institutional validation study of SLN surgery, 125 patients with multicentric cancer underwent ALND after SLN surgery with a false-negative rate of only 4%.[45]

Based on current evidence, SLN surgery may be considered in clinically node-negative patients with multicentric/multifocal disease.[1] However, given the possibility of higher false-negative rates observed in some reports, especially in patients with large tumor burdens, careful intraoperative palpation of the remaining axillary nodes, including excision of any suspicious nodes, should be performed to reduce the possibility of missing axillary metastases in this high-risk group.[49]

NEOADJUVANT CHEMOTHERAPY

In early experience with SLN surgery, patients receiving neoadjuvant chemotherapy (NAC) were excluded from SLN surgery and underwent ALND at the time of their definitive breast cancer surgery after completion of chemotherapy. With increasing use of NAC for operable breast cancer and earlier-stage disease, data have accumulated on SLN surgery after completion of NAC.[52–56] In early smaller series, the SLN identification rates ranged from 85% to 100% and the false-negative rate ranged from 0% to 33%. More recent studies have documented higher identification rates and lower false-negative rates.

In the National Surgical Adjuvant Breast and Bowel Protocol (NSABP) B-27 study evaluating NAC, 420 patients (18%) underwent SLN surgery after completion of chemotherapy. The SLN identification rate was 85% and the false-negative rate 11%.[57] Recent meta-analyses have shown that SLN surgery after NAC is feasible and accurate. The initial meta-analysis in 2006 reported a pooled SLN identification rate of 90% and sensitivity of 88%.[58] A more recent meta-analysis reported an overall SLN identification rate of 90% and false-negative rate of 8.4%.[59]

The nodal status before chemotherapy provides staging information useful in adjuvant treatment planning for chemotherapy as well as adjuvant radiation. Therefore, one of the advantages of axillary staging before chemotherapy is that it may help determine which patients benefit from irradiation to the nodal basins because nodal staging is a strong predictor of local and distant failure. However, when the SLNs are removed before NAC, this limits the ability to evaluate the axillary response to NAC because the SLN, which may be the only positive node, is removed. In addition, this approach requires 2 operations, one at presentation for SLN surgery and the second after completion of NAC for definitive breast surgery. Also, patients who have node-positive disease detected by SLN surgery before chemotherapy undergo ALND after completion of NAC, even though preoperative chemotherapy eradicates nodal disease in up to 40% of patients with axillary nodal disease at initial diagnosis.

Performing SLN surgery after completion of NAC allows assessment of response to NAC. Status of the axillary lymph nodes after NAC has been shown to be the best prognostic indicator for patients with nodal disease. It also allows the nodal staging and definitive breast surgery to be performed at one operation.

In the context of documented node positivity at presentation, ALND remains the recommended procedure after completion of NAC. Studies have reported false-negative rates of 11% to 29.6% in these patients.[54,60–64] A multicenter trial evaluating this question is currently under way. American College of Surgeons Oncology Group ACOSOG Z1071 is a phase 2 prospective study evaluating the reliability of SLN surgery after NAC in women with documented node-positive breast cancer (T1–4, N1–2, M0) at presentation.[65]

In the authors' clinical practice, axillary ultrasound is routinely used with fine-needle aspiration (FNA) of suspicious nodes at the time of presentation. For patients receiving NAC, those who were node positive by FNA before chemotherapy undergo ALND and patients with normal-appearing lymph nodes or negative FNA undergo SLN surgery for axillary staging after NAC.

PREVIOUS BREAST SURGERY

With the increasing number of patients who have breast cancer with previous breast surgery, the question is raised about the feasibility and accuracy of SLN surgery in patients who have had previous breast and/or axillary surgery cosmetically, diagnostically, or therapeutically.

Published evidence in this regard is mostly limited to small, retrospective single-institution case series. Various SLN surgery techniques have been used in these settings with the use of blue dye, isotope, or both, and various injection methods have been described. Preoperative lymphoscintigraphic visualization has been used to ensure identification of SLN mapping before proceeding to SLN surgery.

Excisional Biopsy

SLN surgery has been shown to be reliable after prior excisional breast biopsy with a low false-negative rate, ranging from 0% to 15%, and high identification rate ranging from 81% to 99%.[62,66–68] In the NSABP B-32 trial the false-negative rate was significantly higher in patients who had a prior excisional biopsy (15.3%) compared with those who had FNA or core needle biopsy for diagnosis (8.1%).[62] Where possible, excisional biopsy should be avoided and percutaneous biopsy rather than excisional biopsy of breast lesions is advocated for preoperative diagnosis of malignancy. This option has been shown to increase negative margin resection, and also allows nodal staging with SLN surgery to be performed at the initial operation without a prior excisional biopsy.[69]

Breast Augmentation

Despite the possibility of interruption of the breast and axillary lymphatics, there are several small series reports of successful lymphatic mapping and SLN surgery in the setting of breast implant augmentations. Jakub and colleagues[70] examined the effectiveness of lymphatic mapping and SLN surgery in 49 patients with breast cancer who had prior implant breast augmentation with 100% identification rate, and no clinically detected axillary recurrences in the patients who had a negative SLN. Similar results have been reported in smaller studies.[71] In the largest study to date by Rodriguez Fernandez and colleagues[72] at the European Institute of Oncology in Milan, SLN surgery was performed with a 100% identification rate and no axillary recurrence after 19 months' follow-up in 50 patients with breast cancer who had undergone breast augmentation previously. The augmentations were through inframammary or periareolar approach, which is less likely to cause disruption of the lymphatics to the axilla. There is more concern about the feasibility of SLN surgery in women who have had previous transaxillary breast augmentation. Lymphoscintigraphy has been reported successful in identifying the SLNs in these women, with emphasis of meticulous technique at the time of augmentation to minimize the dissection in the axilla.[73,74] There are more limited data on this approach, with case reports of 2 women undergoing successful SLN surgery after transaxillary breast augmentation.[75]

Breast Reduction

In breast reduction there is greater disruption of the breast tissue and lymphatics than with excisional biopsy or breast augmentation. The data on reliability of SLN surgery in axillary staging of patients with breast cancer who have had previous breast reduction surgery is scarce. Golshan and colleagues[76] described 6 patients who underwent successful SLN surgery for occult carcinomas detected after breast reduction surgery, and concluded that SLN surgery should not be considered a contraindication after breast reduction surgery. In their recent study, Rodriguez Fernandez and colleagues[72] reported on SLN surgery in 20 patients with breast cancer who had previously undergone breast reduction surgery showing a 100% SLN identification rate and no axillary recurrence after 19 months' follow-up.

Overall data regarding SLN surgery after prior breast reduction are significantly limited, and this remains controversial. The use of SLN in these patients should be on a case-by-case basis. If the breast reduction was recent or the tumor is large, then ALND should be considered for accurate staging of the axilla. In women where the breast reduction was many years before the breast cancer, SLN surgery may be an option. Lymphoscintigraphy with mapping to document drainage patterns should be obtained and the patient should be counseled regarding the unknown false-negative rate.

PREVIOUS AXILLARY SURGERY

Reoperative SLN surgery in patients with previous axillary surgery in the form of SLN surgery or ALND has been described. Port and colleagues[77] reported on 117 patients with SLN surgery performed in patients with local recurrence after previous breast conservation surgery and either SLN surgery or ALND. The SLN identification rate was 55% (64 of 117). No axillary recurrences were observed at a median follow-up of 2.2 years. Multiple smaller single-institution series have been reported on SLN surgery in this setting. The SLN identification rate can be much lower than in patients without prior surgery, ranging from 55% to 100%. In addition, drainage of the breast to extra-axillary sites is much more common with reports of drainage to the internal mammary (IM) chain, contralateral axilla, and other sites,[77,78] making lymphoscintig-raphy with mapping important in surgical planning for these cases.

The SLN identification rate is higher when fewer than 10 axillary nodes have been removed previously. Although the SLN identification rate is generally low in these patients, SLN surgery in the setting of recurrent breast cancer can provide additional staging information of the recurrence that can guide adjuvant radiation and medical treatment recommendations.

Overall, data regarding SLN surgery in patients with previous axillary surgery are limited to small series and show higher rates of identification failures.[77,79–82] As the number of lymph nodes removed at prior surgery increases, the likelihood of failure to identify the SLN and the likelihood of extra-axillary drainage increase, and patients should be counseled appropriately.

INTERNAL MAMMARY SLN SURGERY

Advent of SLN surgery allowed focused dissection to evaluate the status of the IM lymph nodes. Historically IM lymph nodes were not routinely sampled at the time of modified radical mastectomy, which raises some debate about the need for IM nodal staging. Information regarding IM nodal status can be used for staging, prognosis, and treatment decisions, and IM nodal involvement has the same significance as axillary nodal involve-ment in adjuvant treatment recommendations. Drainage to the IM lymph nodes is detected on lymphoscintigraphic mapping with use of parenchymal or peritumoral injection. Dermal and subareolar injections are less likely to demonstrate IM drainage. On visualization of the IM node as the first lymphatic drainage site, IM SLN surgery can be performed, provided the surgeon is comfortable with the procedure .[19,68,83]

However, many centers do not perform preoperative mapping and argue against the need for extra-axillary SLN surgery. The issue of IM SLN surgery has been addressed in a recent systematic review by Chen and colleagues.[84] Opponents of IM SLN base their view on the low incidence of isolated IM metastases in early breast cancer (up to 10%), low incidence of clinical recurrence in the IM nodal chain, and the lack of conclusive data on the survival benefits of IM resection or irradiation.[84–87] In addition, as opposed to axillary SLN surgery, the accuracy of IM SLN biopsy has not been as vigorously studied and various injection techniques have been used.[88]

In many recent series, on the other hand, the advocates of preoperative lympho-scintigraphic and IM SLN surgery have reported tailoring individualized treatment decisions, which have included employment of more intensive systemic treatment given the poorer prognosis with positive IM SLN, and addition of IM chain irradiation. However, the results of clinical trials are awaited to show whether these additional interventions can lead to better survival rates.[84,89–92] Alternatively, in the case of nega-tive IM SLN, "unnecessary" IM chain irradiation and its associated morbidities may be avoided.[88]

IM SLN surgery significantly changes the treatment recommendations only in situ-ations where there is a positive IM node and a negative axilla. The ASCO 2005 sentinel node biopsy guidelines leave the decision to perform IM SLN surgery procedure to the clinical judgment of the treating physicians.[1] The 2010 National Comprehensive Cancer Network (NCCN) Clinical Practice Guidelines state that if the preoperative mapping identifies SLNs in the IM chain, IM nodal excision is optional. These guide-lines also state that IM lymph nodes should be irradiated if clinically or pathologically positive, with the caveat that CT-based simulation should be used in radiotherapy planning to reduce cardiac and lung irradiation.[26] At this time, evaluation of IM SLN remains controversial and varies from center to center.

PROPHYLACTIC MASTECTOMY

Women undergoing prophylactic mastectomy (PM) who are found to have invasive cancer in their mastectomy specimen on final pathology will require axillary staging as a second procedure. Axillary staging after mastectomy is generally in the form of ALND, which is associated with greater morbidity than is SLN surgery. Consequently, some surgeons advocate performing the less invasive procedure of SLN surgery at the time of PM, in an attempt to avoid a second and more morbid operation.

The overall frequency of occult invasive cancer in patients who have undergone clinical examination and mammography before undergoing PM is only 1.8%.[93] Boughey and colleagues[93] studied a total of 409 patients (436 PM cases) of whom 382 were contralateral PM (CPM) and 27 were bilateral PM (BPM). Cancer was identified in 5% (22 of 436). Of these, only 8 patients (1.8%) had invasive cancer, with a mean tumor size of 5 mm (range, 2–9 mm), whereas 14 patients had DCIS. There was no difference in the occult cancer rate between those patients with a contralateral breast cancer (ie, those patients undergoing CPM) and those patients without a known breast cancer (ie, those patients undergoing BPM). No cases of invasive cancer were identified in the 23 patients with BRCA mutations. Increased risk of invasive cancer in the PM breast was seen in postmenopausal patients (3.7%), patients older than 60 years

Table 1
Summary of the use of SLN surgery in uncommon clinical scenarios

Clinical Scenarios	Current State of its Use in Clinical Practice
Men with breast cancer	Numerous studies support use of SLN in men with clinically node-negative breast cancer
Pregnant patients with breast cancer	Its use has only been reported in few cases. Full discussion of risks, benefits, and alternative recommended
DCIS in patients undergoing mastectomy	SLN recommended
DCIS in patients undergoing lumpectomy	SLN not recommended unless high risk for harboring occult invasive disease
Multicentric/multifocal tumors	Numerous studies support use of SLN surgery
Patients undergoing preoperative chemotherapy	Feasible and accurate after completion of preoperative chemotherapy
Previous diagnostic or excisional breast surgery	Numerous studies support use of SLN surgery
Previous breast implant augmentation	Successful in several series in selected patients with minimal axillary dissection
Previous breast reduction surgery	Very limited data. SLN remains controversial
Reoperative SLN surgery following recurrence or new primary	Successful in multiple series in selected patients. Generally with lower rates of SLN identification and extra-axillary drainage is more common. Preoperative lymphoscintigraphy seems essential
Internal mammary SLN surgery	If preoperative mapping identifies SLNs in the IM chain, IM sentinel node excision may contribute to the staging and management. Remains controversial and at discretion of surgeon
Prophylactic mastectomy	Routine SLN surgery is not recommended in this setting

(7.5%), and patients with history of invasive lobular carcinoma (9.7%) or lobular carcinoma in situ (7.7%).[93] The investigators concluded that because the frequency of cancer in PM was very low and the majority represented DCIS, routine SLN surgery was not recommended.

Similar results were reported in a more recent study from Moffitt Cancer Center, with no occult cancers in 28 patients who underwent BPM. The incidence of occult cancers in CPM specimens was 4.3% (18 of 420), of which only 1.4% (6 cases) were invasive cancers whereas the majority represented DCIS.[94]

A decision analysis study comparing 2 strategies, routine SLN surgery at the time of PM and ALND for those cases where occult invasive malignancy is identified, found that routine SLN surgery is not warranted given the large number of procedures required to benefit one patient and the potential complications associated with performing SLN surgery in all patients.[95]

Black and colleagues[96] found that the use of magnetic resonance imaging (MRI) before PM failed to identify most occult cancers and also significantly increased the cost. However, in another study by McLaughlin and colleagues[97] at the Memorial Sloan-Kettering Cancer Center, breast MRI accurately ruled out the presence of an invasive cancer in the prophylactic breast, suggesting that MRI can be used to select patients for PM without SLN surgery.

One technique that can be used in PM is routine preoperative isotope injection and intraoperative specimen analysis. If cancer is found, one can proceed to SLN surgery at the same operation.[80]

In summary, routine SLN surgery for patients undergoing prophylactic mastectomy is not recommended.[98] Subgroups of women at higher risk of harboring an occult malignancy for whom SLN surgery may be considered include older postmenopausal women, and patients with invasive lobular cancer or lobular carcinoma in situ.[93]

SUMMARY

Current use of SLN surgery in uncommon scenarios is summarized in **Table 1**. With the ever-increasing experience and use of high-quality preoperative nodal imaging with ultrasound and MRI, along with needle sampling of suspicious nodes, many patients with nodal metastases are identified preoperatively. In the remainder of the patients who have otherwise no obvious evidence of nodal involvement on clinical and imaging examination, the data support the feasibility of SLN surgery in most clinical situations. Preoperative lymphoscintigraphic identification of lymph node drainage basins may identify aberrant drainage patterns in cases where prior breast and/or axillary surgery may have impacted drainage pathways and thus improve SLN identification rates.

Given the rarity of these clinical scenarios, most data are from single-institution studies and long-term follow-up data are lacking. An understanding of the available literature is important to help counsel a patient fully regarding the SLN identification rates and false-negative rates. False-negative SLN results in understaging and may lead to undertreatment, whereas ALND has a higher associated morbidity. Explanation of alternatives and potential benefits and risks remains important for SLN surgery in these less common scenarios where data are less concrete.

REFERENCES

1. Lyman GH, Giuliano AE, Somerfield MR, et al. American Society of Clinical Oncology guideline recommendations for sentinel lymph node biopsy in early-stage breast cancer. J Clin Oncol 2005;23(30):7703–20.

2. Boughey JC, Bedrosian I, Meric-Bernstam F, et al. Comparative analysis of sentinel lymph node operation in male and female breast cancer patients. J Am Coll Surg 2006;203(4):475–80.

3. Mullan MH, Kissin MW. Positive sentinel node biopsy in male breast carcinoma. ANZ J Surg 2001;71(7):438–40.

4. Hill AD, Borgen PI, Cody HS 3rd. Sentinel node biopsy in male breast cancer. Eur J Surg Oncol 1999;25(4):442–3.

5. Gennari R, Renne G, Travaini L, et al. Sentinel node biopsy in male breast cancer: Future standard treatment? Eur J Surg 2001;167(6):461–2.

6. Port ER, Fey JV, Cody HS 3rd, et al. Sentinel lymph node biopsy in patients with male breast carcinoma. Cancer 2001;91(2):319–23.

7. Albo D, Ames FC, Hunt KK, et al. Evaluation of lymph node status in male breast cancer patients: a role for sentinel lymph node biopsy. Breast Cancer Res Treat 2003;77(1):9–14.

8. Goyal A, Horgan K, Kissin M, et al. Sentinel lymph node biopsy in male breast cancer patients. Eur J Surg Oncol 2004;30:480–3.

9. De Cicco C, Baio SM, Veronesi P, et al. Sentinel node biopsy in male breast cancer. Nucl Med Commun 2004;25(2):139–43.

10. Cimmino VM, Degnim AC, Sabel MS, et al. Efficacy of sentinel lymph node biopsy in male breast cancer. J Surg Oncol 2004;86(2):74–7.

11. Rusby JE, Smith BL, Dominguez FJ, et al. Sentinel lymph node biopsy in men with breast cancer: a report of 31 consecutive procedures and review of the literature. Clin Breast Cancer 2006;7(5):406–10.

12. Gentilini O, Chagas E, Zurrida S, et al. Sentinel lymph node biopsy in male patients with early breast cancer. Oncologist 2007;12(5):512–5.

13. Flynn LW, Park J, Patil SM, et al. Sentinel lymph node biopsy is successful and accurate in male breast carcinoma. J Am Coll Surg 2008;206(4):616–21.

14. Wisinski KB, Gradishar WJ. Male breast cancer. In: Harris JR, Lippman ME, Morrow MM, et al, editors. Diseases of the breast. 4th edition. Philadelphia: Lippincott, Williams and Wilkins; 2010. p. 775–80.

15. Pandit-Taskar N, Dauer LT, Montgomery L, et al. Organ and fetal absorbed dose estimates from 99mTc-sulfur colloid lymphoscintigraphy and sentinel node localization in breast cancer patients. J Nucl Med 2006;47(7):1202–8.

16. Keleher A, Wendt R 3rd, Delpassand E, et al. The safety of lymphatic mapping in pregnant breast cancer patients using Tc-99m sulfur colloid. Breast J 2004;10(6): 492–5.

17. Gentilini O, Cremonesi M, Trifirò G, et al. Safety of sentinel node biopsy in pregnant patients with breast cancer. Ann Oncol 2004;15(9):1348–51.

18. International Commission on Radiological Protection Publication 84. Available at: http://icrp.org/docs/ICRP_84_Pregnancy_s.pps. Accessed January 21, 2010.

19. Buscombe J, Paganelli G, Burak ZE, et al. Sentinel node in breast cancer procedural guidelines. Eur J Nucl Med Mol Imaging 2007;34(12):2154–9.

20. Chakera AH, Hesse B, Burak Z, et al. EANM-EORTC recommendations for sentinel node diagnostics in melanoma. Eur J Nucl Med Mol Imaging 2009; 36(10):1713–42.

21. Alkureishi LW, Burak Z, Alvarez JA, et al. Joint practice guidelines for radionuclide lymphoscintigraphy for sentinel node localization in oral/oropharyngeal squamous cell carcinoma. Ann Surg Oncol 2009;16(11):3190–210.

22. Mondi MM, Cuenca RE, Ollila DW, et al. Sentinel lymph node biopsy during pregnancy: initial clinical experience. Ann Surg Oncol 2007;14(1):218–21.

23. Khera SY, Kiluk JV, Hasson DM, et al. Pregnancy-associated breast cancer patients can safely undergo lymphatic mapping. Breast J 2008;14(3):250–4.
24. te Velde EA, Sonke G, Rutgers EJ. Breast cancer and pregnancy: diagnosis and treatment options. Breast Cancer 2009;12(7):e10.
25. Gentilini O, Cremonesi M, Toesca A, et al. Sentinel lymph node biopsy in pregnant patients with breast cancer. Eur J Nucl Med Mol Imaging 2010;37(1):78–83.
26. NCCN practice guidelines. 2010. Available at: http://www.nccn.org/professionals/physician_gls/f_guidelines.asp. Accessed January 25, 2010.
27. Baxter NN, Virnig BA, Durham SB, et al. Trends in the treatment of ductal carcinoma in situ of the breast. J Natl Cancer Inst 2004;96(6):443–8.
28. Jemal A, Siegel R, Ward E, et al. Cancer statistics, 2007. CA Cancer J Clin 2007; 57(1):43–66.
29. Virnig BA, Tuttle TM, Shamliyan T, et al. Ductal carcinoma in situ of the Breast: a systematic review of incidence, treatment, and outcomes. J Natl Cancer Inst 2010;102:170–8.
30. Cox CE, Nguyen K, Gray RJ, et al. Importance of lymphatic mapping in ductal carcinoma in situ (DCIS): why map DCIS? Am Surg 2001;67(6):513–9.
31. Ansari B, Ogston SA, Purdie CA, et al. Meta-analysis of sentinel node biopsy in ductal carcinoma in situ of the breast. Br J Surg 2008;95(5):547–54.
32. Dominguez FJ, Golshan M, Black DM, et al. Sentinel node biopsy is important in mastectomy for ductal carcinoma in situ. Ann Surg Oncol 2008;15(1):268–73.
33. Morrow M. Axillary surgery in DCIS: is less more? Ann Surg Oncol 2008;15(10):2641–2.
34. Mabry H, Giuliano AE, Silverstein MJ. What is the value of axillary dissection or sentinel node biopsy in patients with ductal carcinoma in situ? Am J Surg 2006;192(4):455–7.
35. Zavagno G, Carcoforo P, Franchini Z, et al. Axillary recurrence after negative sentinel lymph node biopsy without axillary dissection: a study on 479 breast cancer patients. Eur J Surg Oncol 2005;31(7):715–20.
36. Camp R, Feezor R, Kasraeian A, et al. Sentinel lymph node biopsy for ductal carcinoma in situ: an evolving approach at the University of Florida. Breast J 2005;11(6):394–7.
37. Chao C, Wong SL, Woo C, et al. Reliable lymphatic drainage to axillary sentinel lymph nodes regardless of tumor location within the breast. Am J Surg 2001; 182(4):307–11.
38. Kim JH, Heerdt AS, Cody HS, et al. Sentinel lymph node drainage in multicentric breast cancers. Breast J 2002;8(6):356–61.
39. Zavagno G, Rubello D, Franchini Z, et al. Italian Study Group on Radioguided Surgery and ImmunoScintigraphy. Axillary sentinel lymph nodes in breast cancer: a single lymphatic pathway drains the entire mammary gland. Eur J Surg Oncol 2005;31(5):479–84.
40. Suami H, Pan WR, Mann GB, et al. The lymphatic anatomy of the breast and its implications for sentinel lymph node biopsy: a human cadaver study. Ann Surg Oncol 2008;15(3):863–71.
41. Schrenk P, Wayand W. Sentinel-node biopsy in axillary lymph-node staging for patients with multicentric breast cancer. Lancet 2001;357(9250):122.
42. Layeeque R, Henry-Tillman R, Korourian S, et al. Subareolar sentinel node biopsy for multiple breast cancers. Am J Surg 2003;186(6):730–5.
43. Kumar R, Jana S, Heiba SI, et al. Retrospective analysis of sentinel node localization in multifocal, multicentric, palpable, or nonpalpable breast cancer. J Nucl Med 2003;44(1):7–10.

44. Gentilini O, Trifirò G, Soteldo J, et al. Sentinel lymph node biopsy in multicentric breast cancer. The experience of the European Institute of Oncology. Eur J Surg Oncol 2006;32(5):507–10.
45. Knauer M, Konstantiniuk P, Haid A, et al. Multicentric breast cancer: a new indication for sentinel node biopsy—a multi-institutional validation study. J Clin Oncol 2006;24(21):3374–80.
46. D'Eredita' G, Giardina C, Ingravallo G, et al. Sentinel lymph node biopsy in multiple breast cancer using subareolar injection of the tracer. Breast 2007; 16(3):316–22.
47. Cipolla C, Vieni S, Fricano S, et al. The accuracy of sentinel lymph node biopsy in the treatment of multicentric invasive breast cancer using a subareolar injection of tracer. World J Surg 2008;32(11):2483–7.
48. Meretoja TJ, Leidenius MH, Heikkilä PS, et al. Sentinel node biopsy in breast cancer patients with large or multifocal tumors. Ann Surg Oncol 2009;16(5): 1148–55.
49. Fearmonti RM, Batista LI, Meric-Bernstam F, et al. False negative rate of sentinel lymph node biopsy in multicentric and multifocal breast cancers may be higher in cases with large additive tumor burden. Breast J 2009;15(6):645–8.
50. Ozmen V, Muslumanoglu M, Cabioglu N, et al. Increased false negative rates in sentinel lymph node biopsies in patients with multi-focal breast cancer. Breast Cancer Res Treat 2002;76(3):237–44.
51. Bergkvist L, Frisell J, Swedish Breast Cancer Group, et al. Multicentre validation study of sentinel node biopsy for staging in breast cancer. Br J Surg 2005;92(10): 1221–4.
52. van Deurzen CH, Vriens BE, Tjan-Heijnen VC, et al. Accuracy of sentinel node biopsy after neoadjuvant chemotherapy in breast cancer patients: a systematic review. Eur J Cancer 2009;45(18):3124–30.
53. Neuman HB, Ollila DW. Sentinel lymph node biopsy controversy: before or after neoadjuvant chemotherapy. Curr Breast Canc Rep 2009;1(2):71–7.
54. Classe JM, Bordes V, Campion L, et al. Sentinel lymph node biopsy after neoadjuvant chemotherapy for advanced breast cancer: results of Ganglion Sentinelle et Chimiotherapie Neoadjuvante, a French prospective multicentric study. J Clin Oncol 2009;27(5):726–32.
55. Hunt KK, Yi M, Mittendorf EA, et al. Sentinel lymph node surgery after neoadjuvant chemotherapy is accurate and reduces the need for axillary dissection in breast cancer patients. Ann Surg 2009;250:558–66.
56. Schwartz GF, Tannebaum JE, Jernigan AM, et al. Axillary sentinel lymph node biopsy after neoadjuvant chemotherapy for carcinoma of the breast. Cancer 2010;116:1243–51.
57. Mamounas EP, Brown A, Anderson S, et al. Sentinel node biopsy after neoadjuvant chemotherapy in breast cancer: results from National Surgical Adjuvant Breast and Bowel Project Protocol B-27. J Clin Oncol 2005;23(12):2694–702.
58. Xing Y, Foy M, Cox DD, et al. Meta-analysis of sentinel lymph node biopsy after preoperative chemotherapy in patients with breast cancer. Br J Surg 2006;93(5): 539–46.
59. Kelly AM, Dwamena B, Cronin P, et al. Breast cancer sentinel node identification and classification after neoadjuvant chemotherapy—systematic review and meta analysis. Acad Radiol 2009;16(5):551–63.
60. Shen J, Gilcrease MZ, Babiera GV, et al. Feasibility and accuracy of sentinel lymph node biopsy after preoperative chemotherapy in breast cancer patients with documented axillary metastases. Cancer 2007;109(7):1255–63.

61. Newman EA, Sabel MS, Nees AV, et al. Sentinel lymph node biopsy performed after preoperative chemotherapy is accurate in patients with documented node-positive breast cancer at presentation. Ann Surg Oncol 2007;14(10): 2946–52.

62. Krag DN, Anderson SJ, Julian TB, et al. Technical outcomes of sentinel-lymph-node resection and conventional axillary-lymph-node dissection in patients with clinically node-negative breast cancer: results from the NSABP B-32 randomised phase III trial. Lancet Oncol 2007;8(10):854–5.

63. Krag D, Weaver D, Ashikaga T, et al. The sentinel node in breast cancer—a multi-center validation study. N Engl J Med 1998;339(14):941–6.

64. Gimbergues P, Abrial C, Durando X, et al. Sentinel lymph node biopsy after neo-adjuvant chemotherapy is accurate in breast cancer patients with a clinically negative axillary nodal status at presentation. Ann Surg Oncol 2008;15(5): 1316–21.

65. Surgery to remove the sentinel lymph node and axillary lymph nodes after chemotherapy in treating women with stage II, stage IIIA, or stage IIIB breast cancer. Available at: http://clinicaltrials.gov/ct2/show/record/NCT00881361. Accessed January 21, 2010.

66. Haigh PI, Hansen NM, Qi K, et al. Biopsy method and excision volume do not affect success rate of subsequent sentinel lymph node dissection in breast cancer. Ann Surg Oncol 2000;7(1):21–7.

67. Luini A, Galimberti V, Gatti G, et al. The sentinel node biopsy after previous breast surgery: preliminary results on 543 patients treated at the European Institute of Oncology. Breast Cancer Res Treat 2005;89(2):159–63.

68. Heuts EM, van der Ent FW, Kengen RA, et al. Results of sentinel node biopsy not affected by previous excisional biopsy. Eur J Surg Oncol 2006;32(3): 278–81.

69. Smitt MC, Horst K. Association of clinical and pathologic variables with lumpec-tomy surgical margin status after preoperative diagnosis or excisional biopsy of invasive breast cancer. Ann Surg Oncol 2007;14(3):1040–4.

70. Jakub JW, Ebert MD, Cantor A, et al. Breast cancer in patients with prior augmen-tation: presentation, stage, and lymphatic mapping. Plast Reconstr Surg 2004; 114(7):1737–42.

71. Gray RJ, Forstner-Barthell AW, Pockaj BA, et al. Breast-conserving therapy and sentinel lymph node biopsy are feasible in cancer patients with previous implant breast augmentation. Am J Surg 2004;188(2):122–5.

72. Rodriguez Fernandez J, Martella S, Trifirò G, et al. Sentinel node biopsy in patients with previous breast aesthetic surgery. Ann Surg Oncol 2009;16(4): 989–92.

73. Munhoz AM, Aldrighi C, Buschpiegel C, et al. The feasibility of sentinel lymph node detection in patients with previous transaxillary implant breast augmenta-tion: preliminary results. Aesthetic Plast Surg 2005;29(3):163–8.

74. Sado HN, Graf RM, Canan LW, et al. Sentinel lymph node detection and evidence of axillary lymphatic integrity after transaxillary breast augmentation: a prospective study using lymphoscintigraphy. Aesthetic Plast Surg 2008; 32(6):879–88.

75. Mottura AA, Del Castillo R. Transaxillary breast augmentation: two breast cancer patients with successful sentinel lymph node diagnosis. Aesthetic Plast Surg 2007;31(5):544–9.

76. Golshan M, Lesnikoski BA, Lester S. Sentinel lymph node biopsy for occult breast cancer detected during breast reduction surgery. Am Surg 2006;72(5):397–400.

77. Port ER, Garcia-Etienne CA, Park J, et al. Reoperative sentinel lymph node biopsy: a new frontier in the management of ipsilateral breast tumor recurrence. Ann Surg Oncol 2007;14(8):2209–14.

78. Boughey JC, Ross MI, Babiera GV, et al. Sentinel lymph node surgery in locally recurrent breast cancer. Clin Breast Cancer 2006;7(3):248–53.

79. Intra M, Trifirò G, Galimberti V, et al. Second axillary sentinel node biopsy for ipsilateral breast tumour recurrence. Br J Surg 2007;94(10):1216–9.

80. Boughey JC, Hunt KK. Expanding the indications for sentinel lymph node surgery in breast cancer. Future Oncol 2007;3(1):9–14.

81. Karam A, Stempel M, Cody HS 3rd, et al. Reoperative sentinel lymph node biopsy after previous mastectomy. J Am Coll Surg 2008;207(4):543–8.

82. Schrenk P, Tausch C, Wayand W. Lymphatic mapping in patients with primary or recurrent breast cancer following previous axillary surgery. Eur J Surg Oncol 2008;34(8):851–6.

83. Madsen E, Gobardhan P, Bongers V, et al. The impact on post-surgical treatment of sentinel lymph node biopsy of internal mammary lymph nodes in patients with breast cancer. Ann Surg Oncol 2007;14(4):1486–92.

84. Chen RC, Lin NU, Golshan M, et al. Internal mammary nodes in breast cancer: diagnosis and implications for patient management—a systematic review. J Clin Oncol 2008;26(30):4981–9.

85. Lacour J, Bucalossi P, Cacers E, et al. Radical mastectomy versus radical mastectomy plus internal mammary dissection. Five-year results of an international cooperative study. Cancer 1976;37(1):206–14.

86. Veronesi U, Paganelli G, Viale G, et al. Sentinel lymph node biopsy and axillary dissection in breast cancer: results in a large series. J Natl Cancer Inst 1999; 91(4):368–73.

87. van Geel AN, Wouters MW, van der Pol C, et al. Chest wall resection for internal mammary lymph node metastases of breast cancer. Breast 2009; 18(2):94–9.

88. Bourre JC, Payan R, Collomb D, et al. Can the sentinel lymph node technique affect decisions to offer internal mammary chain irradiation? Eur J Nucl Med Mol Imaging 2009;36(5):758–64.

89. Noushi F, Spillane AJ, Uren RF, et al. Internal mammary node metastasis in breast cancer: predictive models to determine status & management algorithms. Eur J Surg Oncol 2010;36(1):16–22.

90. Zhang YJ, Oh JL, Whitman GJ, et al. Clinically apparent internal mammary nodal metastasis in patients with advanced breast cancer: incidence and local control. Int J Radiat Oncol Biol Phys, December 11, 2009. [Epub ahead of print].

91. Oh JL, Buchholz TA. Internal mammary node radiation: a proposed technique to spare cardiac toxicity. J Clin Oncol 2009;27(31):e172–3.

92. Coombs NJ, Boyages J, French JR, et al. Internal mammary sentinel nodes: ignore, irradiate or operate? Eur J Cancer 2009;45(5):789–94.

93. Boughey JC, Khakpour N, Meric-Bernstam F, et al. Selective use of sentinel lymph node surgery during prophylactic mastectomy. Cancer 2006;107(7): 1440–7.

94. Laronga C, Lee MC, McGuire KP, et al. Indications for sentinel lymph node biopsy in the setting of prophylactic mastectomy. J Am Coll Surg 2009; 209(6):746–52.

95. Boughey JC, Cormier JN, Xing Y, et al. Decision analysis to assess the efficacy of routine sentinel lymphadenectomy in patients undergoing prophylactic mastectomy. Cancer 2007;110(11):2542–50.

96. Black D, Specht M, Lee JM, et al. Detecting occult malignancy in prophylactic mastectomy: preoperative MRI versus sentinel lymph node biopsy. Ann Surg Oncol 2007;14(9):2477–84.

97. McLaughlin SA, Stempel M, Morris EA, et al. Can magnetic resonance imaging be used to select patients for sentinel lymph node biopsy in prophylactic mastectomy? Cancer 2008;112(6):1214–21.

98. Giuliano AE, Boolbol S, Degnim A, et al. Society of surgical oncology: position statement on prophylactic mastectomy. Ann Surg Oncol 2007;14(9):2425–7.

Total Skin Sparing (Nipple Sparing) Mastectomy: What is the Evidence?

Amar Gupta, MD[a], Patrick Ivan Borgen, MD[b],*

KEYWORDS

- Nipple sparing mastectomy • Total skin sparing mastectomy
- Breast cancer

Physicians endeavoring to treat cancer have struggled to strike a balance between the efficacy of a particular treatment and the quality of life after that treatment. Nowhere has this struggle had a more varied and tortuous course, or been more controversial, than in the treatment of breast cancer.[1]

Nothing has been as *constant* in the field of breast cancer treatment as *change*. The past two decades have witnessed dramatic conceptual changes in strategic and practical approaches to virtually all forms of breast cancer. These sea changes have been driven by improvements in technology, improvements in public awareness resulting in earlier stage at diagnosis, and improvements in our understanding of fundamental biologic mechanisms of the disease, most importantly, better understanding of disease subsets. The surgical treatment of breast cancer has evolved from radical mastectomy with routine removal of the nipple-areolar complex (NAC) to breast conservative therapy with preservation of the breast and NAC. Each step along this evolutionary process was met with criticism, skepticism, controversy, anger, emotion, and often bitter and impassioned debate. Today we find ourselves at yet another therapeutic decision point: the management of the skin of the nipple-areolar complex in mastectomy. Enhanced understanding of the pathogenesis of breast cancer coupled with rising interest in improved cosmesis has led to the investigation of the skin-sparing (SSM) and nipple-sparing mastectomy (NSM) as potential modifications to conventional mastectomy. There has been much debate regarding the oncologic safety of

This work was supported by a grant from the Breast Cancer Alliance.
The authors have nothing to disclose.
[a] Department of Surgery, Mount Sinai Hospital, University of Toronto, Toronto, Canada
[b] Department of Surgery, Maimonides Medical Center, Brooklyn, 4802 Tenth Avenue, Brooklyn, New York 11219, USA
* Corresponding author.
E-mail address: pborgen@maimonidesmed.org

these procedures. Purists argue that leaving the skin of the NAC behind may increase the chance for local recurrence and is therefore contraindicated. A growing number of clinicians argue that the nipple is a rare site for end-organ carcinogenesis and think that leaving the skin of the nipple in-situ (after removing lactiferous ducts) adds little or no risk. What is the clinical evidence that suggests that a total skin-sparing approach is oncologically safe?

LITERATURE REVIEW

There have been a growing number of series of total skin sparing mastectomy (TSSM) in recent years.[2–6] Although all reported series lack the statistical power to reach definitive conclusions, taken in the aggregate they form the basis for continued clinical study and rational clinical practice. This information is important insofar as a randomized clinical trial will never be achievable. There is no evidence to date that suggests an increased oncologic risk associated with sparing the skin of the NAC.

In reviewing the efficacy of bilateral prophylactic mastectomy, Hartmann and colleagues[7] conducted a retrospective study of 639 women at moderate-high risk for breast cancer undergoing prophylactic mastectomy. A total of 575 (90%) of these women underwent bilateral subcutaneous mastectomy, sparing residual breast tissue beneath an intact NAC, whereas the remaining 64 underwent bilateral total mastectomy. After 14 years of median follow-up, seven subjects (1.2%) versus no subjects (0%) developed breast cancer after prophylactic subcutaneous mastectomy and total mastectomy, respectively ($P = .32$). Six tumors were found in the chest wall, whereas one subject was found to have bone metastases with no evidence of local disease. No subject developed breast cancer in the residual NAC. Although not their primary goal, this group's data demonstrates the exceedingly low rate of breast cancer in the NAC, even in patients with a moderate-high risk.

Margulies and colleagues[8] described their experience with 31 subjects undergoing 50 mastectomies, including four cases with centrally located tumors. Six attempted NSMs had to have the NAC excised because of tumor involvement on touch-preparation cytology (n = 4) or nipple necrosis (n = 2). Although this group reported a short follow-up time, no local or distant recurrences were observed in this series.

In 2006, Sacchini and colleagues[9] reported a multi-institutional review of 123 subjects undergoing 192 TSSM, including 20 mastectomies for ductal carcinoma in situ (DCIS) and 44 for invasive cancer. All tumors were peripherally located and none showed preoperative evidence of disease less than 1cm from the areolar margins. After a median follow-up of 98.4 weeks, four subjects presented with a local recurrence, two after TSSM for invasive cancer, and two after prophylactic mastectomy. All recurrences were distant from the NAC, with three in the upper-outer quadrant and one in the axillary tail. A fifth subject succumbed to distant metastatic disease without evidence of loco-regional recurrence.

Crowe and colleagues[10] selected 110 subjects to undergo NSM in 149 breasts as a procedure for treatment (73%) or prophylaxis (27%) of breast cancer. Of the 149 procedures, a total of 9 (6%) were eventually converted to total mastectomy secondary to tumor involvement of the NAC as demonstrated by intraoperative frozen section. Four subjects treated for invasive breast cancer developed recurrences, two local recurrences (LR) and two distant recurrences (DR), with no disease seen in the NAC after a median of 164 weeks of follow-up. Only three (2.7%) of the subjects with NSM experienced significant complications, including one subject who required subsequent removal of the NAC because of infection.

One of the earliest studies was conducted by the Karolinska group[11] in Stockholm, Sweden in the late 1980s. Their prospective series included 216 subjects who underwent 184 NSM and 32 SSM with NAC. They enjoyed a robust follow-up of 676 weeks to evaluate recurrence rates. In general these were subjects with large tumors and extensive axillary metastases. The high LR and DR rates (24% and 20% respectively) seen in this study may stem from the fact that only 47 (22%) of enrolled subjects received radiation therapy (RT); in fact, the LR rate for these 47 subjects was only 8.5%. This group left a 2 cm plate of breast tissue of 5 mm thickness behind in an attempt to preserve NAC blood supply. Despite this technical point, no LRs were seen in the preserved NAC tissue.

Garwood and colleagues[12] have prospectively reported two cohorts of 115 subjects undergoing 170 NSMs for prophylaxis and treatment of invasive breast cancer. This study used the results of early NSMs, grouped into cohort one, to expand subject selection and improve surgical technique. The second cohort of subjects included more subjects receiving adjuvant chemotherapy or radiotherapy, which was as expected considering 37 of 48 (54%) of the subjects had stage 2 or 3 disease. Despite this, necrotic complication rates dropped from 30% to 13% from cohort one to cohort two, respectively. Additionally, only 5% of cohort two subjects experienced nipple loss, which was significantly less than the 15% nipple loss seen in cohort one. The investigators contribute these differences to surgical-technique lessons learned from the first cohort of subjects. The second group had significantly fewer incisions crossing more than 30% of the NAC as these subjects seemed to have a lower rate of nipple necrosis. Also, this group identified reconstruction with immediate implants as a risk factor for skin flap necrosis and implant loss, presumably because of increased skin tension and ischemia. Significantly more subjects had tissue expander reconstructions in the second cohort when compared with cohort one, probably contributing to the decrease in complications. Fifty-two weeks of median follow-up revealed only one LR (0.6%) discovered in the axillary tail following NSM. Two subjects developed metastatic disease without evidence of local recurrence. No NAC recurrences were identified by this group.

Petit and colleagues[13–16] have introduced a novel method of delivering intraoperative, single fraction electron boost radiotherapy, dubbed ELIOT. Patients are treated while under anesthesia at the time of TSSM. The surgeons reportedly preserve 5 to 10mm of breast tissue beneath the NAC to preserved vascular supply. A 2009 review of 1001 subjects has provided the largest single-institution experience of TSSM for invasive cancer (82%) and DCIS (18%). After a median follow-up of 80 weeks, only 14 (1.4%) local recurrences were documented, and 36 subjects developed distant metastasis, with 4 succumbing to their disease. No local recurrence was identified at the NAC. This finding is surprising considering final pathology showed cancer cells in 79 cases in which the NAC was ultimately preserved. Of the 1001 subjects, 800 underwent ELIOT and 201 received delayed radiotherapy, with no significant difference seen in the complication rates between these two groups. Total or partial NAC necrosis was seen in 30 (3%) and 55 (5.5%) of the subjects respectively, with 50 (5%) requiring subsequent NAC removal. Although the short follow-up time in this series precludes any definitive conclusions, the early results from this group are quite promising and extended follow-up will provide valuable insight into the oncologic safety of NSM with radiotherapy to the breast.

Gerber and colleagues[17,18] reported a prospective series of 238 subjects with indications for mastectomy. A total of 112 NSM were attempted, however, 51 (45.5%) were converted to SSM because of NAC involvement by intraoperative frozen section (FS), resulting in 61 (54.5%) cases of NSM. The remaining 134 subjects underwent standard modified radical mastectomy (MRM). Despite no significant differences in the indications for surgery, overall disease stage, axillary node involvement, or adjuvant treatment in these three groups, LR rates were virtually indistinguishable at 11.7% (NSM), 10.4% (SSM), and 11.5% (MRM) at mean follow-up of 404 weeks. This series includes a rare subject with local recurrence in preserved NAC tissue that underwent nipple resection with areola preservation, and remained disease free at 364 weeks of follow-up. Aesthetic results as reported by subjects and surgeons were comparable among TSSM and SSM subjects.

Paepke and colleagues[19] recently reported their prospective experience with 109 attempted NSM in 96 subjects, including 33 (30%) centrally located tumors and 36 of 78 invasive cancers of stage 2 or greater. All duct tissue was removed by nipple inversion and sharp dissection, with FS performed to evaluate for occult disease. Thirteen cases were found to have NAC involvement, and 12 of these subjects underwent SSM as the definitive procedure. One subject refused removal of the NAC and underwent NSM despite the positive FS; she remained disease free after 160 weeks of follow-up. Overall, two (2%) local recurrences were observed, neither within the NAC. Two (2%) other subjects developed distant recurrence. Only one (1%) subject had NAC necrosis severe enough to warrant surgical intervention. Based on the higher-risk subject profile presented in their series, the investigators offer clinical suspicion of skin or nipple involvement and inflammatory breast cancer as the remaining absolute contraindications for TSSM.

A thorough review of the literature provides many examples of high-volume surgeons performing NSM for prophylaxis and for the treatment of breast cancer in carefully selected patients (**Table 1**). The oncologic and cosmetic outcomes of these series often recapitulate those seen for SSM and MRM while allowing for a more natural reconstruction. Although many of the aforementioned studies require further subject accrual and extended follow-up, these promising early results will no doubt increase the interest in this controversial arena.

TECHNICAL CONSIDERATIONS

The most important caveat is that the term nipple sparing mastectomy is a misnomer. The preserved tissue is the skin of the nipple-areolar complex. The major lactiferous

Table 1 Summary of NSM review						
Author	Year	NSM (n)	SSM (n)	Total (n)	LR (%)	Complications (%)
Paepke et al[19]	2009	96	13	109	2.0	0.9
Gerber et al[17,18]	2009	60	48	108	11.7[a], 10.4[b]	NR
Petit et al[15,16]	2009	1001	0	1001	1.4	13.3
Garwood et al[12]	2009	170	0	170	0.6	5
Benediktsson & Perbeck[11]	2008	184	32	216	24.1	NR
Crowe et al[10]	2008	140	0	140	1.4	2.7
Sacchini et al[9]	2006	192	0	192	0.0	8
Margulies et al[8]	2005	44	6	50	7.9	NR

Abbreviation: NR, not reported.
[a] LR of NSM
[b] LR of SSM

ducts are removed from the lumen of the nipple and are always sent as a separate surgical specimen for pathologic analysis. Therefore the terminology total skin sparing mastectomy may be preferable to nipple sparing mastectomy and is the terminology used herein. It is also important to distinguish between TSSM in the setting of a risk-reducing mastectomy versus TSSM in the setting of cancer treatment.

PATIENT SELECTION FOR TOTAL SKIN SPARING MASTECTOMY

In the setting of risk reducing surgery, the issue of TSSM becomes largely a cosmetic issue. The fundamental question centers on the location of the native NAC in the reconstructed breast. Large, pendulous breasts are a relative contraindication to this technical approach as are patients who wish to greatly enhance the breast cup size in the process of risk reduction. Unilateral TSSM is also a relative contraindication because matching the location and orientation of the native nipple in the contralateral breast can be technically difficult. Contrary to the thinking of some authors, BRCA mutation is not a contraindication to a TSSM approach. Location of the primary tumor in these high-risk patients is in the upper-outer quadrant of the breast in 85% of cases, similar to rates seen in patients with sporadic breast cancer. There is no evidence that the NAC is a more frequent site of end-organ carcinogenesis in these mutation carriers than in the general population. If one were to espouse the thought that removing the skin of the NAC would significantly reduce the chance of breast cancer development, one would then need to recommend removing the skin of the breast in the upper-outer quadrant, over the area at greatest risk. This, of course, is not reasonable.

TECHNICAL APPROACHES: INCISION PLANNING

There are a variety of incisions that have been advocated for a TSSM. The most popular include lateral radial incision, circumareolar incision with lateral extension, and inferolateral inframammary crease incision.

The lateral radial incision has become the incision of choice for the investigators in the majority of cases. It provides excellent access to glandular breast tissue in all four quadrants, affords excellent exposure for the excision of the major ducts, allows for axillary exploration (and removal of axillary breast tissue), and preserves flap-skin sensation. This incision also provides excellent access for implant placement and tissue expander exchange.

Some investigators have advocated a circumareolar incision with a lateral extension. (**Figs. 1–4**) There does not appear to be any significant advantage to adding the circumareolar component of the incision, although results can be excellent.

The inframammary crease approach (**Figs 5** and **6**) offers a chance to remove the skin scar from the breast proper and hide it in a natural skin fold. This incision works best in patients with a small breast cup size, little ptosis, and a manageable distance between the incision site and the upper-inner extent of the glandular breast tissue. In the authors' experience this distance should be less than 15 to 20 cm to allow for complete tissue excision and maximize flap viability.

TECHNICAL CONSIDERATIONS: CREATING SKIN FLAPS

With all three of the aforementioned approaches the skin flaps are typically longer and more vulnerable than conventional mastectomy flaps. Therefore, it is critical that dissection should be done expeditiously by a skilled surgeon. Flap-loss rates are directly related to counter traction time. It is venous congestion (more than arterial blockage) that leads to devastating flap loss. Flaps should be raised as quickly as

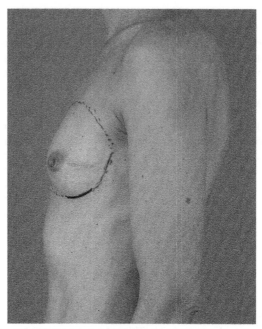

Fig 1. Circumareolar incision with a lateral extension, lateral preoperative view.

expertise will allow. For more difficult dissections it is prudent to periodically relax tension on the flaps. Application of warm saline compresses will also aid in flap viability. The authors prefer to raise the superior, medial, and lower flap completely, followed by reflecting the breast off of the pectoralis and serratus muscles. The breast specimen is then delivered out of the incision and the superior and lateral flaps are created (**Fig. 7**). The dissection behind the NAC is continued without interruption as the anterior flaps is constructed. This residual tissue is then carefully dissected (sharply) and the major ducts are removed from the lumen of the NAC. This tissue is sent as a separate surgical specimen for pathologic analysis. It is often helpful to place a small stay suture at the base of the nipple to prevent inversion.

DISCUSSION

The first step in the process of evaluating a proposed evolutionary modification to the management of any disease necessarily involves addressing common misconceptions or myths about the derivation and source of data that have historically impacted treatment changes.

The first and most important historic myth concerning the evolution of breast cancer treatment is that every step along the changing treatment paradigm in mastectomy was based upon the results of randomized clinical trials. This is not the case and will not be the case in the future. Halsted[20] and Meyer[21] independently reported their individual techniques for the successful therapy of breast cancer with radical mastectomy in 1894 (Bland p881 7 and 8). Their method, which reduced local recurrences tenfold when compared with historical controls, became the gold standard operative procedure for breast cancer. However, American and British surgeons began to develop more conservative procedures almost immediately. In 1912 Murphy reported that he had abandoned Halsted's radical mastectomy in favor of preserving both

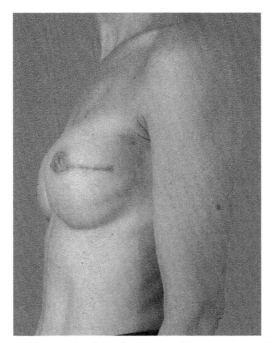

Fig 2. Circumareolar incision with a lateral extension, lateral postoperative view.

muscles. Bryant of London, over a 40-year period, encountered only a single patient who recurred in preserved pectoral muscles. Nevertheless, 50 years would pass before the landmark reports of modified radical mastectomy of McWhirter, Patey, and Dyson in the late 1940s and another 30 years would pass before two randomized

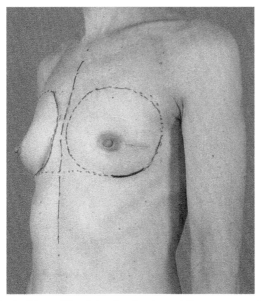

Fig 3. Circumareolar incision with a lateral extension, oblique preoperative view.

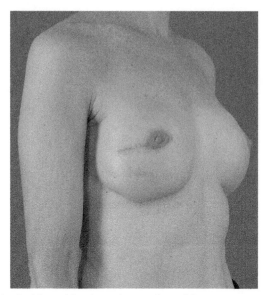

Fig 4. Circumareolar incision with a lateral extension, oblique postoperative view.

clinical trials would put the question to rest.[22] Before the report of the Manchester and Alabama clinical trials, more than 70% of clinicians had already adopted the modified radical mastectomy.

There was never a randomized trial to assess the safety of a breast-conserving approach to DCIS that included a mastectomy arm. There was never a randomized trial that clearly defined the role of surgical margins in conservative approaches to breast cancer. Virtually all major surgical oncology groups adopted the practice of

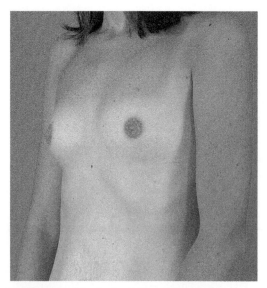

Fig 5. The inframammary crease approach, preoperative view.

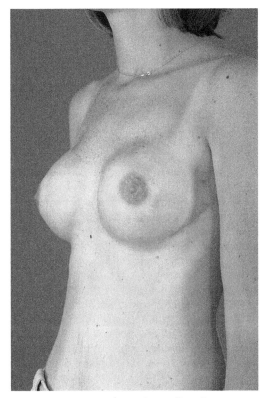

Fig 6. The inframammary crease approach, postoperative view.

sentinel node biopsy well before the trials of Veronesi or the National Surgical Adjuvant Breast Project (NSABP) were published. The American College of Surgeons Z-10 trial included a control arm of no further intervention in the sentinel node negative group, despite a lack of trial data that sentinel node mapping techniques were equal to axillary clearance. Techniques of accelerated partial breast irradiation have been employed for nearly a decade despite an absence of trial results. Not a single aspect

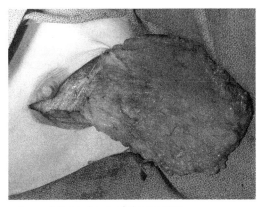

Fig 7. The breast specimen delivered out of the incision.

of the treatment of male breast cancer finds its foundation in clinical trial data. Finally, techniques that preserved much or all of the skin of the breast during mastectomy (skin sparing mastectomy) have been adopted and integrated into routine clinical practice without trial evidence.

The second historical myth that is worth addressing is that all confirmatory clinical trial results are eventually incorporated into clinical practice. The conceptual evolution away from axillary clearance and toward total mastectomy (with and without) radiation therapy was driven by the landmark NSABP B-04 trial, which included an arm of no axillary treatment. Despite showing no apparent survival benefit to axillary treatment in this underpowered trial, axillary clearance remained the standard of care and was included as standard management in all ensuing NSABP trials. Harris and Osteen were the first to demonstrate that this trial could not have possibly addressed the survival question that the study embraced.[23] The results of this trial were largely ignored and clinicians continued to remove axillary nodes in subjects with invasive mammary cancer until the era of sentinel node biopsy.

It is clear therefore that clinical interventions, such as total skin sparing mastectomy, with no chance of a survival impact and negligible impact on local-regional recurrence rates will not lend themselves to a randomized, prospective clinical trial. It is naïve to suggest that sparing the skin of the NAC during TSSM should be avoided pending the results of randomized trials. Rather, it is reasonable to derive cumulative safety confirmation from the recently reported 2000 cases. Mastectomy has historically provided good but not perfect local control of breast cancer. Assuming that local control is improved substantively by removing the skin of the nipple areolar complex is illogical. The reported series share common observations, including the fact that the skin of the NAC is a rare site for end organ carcinogenesis in breast cancer.

As a discipline, breast oncology has never been satisfied accepting the status quo. Much of the credit for creating a culture that expects and demands continual improvement in outcomes must be given to patients and advocates who have demanded and have successfully campaigned for progress and meaningful funding for research. The end result of these efforts is a constantly changing landscape of treatment strategies and approaches. Again, clinicians are polarized: either in favor of a nipple sparing approach or opposed to this minor technical innovation. Again, debate will center, as it should, on the safety of this procedure. However, unlike previous treatment paradigmatic shifts, this one will not lend itself to randomized clinical trials. Rather, clinicians will have to extrapolate from growing datasets and a common-sense understanding of the disease.

Nearly 100 years ago James Ewing presaged the events of the coming century of breast cancer treatment when he stated that "….in mammary cancer, surgery meets with more peculiar difficulties and uncertainties than with almost any other form of the disease." He concluded that it was impossible to render "…in the majority of cases a reasonably accurate adjustment of a means to an end.[23]" Veronesi described this as a quest for the "ideal treatment for breast cancer," (personal communication, 1990) one that represented the best compromise between treatments that were unnecessarily mutilating and those that were dangerously inadequate. Veronesi described this as a virtually never-ending process of doubt engendering debate followed by study and resolution. It is difficult to conceive that anyone familiar with the history of breast cancer treatment would reject out of hand the next logical area for clinical investigation and treatment improvement: the total skin sparing mastectomy.

REFERENCES

1. Patrick IB. Role of mastectomy in breast cancer. Surg Clin North Am 1990;70(5): 1023–46.
2. Sookhan N, Boughey JC, Walsh MF, et al. Nipple-sparing mastectomy–initial experience at a tertiary center. Am J Surg 2008;196(4):575–7.
3. Voltura AM, Tsangaris TN, Rosson GD, et al. Nipple-sparing mastectomy: critical assessment of 51 procedures and implications for selection criteria. Ann Surg Oncol 2008;15(12):3396–401.
4. Wijayanayagam A, Kumar AS, Foster RD, et al. Optimizing the total skin-sparing mastectomy. Arch Surg 2008;143(1):38–45 [discussion: 45].
5. Garcia-Etienne CA, Cody Iii HS 3rd, Disa JJ, et al. Nipple-sparing mastectomy: initial experience at the Memorial Sloan-Kettering Cancer Center and a comprehensive review of literature. Breast J 2009;15(4):440–9.
6. Munhoz AM, Aldrighi C, Montag E, et al. Optimizing the nipple-areola sparing mastectomy with double concentric peri-areolar incision and biodimensional expander-implant reconstruction: aesthetic and technical refinements. Breast 2009;18(6):356–67.
7. Hartmann LC, Schaid DJ, Woods JE, et al. Efficacy of bilateral prophylactic mastectomy in women with a family history of breast cancer. N Engl J Med 1999;340(2):77–84.
8. Margulies AG, Hochberg J, Kepple J, et al. Total skin-sparing mastectomy without preservation of the nipple-areola complex. Am J Surg 2005;190(6):907–12.
9. Sacchini V, Pinotti JA, Barros AC, et al. Nipple-sparing mastectomy for breast cancer and risk reduction: oncologic or technical problem? J Am Coll Surg 2006;203(5):704–14.
10. Crowe JP, Patrick RJ, Yetman RJ, et al. Nipple-sparing mastectomy update: one hundred forty-nine procedures and clinical outcomes. Arch Surg 2008;143(11): 1106–10 [discussion: 1110].
11. Benediktsson KP, Perbeck L. Survival in breast cancer after nipple-sparing subcutaneous mastectomy and immediate reconstruction with implants: a prospective trial with 13 years median follow-up in 216 patients. Eur J Surg Oncol 2008;34(2):143–8.
12. Garwood ER, Moore D, Ewing C, et al. Total skin-sparing mastectomy: complications and local recurrence rates in 2 cohorts of patients. Ann Surg 2009;249(1):26–32.
13. Petit JY, Veronesi U, Orecchia R, et al. The nipple-sparing mastectomy: early results of a feasibility study of a new application of perioperative radiotherapy (ELIOT) in the treatment of breast cancer when mastectomy is indicated. Tumori 2003;89(3):288–91.
14. Petit JY, Veronesi U, Orecchia R, et al. Nipple-sparing mastectomy in association with intra operative radiotherapy (ELIOT): A new type of mastectomy for breast cancer treatment. Breast Cancer Res Treat 2006;96(1):47–51.
15. Petit JY, Veronesi U, Rey P, et al. Nipple-sparing mastectomy: risk of nipple-areolar recurrences in a series of 579 cases. Breast Cancer Res Treat 2009;114(1):97–101.
16. Petit JY, Veronesi U, Orecchia R, et al. Nipple sparing mastectomy with nipple areola intraoperative radiotherapy: one thousand and one cases of a five years experience at the European institute of oncology of Milan (EIO). Breast Cancer Res Treat 2009;117(2):333–8.
17. Gerber B, Krause A, Reimer T, et al. Skin-sparing mastectomy with conservation of the nipple-areola complex and autologous reconstruction is an oncologically safe procedure. Ann Surg 2003;238(1):120–7.

18. Gerber B, Krause A, Dieterich M, et al. The oncological safety of skin sparing mastectomy with conservation of the nipple-areola complex and autologous reconstruction: an extended follow-up study. Ann Surg 2009;249(3):461–8.
19. Paepke S, Schmid R, Fleckner S, et al. Subcutaneous mastectomy with conservation of the nipple-areola skin: broadening the indications. Ann Surg 2009; 250(2):288–92.
20. Halsted WS. The results of operations for the cure of cancer of the breast performed at the John Hopkins Hospital from June 1889 to January 1894. Arch Surg 1894;20:497.
21. Meyer W. An improved method for the radical operation for carcinoma of the breast. Med Rec NY 1894;46:746.
22. Bland K, Chang H, Chandler G, et al. In: Kirby B, Edward C, editors, Modified radical mastectomy and total (Simple mastectomy) in THE BREAST, vol 2. St Louis (MO): Saunders; 2004. p. 865–83. Chapter 41.
23. Osborne MP, Borgen PI. Role of mastectomy in breast cancer. Surg Clin North Am 1990;70(5):1023–46.

Oncoplastic Surgery: A Creative Approach to Breast Cancer Management

Gail S. Lebovic, MA, MD

KEYWORDS

- Oncoplastic surgery • Breast cancer
- Skin-sparing mastectomy • Reconstruction

HISTORICAL PERSPECTIVE

History has proved that in most cases, the treatment of breast cancer requires surgical intervention. Since Halsted's[1] original work in the late 1880s, the surgical management of breast cancer has instilled fear in women throughout the world, and breast surgery has been considered unpleasant but a necessary evil.[2] Although the radical mastectomy accomplished local control, the advanced stage of disease often led to poor survivability; thus, surgical change was not possible until the era of screening mammography and the subsequent shift to the detection of earlier, often nonpalpable, tumors. Fortunately, since that time, significant progress has been made in the surgical management of breast cancer.

Much of this work began in the mid to late 1970s, and after decades of diligent scientific research, surgeons were able to show that less-extensive tissue resection was possible without endangering a woman's life. The two most widely recognized clinical trials supporting this hypothesis are the Milan trials and the National Surgical Adjuvant Breast and Bowel Project. After more than 20 years of follow-up for each of these studies, clinicians have learned that various portions of the breast and surrounding structures can be preserved without having an impact on survival in a negative manner. During the course of these studies, however, it also became evident that surgery alone was not sufficient, and adjuvant treatment was necessary in order to achieve success with breast conservation surgery.[3,4] **Fig. 1** illustrates the dramatic differences that result from various surgical approaches for resection of primary breast tumors, ranging from radical mastectomy to lumpectomy. Combining the process of early tumor detection with less-extensive tissue resection and adjuvant therapies allowed for the first major changes in breast cancer surgery to occur. In the

American Society of Breast Disease, PO Box 1620, Frisco, TX 75034, USA
E-mail address: oper8n@gmail.com

Surg Oncol Clin N Am 19 (2010) 567–580
doi:10.1016/j.soc.2010.04.003   surgonc.theclinics.com
1055-3207/10/$ – see front matter © 2010 Elsevier Inc. All rights reserved.

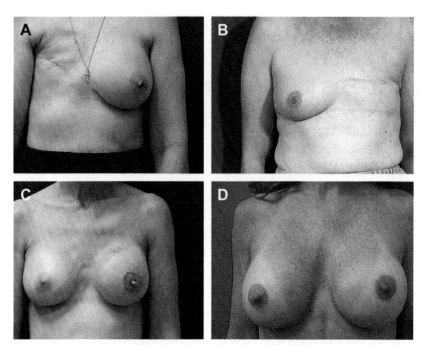

Fig. 1. (*A*) Standard radical mastectomy (note vertical skin incision). (*B*) Standard modified radical mastectomy (note horizontal skin incision, preservation of additional skin, and pectoralis major muscle). (*C*) Patient after left skin-sparing mastectomy, implant reconstruction, nipple reconstruction, and right breast augmentation mammoplasty for symmetry. (*D*) Patient after left breast lumpectomy (periareolar incision). Patient had subglandular augmentation mammoplasty many years prior to lumpectomy.

years that followed, these same advances contributed to the genesis of the field of oncoplastic, surgery, allowing for more and more creative, yet safe, surgical solutions (**Fig. 2**).[5–8]

The idea of combining knowledge from various subspecialties to create a comprehensive, individualized treatment plan was the modest beginning of the multidisciplinary patient-centered model.[9] When considered separately, the advancements over the past several decades in each field, such as radiology, surgery, medical oncology, radiation therapy, and other fields, are impressive. When taken together collectively, however, the progression within each field allowed for clinical changes that are nothing less than extraordinary.

Given the widespread implementation of less-aggressive surgical resections (such as lumpectomy and sentinel lymph node biopsy), the interaction between surgeon, radiation oncologist, radiologist, pathologist, and oncologist has become essential to achieving a good outcome. First and foremost, the objective is to design a surgical plan that does not compromise tumor resection or place patients at undo risk of local recurrence that might result in the need for multiple surgeries. The determination for how much tissue must be removed (from an oncologic perspective) cannot be separated from a thorough and complete preoperative assessment of both breasts, including consideration of breast size and shape and patient desires. In this regard, the basic principles of aesthetic and reconstructive surgery must be understood by the surgeon performing the extirpative procedure because placement of incisions

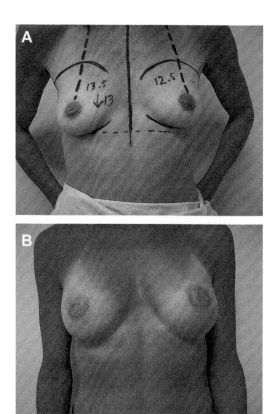

Fig. 2. (*A*) Preoperative photograph of patient with early breast cancer and positive for BRCA mutation. (*B*) Postoperative photograph of same patient after bilateral skin-sparing mastectomy, immediate breast reconstruction with saline implants (submuscular), and bilateral nipple reconstruction.

influences later options for reconstruction. Once full consideration is given to the surgical options and possible need for postoperative adjuvant therapy, an extensive discussion with patients helps define the most appropriate surgical plan.

Although studies show that local recurrence may not ultimately have an impact on overall survival rates, mortality is not the ultimate endpoint most women are trying to beat. Most women who have faced the reality of a diagnosis of breast cancer find it challenging to go through the experience, and most of them prefer not to endure the experience again. Thus, although the option of breast conservation brings with it the alluring possibility of avoiding bodily disfigurement (discussed previously), local resection alone is not as effective as mastectomy in reducing the risk of local recurrence. Thus, even in cases of early-stage breast cancer, radiation therapy and often chemotherapy are necessary when breast conservation is chosen instead of mastectomy. Given the widespread and long-standing aversion to mastectomy, however, breast conservation quickly became adopted by surgeons and women alike, and the addition of adjuvant therapies has been accepted when necessary. The reality and fear of local recurrence, however, remains a significant concern for many women, and many of these women opt for mastectomy instead of lumpectomy. Oncoplastic surgery can offer dramatic surgical improvements in this group of women, because often methods of skin sparing, and sometimes even nipple-areolar sparing, can be offered in a safe and effective manner (see **Fig. 2**).[7,8,10]

With the adoption of breast conservation, physicians soon found clinical follow-up of these patients challenging because lumpectomy and radiation can result in significant scarring of the breast. This resulted in the unfortunate dilemma of making clinical or mammographic examination of the breast difficult and, in some cases, almost impossible. In addition, the aesthetic outcomes after breast conservation vary widely, and the results are often unpredictable after postoperative radiation therapy. When poor outcomes occur (**Fig. 3**), surgical intervention with salvage mastectomy is often required to alleviate painful retraction from scarring, and the options for various methods of reconstruction may be limited given the commonly seen damage to the skin and underlying tissues secondary to postlumpectomy radiation.

DEFINITION OF ONCOPLASTIC SURGERY

The issues (discussed previously) helped spark the notion for a surgical subspecialty focused on breast surgery. Ultimately, in 2000 this led to the establishment of breast fellowship training programs, and in all likelihood, this subspecialty training will soon include training in oncoplastic surgery. The term, *oncoplastic surgery*, is fitting and was coined by Dr Werner Audretsch in an attempt to described the blending of surgical techniques from the fields of surgical oncology and plastic and reconstructive surgery. The premise is that whenever surgery is to be performed on the breast, consideration for cancer and aesthetics must be included. A handful of surgeons scattered over many countries began practicing in this manner in the early 1990s; however, only in the past decade has this approach gained widespread acceptance and enthusiasm in the United States. No doubt, this slow process of adoption was necessary in order to ensure that new techniques would not jeopardize patient safety. It is well recognized that oncoplastic surgery can improve surgical outcomes in a safe and effective manner as long as patient selection is appropriate.[5-8,11-13] It is for this reason that multidisciplinary approach to the preoperative work-up is key to the practice of oncoplastic surgery.

Oncoplastic surgery does not refer to any given procedure; rather, it describes a surgical mindset in the approach of a patient facing various types of breast surgery. For example, a woman who presents for breast reduction surgery (commonly considered an aesthetic procedure) should be questioned about her risk for breast cancer and should undergo a preoperative work-up, including appropriate breast examination and imaging. This is done as a preoperative baseline and as a way to detect any potentially occult lesions within the breast. Any abnormalities are worked up prior to surgery, which may include mammography, ultrasound, MRI, and even minimally invasive biopsy if necessary.

Similarly, a patient presenting with a diagnosis of breast cancer in the setting of large pendulous breasts may be an ideal candidate for a large tumor resection performed using standard techniques for breast reduction. Both of these examples illustrate how the oncoplastic approach can be applied to various clinical situations. Furthermore, the utility of breast reduction as a method for resection of breast cancer offers broad applications in oncoplastic surgery (**Fig. 4**).[10,13,14]

ONCOPLASTIC SURGERY AND BREAST CANCER

Care of breast cancer patients can vary widely depending on the clinical environment. At times, patients may experience a fragmented approach to their care, requiring them to visit multiple different physicians at various institutions. Sometimes, these clinicians

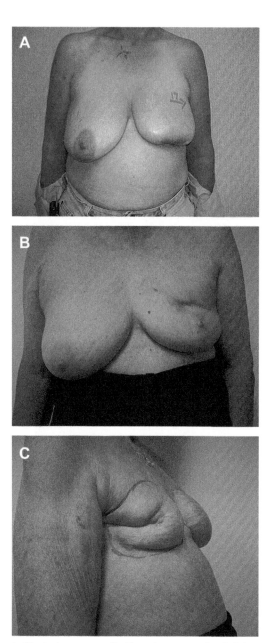

Fig. 3. These patients illustrate poor aesthetic outcomes and painful scar contractures that can occur in some cases after breast conservation surgery followed by radiation therapy. (*A*) Severe scar contracture following excision of tumor from inferior segment of large pendulous breast. (*B*) Large glandular deformity with scar contracture adherent to chest wall following lumpectomy in superior central portion of the breast. (*C*) Scar contracture with lateral rotation of nipple-areolar complex following lumpectomy at lateral aspect of breast.

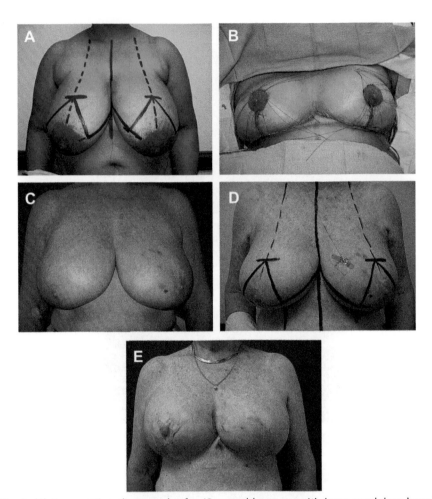

Fig. 4. (*A*) Preoperative photograph of a 43-year-old woman with large pendulous breast and small invasive cancer found on screening mammogram. Lesion was located in the inferior aspect of left breast. Markings illustrate skin markings standard for reduction mammoplasty techniques. (*B*) Immediate surgical result after breast reduction, sentinel node biopsy, and reconstruction using standard breast reduction techniques and free nipple-areolar transfers. (*C*) Preoperative photograph of patient with multiple central tumors in left breast. (*D*) Preoperative photograph showing patient with skin markings and wire-localization to confirm area of tumor. (*E*) Immediate postoperative photograph showing central lumpectomy technique to remove central tumors and reconstruction using standard reduction mammoplasty techniques.

may not even communicate with one another about a given patient. The multidisciplinary model has helped encourage a team approach, however, and has more commonly become an integral part of patient care in many centers. This model provides structure for comprehensive review within a multidisciplinary tumor board conference, where individual patients are reviewed by the different specialty teams providing care. This helps coordinate and optimize a plan for each patient and allows physicians and patients a more comprehensive approach.[9]

The practice of oncoplastic surgery requires that surgeons obtain a level of understanding of each of the critical components of cancer care, including those of other disciplines, in order to integrate the knowledge when devising a surgical plan. This can be accomplished in a variety of practice settings but is important particularly if surgeons are in an environment that does not have access to a multidisciplinary clinic or team. Often there is a surgical oncologist working in concert with a plastic and reconstructive surgeon. Even in this situation, it is crucial for the two surgical teams to confer prior to surgery in order to optimize the oncologic and aesthetic outcomes. In some environments, breast surgeons need to be able to integrate this knowledge independently and even perform both aspects of the surgery. Thus, the need for changes in the training curriculum for oncologic breast surgeons becomes obvious and should include the addition of aesthetic and reconstructive techniques. Currently, an international steering committee has been challenged with the task of developing standardized recommendations for training, and a preliminary outline of proposed skills for various levels of training is listed in (**Table 1**).

PREOPERATIVE ASSESSMENT

As discussed previously, a thorough preoperative assessment is critical when practicing oncoplastic surgery so as to insure appropriate patient selection. This evaluation begins with a comprehensive history and physical examination that pays particular attention to details that may indicate an increased risk for breast cancer or an increased risk for a recurrence. Often, patients present with a known history or recent diagnosis of breast cancer, but some may seek surgical consultation for other reasons, such as a strong family history of breast cancer. In each instance, a complete evaluation should be performed, including

- Complete personal and family medical history
- BRCA testing if indicated
- Evaluation of additional risk factors, such as hormone replacement therapy, history of radiation treatment for Hodgkin's disease, etc

Table 1	
Preliminary guidelines for standardized training in oncoplastic surgery	
Level I	Thorough knowledge and understanding of risk assessment within the multidisciplinary framework
	Thorough knowledge and understanding of aesthetic principles and reconstructive options
	Devise comprehensive surgical approach without compromise of oncologic or aesthetic principles
	Ability to perform large resections with breast conservation surgery
	Ability to design and implement glandular resections and use local tissue for reconstruction
Level II	Ability to perform skin-sparing mastectomy
	Ability to perform breast reduction with/without nipple transfer
	Ability to perform mastopexy
Level III	Ability to perform augmentation mammoplasty
	Ability to perform mastopexy with implants
	Ability to perform nipple-areolar–sparing mastectomy
	Ability to perform capsulectomy/implant removal and reconstruction
	Ability to perform various types of implant/expander reconstruction
	Ability to perform nipple reconstruction
Level IV	Specialty training to include myocutaneous flaps

- General medical condition
- Smoking history
- History of previous breast surgery, biopsies, implants (including size/type), and so forth
- Multimodality breast imaging (review films: mammography, ultrasound, MRI)
- Patient desires in regards to breast shape, size, symmetry.

Particular attention to details from prior surgical procedures should be obtained and a thorough review of all previous medical records, imaging studies, and pathology (actual films and slides) should be completed.[9,10,15]

SURGICAL PLANNING

Under the best circumstances, surgeons function as patient advocates in developing a surgical plan in order to achieve the objectives of surgical treatment. These objectives include (1) obtaining optimal local control of the tumor with wide margins free of disease; (2) prevention of local recurrence, because 80% of tumor recurrences ultimately occur at the site of the original tumor and a significant number of women may have multicentric/multifocal disease; and (3) maintaining or improving the aesthetic appearance of the breast. In addition to the preoperative assessment (discussed previously), **Table 2** provides clinical indications and rationale for the use of

Table 2
Clinical indications and rationale for preoperative MRI

Clinical Indication	Rationale for Preoperative MRI
Newly diagnosed patients with breast cancer	Define extent of disease, multifocality, contralateral lesions, etc. Helps to refine surgical plan
Yearly follow-up for breast cancer patients including those post reconstruction	May help to identify lesions difficult to detect postoperatively by mammography/ultrasound
Cancer screening in high risk patients	Adjunct to screening mammography for women with dense breasts, BRCA positive, etc.
Evaluation of indeterminate lesions after mammography and ultrasound	When high index of clinical suspicion and lesion is not visualized with other imaging methods
Cancer screening in women with breast implants in addition to mammography	May help to identify lesions underneath or blocked by implant placement
Monitor response to neoadjuvant therapy	Helps determine length of preoperative course of chemotherapy and defines area for surgical resection
Locate primary disease in patients with axillary nodal disease and unknown primary	Adjunct to mammography and ultrasound if primary not located by these methods
Evaluation of silicone gel implants (as recommended by the Food and Drug Administration)	Can distinguish intracapsular versus extracapsular gel implant rupture
Adjunct to screening mammography in women with dense breasts	In particular, those women with dense breasts and at increased risk for breast cancer
Preoperative assessment in patients undergoing elective breast procedures	As baseline and to identify any possible occult lesions

preoperative MRI as it pertains to surgical management/follow-up. Although a standard role for MRI in breast surgery remains controversial, the use of MRI in oncoplastic surgery is essential.[16,17]

In exploring the role of oncoplastic surgery and breast conservation, several comprehensive articles have been published describing level I (listed in **Table 1**) oncoplastic techniques for lumpectomy and reconstruction of the breast using local tissue flap advancement to minimize breast deformities.[18,19] The most recent and thorough publication has been presented by Clough and colleagues.[13] This monograph provides a detailed quadrant-by-quadrant atlas for oncoplastic surgery and illustrates the importance of defining the volume of tissue to be excised compared to patients' overall breast size. When contemplating the decision between breast conservation and mastectomy, it becomes imperative to consider factors, such as skin laxity, degree of ptosis (sagging), and nipple-areolar position.

Given the limitations of this brief review, a few of the creative techniques in oncoplastic surgery that offer an opportunity to improve outcomes after mastectomy are focused on. This discussion is separated into two parts, depending on patient breast size, because the surgical approaches differ completely for patients with small versus large breasts. Any and all of these procedures can be combined with other important techniques such as sentinel lymph node biopsy and wire localization.

THE SMALL BREAST

In many cases, surgeons find that patients with small breasts often choose mastectomy rather than breast conservation. These patients frequently make excellent candidates for using creative surgical techniques for mastectomy, and they tend to share some common factors. Often these patients present with an early stage of disease, but the tumor may require a relatively large excision in comparison to the volume of existing breast tissue. These patients may also present at a young age and they frequently lead active lifestyles. In addition, they may fear or truly be faced with an increased risk for cancer recurrence due to several factors, such as histologic subtype, family history of breast cancer, extended longevity, and/or other factors. Consequently, many of these patients seek mastectomy, and often they desire immediate reconstruction. In this setting, skin-sparing mastectomy with immediate implant reconstruction can be the ideal solution, and a pleasing aesthetic appearance of the breast can be achieved without compromise as shown here in **Fig. 5**, this is a staged procedure. The first stage consists of a skin-sparing mastectomy, sentinel node biopsy (axillary dissection if indicated), and first-stage breast reconstruction. The second stage achieves the nipple-areolar reconstruction and is typically performed as an outpatient procedure after completion of any necessary adjuvant therapy. Aesthetic changes, such as adjusting implant size and position, breast shape, and nipple-areolar reconstruction are achieved.

In some cases, it may be appropriate to preserve the nipple-areolar complex. This can be achieved using similar techniques and is often a viable surgical option for high-risk patients (ie, BRCA positive) prior to any evidence of disease (**Fig. 6**).

THE LARGE BREAST

Patients with large breasts afford oncoplastic surgeons more options for surgical creativity. The most important aspect of these procedures is the use of the Wise pattern for the skin incision. This technique is widely applicable and can be used for procudures such as mastectomy, partial mastectomy (removal of the inferior segment of the breast) as well as central lumpectomy. Again, use of these techniques does not

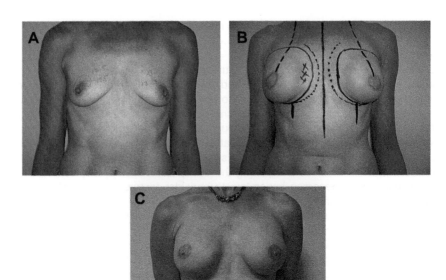

Fig. 5. (*A*) Preoperative photograph of patient with *ductal carcinoma in situ* right breast and positive for BRCA mutation. (*B*) Photograph showing same patient after bilateral skin-sparing mastectomy, first-stage immediate reconstruction with submuscular saline implants. Markings show areas for improvement in final aesthetic outcome for second-stage reconstruction. (*C*) Postoperative photograph of same patient after second-stage reconstruction and bilateral nipple-areolar reconstruction.

preclude the addition of wire localization, and/or sentinel node biopsy. Many of these techniques follow the standard approach to breast reduction but extend resection to include the nipple-areolar complex if involved or close to the primary tumor (central lumpectomy). These techniques can be used in a multitude of clinical situations lending excellent results for breast conservation or mastectomy with or without reconstruction. If the nipple-areolar complex is removed, it can be reconstructed at a later, second stage after adjuvant therapy is completed. If necessary, radiation therapy can

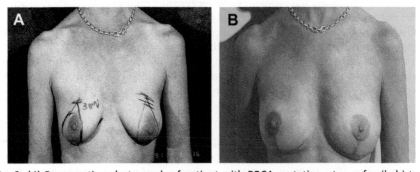

Fig. 6. (*A*) Preoperative photograph of patient with BRCA mutation, strong family history, and desire for bilateral prophylactic mastectomy with immediate reconstruction. (*B*) Postoperative photograph of same patient after bilateral mastectomy with reconstruction.

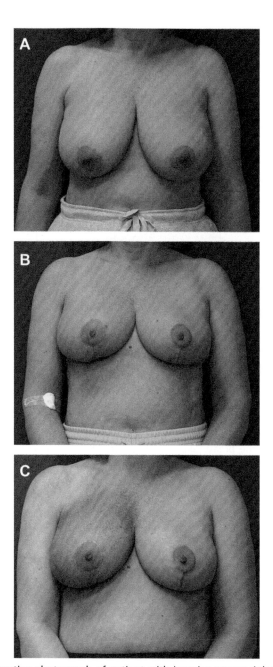

Fig. 7. (A) Preoperative photograph of patient with invasive cancer right breast and large pendulous breasts. (B) Postoperative photograph of same patient. (C) Same patient after postoperative radiation therapy illustrating skin changes. Shrinkage of the breast can occur as well.

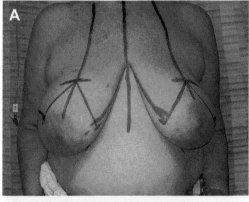

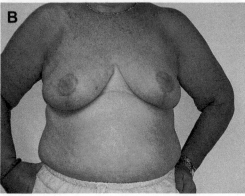

Fig. 8. (*A*) Preoperative photograph of patient with invasive cancer right breast located in inferior segment of the breast. Skin markings for standard reduction mammoplasty are shown. (*B*) Postoperative photograph of same patient after reduction mammoplasty for resection of tumor and bilateral nipple-areolar transfer.

be added after completion of postsurgical healing, and once complete, the nipple-areolar reconstruction can be performed. As with all patients undergoing breast surgery, a thorough review of the potential risks and complications should be completed, and patients should be aware of the likelihood for asymmetry, particularly if radiation therapy is administered (**Fig. 7**).

Because the principles of breast reduction surgery lend tremendous versatility to the breast cancer surgeons' repertoire, it is perhaps the first and most important procedure for oncoplastic surgeons to learn (**Fig. 8**). Once mastered, techniques such as mastopexy and skin-sparing mastectomy will follow more easily and the ability to develop comprehensive surgical approaches unique to each patient becomes second nature.

SUMMARY

In many circumstances, historical turf issues have delineated which procedures belong to a given specialty. The case for oncoplastic surgery, however, is different. The breast has long been regarded in many societies as a symbolic anatomic structure—one that embodies motherhood, femininity, and grace. Because this highly regarded female organ is so often the unfortunate victim of cancer, surgeons must change their approach, combining academic life-saving surgical techniques with a woman's sensitivity to preserving the aesthetics of the breast, in order to be effective patient advocates in the fight against breast cancer. Therein lies the foundation for the field of oncoplastic surgery.

The cross-fertilization that occurs when specialists from different fields convene to devise a treatment plan for given patients is formidable. There is no doubt that maintaining the multidisciplinary approach is paramount to the successful outcomes in oncoplastic surgery, and the benefits include improved aesthetic results after cancer surgery. As these procedures are adopted by surgeons throughout the world (teams of surgeons working together or individual surgeons), oncoplastic surgical training combined with appropriate patient selection will ultimately lead to achieving safe and aesthetically pleasing outcomes for breast cancer patients. Hopefully with time, the practice of oncoplastic surgery will help to alleviate some of the long-standing fear and hatred associated with the surgical treatment of this disease.

REFERENCES

1. Halsted WS. The results of radical operations for the cure of carcinoma of the breast. Ann Surg 1907;46:1.
2. Patey DH, Dyson WH. The prognosis of carcinoma of the breast in relation to the type of operation performed. Br J Cancer 1948;2:7.
3. Fisher B, Anderson S, Bryant J, et al. Twenty-year follow-up of a randomized trial comparing total mastectomy, lumpectomy, and lumpectomy plus irradiation for the treatment of invasive breast cancer. N Engl J Med 2002;347:1233–41.
4. Veronesi U, Cascinelli N, Mariani L, et al. Twenty-year follow-up of a randomized study comparing breast-conserving surgery with radical mastectomy for early breast cancer. N Engl J Med 2002;347:1227–32.
5. Brown IM, Wilson CR, Doughty JC, et al. The future of breast surgery: a new sub-speciality of oncoplastic breast surgeons? Breast 2004;13:82.
6. Skillman JM, Humzah MD. The future of breast surgery: a new subspecialty of oncoplastic breast surgeons? Breast 2003;12:161–2.
7. Singletary SE, Robb GL. Oncologic safety of skin-sparing mastectomy. Ann Surg Oncol 2003;10:95–7.
8. Chen CY, Calhoun KE, Masetti R, et al. Oncoplastic breast conserving surgery: a renaissance of anatomically-based surgical technique. Minerva Chir 2006;61: 421–34.
9. Anderson BO, Kaufman CS, Kiel KD, et al. Interdisciplinary coordination for breast healthcare: a rational approach to detection, diagnosis and treatment. Dis Manage Health Outcomes 2008;16:7–11.
10. Lebovic GL, Anderson BO. Oncoplastic breast surgery: current status and best candidates for treatment. Current Breast Cancer Reports 2009;1:118–23.
11. Rew DA. Towards a scientific basis for oncoplastic breast surgery. Eur J Surg Oncol 2003;29:105–6.
12. Kaur N, Petit JY, Rietjens M, et al. Comparative study of surgical margins in onco-plastic surgery and quadrantectomy in breast cancer. Ann Surg Oncol 2005;12: 539–45.
13. Clough KB, Kaufman GJ, Nos C, et al. Improving breast cancer surgery: a classi-fication and quadrant per quadrant atlas for oncoplastic surgery. Ann Surg Oncol 2010;17:1375–91.

14. Lebovic GS. Utility of breast reduction in breast cancer surgery. In: Klimberg SV, editor. Atlas of breast surgical techniques. Philadelphia: WB Saunders; 2009. p. 332–50 Chapter 20.

15. Carlson RW, Anderson BO, Burstein HJ, et al. Invasive breast cancer. J Natl Compr Canc Netw 2007;5:246–312.

16. Beatty JD, Porter BA. Contrast-enhanced breast magnetic resonance imaging: the surgical perspective. Am J Surg 2007;193:600–5 [discussion: 605].

17. Lehman CD, Gatsonis C, Kuhl CK, et al. MRI evaluation of the contralateral breast in women with recently diagnosed breast cancer. N Engl J Med 2007;356: 1295–303.

18. Anderson BO, Masetti R, Silverstein MJ. Oncoplastic approaches to partial mastectomy: an overview of volume-displacement techniques. Lancet Oncol 2005;6:145–57.

19. Clough KB, Lewis JS, Couturaud B, et al. Oncoplastic techniques allow extensive resections for breast-conserving therapy of breast carcinomas. Ann Surg 2003; 237:26–34.

Clinical Application of Gene Expression Profiling in Breast Cancer

Joseph A. Sparano, MD[a],*, Melissa Fazzari, PhD[b],
Paraic A. Kenny, PhD[c]

KEYWORDS

- Gene expression profiling • Breast cancer
- Multiparameter assay • Prognostic factor • Predictive factor

Genomics is defined as the study of all of the nucleotide sequences in an organism (see **Table 1** for definition and glossary of other terms). Sequencing of the human genome in tumors is technically daunting, but is currently being performed as part of the Human Cancer Genome Atlas project.[1] One report describing an analysis including 11 breast cancers concluded that the genomic landscape of breast cancer is characterized by a handful of commonly mutated gene mountains and a larger number of gene hills that are mutated at a low frequency.[2] In addition to mutation of individual genes, it has recently become apparent that the genomes of breast tumors harbor many more somatic genomic rearrangements than had previously been identified, suggesting that novel fusion genes found at these translocations may also play a role in disease progression.[3] These methods are being used to identify specific genetic changes that may contribute to the pathogenesis of breast cancer and that may be targeted with specific therapeutic interventions, similar to targeting mutated c-KIT with imatinib in gastrointestinal stromal tumor.[4] These methods are not yet

Supported in part by grants from the National Institute of Health (P30-13330), Susan G. Komen for the Cure (KG091136), and the Department of Defense CDMRP Breast Cancer Research Program (W81XWH-09-46-0680).

[a] Department of Medicine and Oncology, Albert Einstein College of Medicine, Montefiore Medical Center, 1825 Eastchester Road, Bronx, NY 10461, USA

[b] Department of Epidemiology & Population Health, Albert Einstein College of Medicine, 1301 Morris Park Avenue, Bronx, NY 10461, USA

[c] Department of Development and Molecular Biology, Albert Einstein College of Medicine, 1301 Morris Park Avenue, Bronx, NY 10461, USA

* Corresponding author. Department of Medicine and Oncology, Albert Einstein College of Medicine, Montefiore Medical Center, 1825 Eastchester Road, Bronx, NY 10461.
E-mail address: jsparano@montefiore.org

Table 1
Glossary of terms commonly used in describing microarray studies

Term	Definition
Gene Expression Analysis	
Genomics	Study of all of the nucleotide sequences, including structural genes, regulatory sequences, and noncoding DNA segments, in the chromosomes of an organism
DNA microarray	A glass slide or silicon chip with DNA sequences complementary to thousands of genes arrayed at precise locations
qRT-PCR	Quantitative reverse transcriptase polymerase chain reaction: method used for quantitative RNA expression in RNA extracted from specimens, including degraded RNA extracted from formalin-fixed paraffin-embedded tissues
Analysis of Gene Expression Data	
Hierarchical clustering	Commonly used method for performing unsupervised analysis of gene expression data
PAM or SAM	Prediction analysis of microarray or significance analysis of microarray: commonly used methods to analyze gene expression data
Centroid	Average gene expression profile defining a classifier
Regulation of Gene Expression Assays	
CLIA	Clinical Laboratory Improvement Amendments: regulations that cover approval of diagnostic tests, including multiparameter assays
IVDMIA	In vitro diagnostic multivariate index assay: term used by the FDA to describe certain types of multiparameter assays that are regulated as medical devices

510(k) clearance	Regularly approval by the FDA for medical devices characterized as an IVDMIA
Standards	
MAQC	Microarray quality control: effort initiated by the FDA to standardize methods for clinical application of microarray and other genomic assays
REMARK Guidelines	Reporting recommendations for tumor marker prognostic studies: standard criteria for reporting publications about tumor markers, including multiparameter gene expression assays
MIAME	Minimal information about a microarray experiment: set of standards for release of gene expression ion
GEO	Genomic Expression Omnibus (http://www.ncbi.nlm.nih.gov/geo): publicly available repository for gene expression data
Interpretation of Published Literature	
Hazard ratio	Relative risk of an event in a high- versus low-risk population
Sensitivity	Proportion of actual positives which are correctly identified as such (TP/TP+FN)
Specificity	Proportion of negatives which are correctly identified (TN/TN+FP)
Positive predictive value (precision)	Proportion of patients with positive test results who are correctly diagnosed (TP/TP+FP)
Negative predictive value	Proportion of patients with negative test results who are correctly diagnosed (TN/TN+FN)
Accuracy	Proportion of true results (positive and negative) in a population (TP+TN/TP+PF+FN+TN)
Receiver operator curve	Graphical plot of the sensitivity versus (1 − specificity) for binary classifier as its discrimination threshold is varied (fraction of TP versus fraction of FP)

Abbreviations: FN, false-negative; FP, false-positive; TN, true-negative; TP, true-positive.

available for routine clinical application, however. For the most part, genomic profiling has focused on the evaluation of gene expression, or the translation of the information encoded in genomic DNA into an RNA transcript. RNA transcripts include messenger RNAs (mRNAs), which are translated into proteins, and various other RNAs (eg, transfer RNA, ribosomal RNA, micro RNA, and noncoding RNA) that have important biologic functions. For the most part, gene expression profiling in breast cancer has focused on the evaluating expression of mRNA. However, the same principles may be applied to the study of the epigenome,[5,6] micro RNAs,[7] proteins,[8] or integrative approaches that evaluate combinations of profiling methods.[9]

Substantial technical advances within the past decade have facilitated high-throughput analysis of clinical specimens for gene expression, a process that has been referred to as genomic profiling, although gene expression profiling is the more accurate term.[10] There have likewise been important advances in bioinformatics that permit analysis and interpretation of the huge of amount of data generated by expression profiling.[11] By combining high-throughput specimen evaluation and sophisticated bioinformatics analysis, one can identify distinctive patterns of expression that correlate with clinical behavior or response to specific therapies. Some have referred to these distinctive expression patterns as molecular portraits[12] or signatures,[13] and the assays used to detect these patterns as multiparameter assays; the latter term has been used because rather than relying on expression of a single gene or protein, these assays typically incorporate information from measuring expression of multiple genes by using mathematical algorithms to derive a qualitative (eg, high vs low risk) or quantitative (eg, score) test result.[14] These assays may also be categorized as a tumor marker, a clinical assay that serves as a surrogate for defining clinical end points, such as disease response or progression, or predicting clinical end points, such as prognosis or response to therapy.[14,15] Although the term tumor marker in the past has usually referred to a substance released from a tumor into the blood or other body fluids (eg, CA27-29, CEA, PSA), it more recently has been defined more broadly to include tissue-derived markers including multiparameter assays.

The promise and pitfalls in developing multiparameter assays have been reviewed elsewhere,[16–19] and specific criteria have been proposed for the level of evidence required to define and support their clinical usefulness.[15] Several multiparameter assays are currently approved for clinical use, including some which have been recommended by expert panels for clinical decision making.[14,20] This article focuses on principles of gene expression profiling, and multiparameter assays that have been developed for breast cancer. The term multiparameter assay is used interchangeably with the terms assay, tumor marker, and marker.

PROGNOSTIC AND PREDICTIVE MARKERS

A tumor marker is valuable only if it provides information above and beyond that provided by classic clinicopathologic features. A prognostic marker is one that is associated with clinical outcome, usually irrespective of the treatment given. Examples of prognostic markers include tumor size, number of positive lymph nodes, and tumor grade. A predictive marker is one that predicts clinical benefit from a specific therapy. Examples include estrogen receptor (ER) expression (predictive of benefit from endocrine therapy) and HER2/neu overexpression (predictive of benefit from anti-HER2 directed therapies). Some predictive markers are also prognostic, particularly when the therapy predicted to be beneficial is not used (eg, ER, HER2 expression). Predictive markers are more difficult to develop and validate, but are of intrinsically greater value because they are essential in selecting patients for beneficial therapies, more difficult to identify, and fewer.

PROCESS FOR DEVELOPMENT OF A MULTIPARAMETER ASSAY

There are several steps in the development of a marker, and a typical roadmap is summarized in **Box 1**. Steps included in the process may be broadly classified as (1) conceptualization, (2) clinical development, (3) technical development, (4) validation, and (5) application. For the purpose of maker validation, prospective trials may be performed by retrospectively evaluating samples from completed clinical trials with mature clinical outcomes. Models have been proposed for appropriate strategies to validate markers prospectively in either newly initiated clinical trials, or in completed clinical trials.[21] A critical issue is to ensure that there is sufficient sample size to conduct training and validation studies, and in particular a sufficient number of patients with the clinical event of interest (eg, recurrence).[17] Development of an accurate marker is largely a function of the interplay between sample size and classification difficulty.[22] It is not uncommon to find that several statistically equally good predictors can be developed for any given classification problem.[23] In the postdevelopment process, there is potential for the assay to be less accurate and informative as a result of bias in clinical application of the assay. For example, clinicians may be more apt to use an assay in patients with intermediate clinical features, and not to use it in those with good or poor risk clinical features.[24]

METHODS FOR ANALYZING GENE EXPRESSION

There are several methods for analyzing gene expression, which have been reviewed extensively elsewhere and which are illustrated in **Fig. 1** and summarized in **Table 2**.[25,26] Irrespective of the analysis platform used, messenger RNA (mRNA) is first extracted from the tissues of interest (see **Fig. 1A–C**). Because mRNA is highly vulnerable to degradation, sample handling at this step is critical; surgical specimens should be frozen as soon as possible when used for analysis, or placed in appropriate preservative (eg, RNA Later, Qiagen, Valencia, CA, USA). Following mRNA purification, several platforms exist for gene expression profiling. The first gene expression microarray technology to enter widespread use was the 2-color microarray (see **Fig. 1D**). mRNA from 2 samples (an experimental sample and a reference sample) is converted to fluorescently labeled cDNA. Each sample is labeled with a different color (red or green) and the samples are pooled at a 1:1 ratio and hybridized to the same microarray. For all microarrays, each spot on the microarray represents 1 gene and the fluorescence intensity at each spot is proportional to the expression level of that gene in the sample. In a single-color array (see **Fig. 1E**), each tumor sample is labeled with the same fluorescent dye and hybridized to its own microarray. For both array types, after removal of nonhybridized material by washing, images are obtained using laser scanning, which detects the relative fluorescent intensity of the hybridized probe at each spot. Before statistical analysis, the data must be normalized (see **Fig. 1H**) to compensate for variation in labeling, hybridization, and fluorescent detection, and filtered using specific criteria to reduce the likelihood of detecting noise. In the example shown (see **Fig. 1H**), array 3 had a higher average signal intensity (red) than array 1, which, in turn, was higher than array 2. Mathematical correction by normalization results in each array having the same average signal intensity, thereby largely eliminating variation caused by technical issues and allowing detection of biologically relevant differences in gene expression between samples. When many samples are analyzed, it is often convenient to summarize the data in a heatmap (see **Fig. 1I**). In this format, the patient samples are

Box 1
Roadmap for development of a multiparameter marker or other markers

1. Conceptualization: identify clinical need and how marker addresses the clinical need
   - Identify clinical problem
   - Identify treatment options and costs of misclassification using standard clinicopathologic criteria, and potential costs of misclassification with standard criteria (eg, over treatment, under treatment)
   - Identify potential clinical relevance of information provided by marker (prognostic, predictive, or both)

2. Clinical development: marker developed (trained) in an appropriate population, typically referred to as a training set
   - Population sufficiently homogeneous and receiving uniform treatment
   - Perform internal validation of classifier to assess whether it seems sufficiently accurate relative to standard prognostic factors that it is worth further development

3. Technical development: establish technical specifications of marker to ensure reproducible performance in clinical samples
   - Establish reproducibility and reliability of assay
   - Identify and minimize sources of preanalytic variability that may occur in sample collection and processing in the clinic
   - Identify and minimize sources of analytical variability in the laboratory that is conducting the assay

4. Validation: validation of marker in other independent data sets in prospectively planned studies
   - Identify appropriate subject population for marker validation

     Population appropriate for prognostic (no treatment or uniform treatment) or predictive assay (2 or more treatment regimens administered with differing therapeutic outcomes)

     Sufficient sample size and sufficient number of events of interest
   - Identify relevant clinical end point

     Distant recurrence, local recurrence, organ-specific recurrence, all recurrences

     Other clinically relevant end points (eg, specific toxicities)

     Death (eg, from primary cancer, other cancers, toxicity, or other causes)
   - Establish reliability of marker in correlating with clinical end points of interest in different populations

5. Application: establishment or confirmation of clinical usefulness of the assay
   - Prospective testing of marker in data sets that are independent of data sets used for initial validation
   - Postmarking experience

     Evaluate potential biased used of assay in clinical practice (eg, use preferentially in patients with intermediate-grade tumors)

     Evaluate how test information influences clinical decision making

Adapted from Simon R. Roadmap for developing and validating therapeutically relevant genomic classifiers. J Clin Oncol 2005;23:7332.

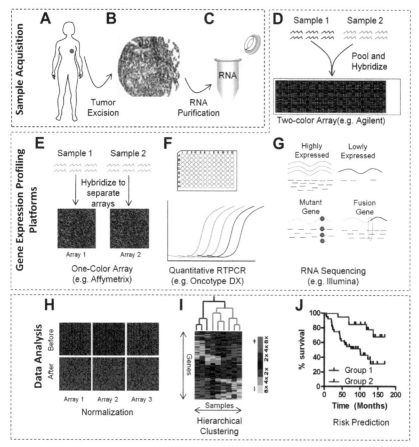

Fig. 1. Summary of steps involved in sample preparation and analysis using high-throughput genomic technologies (A–J).

typically represented in columns, and genes in rows. Genes that are expressed at levels above the median are colored in red, close to the median in black, and below the median in green. Other color schemes are also commonly used (eg, blue-yellow), which may be especially helpful for individuals with red-green color blindness. By comparing the expression level of a large number of genes in each of the samples, the technique of hierarchical clustering can be used to determine which samples are most similar in gene expression. For example, in **Fig. 1I**, the samples from 2 distinct clusters are indicated by the blue and purple branching in the dendrogram at the top of the heatmap. These groups may correspond to samples with different biologic properties (eg, ER-positive vs ER-negative tumors, or high-grade vs low-grade tumors) or groups with different clinical outcomes (see **Fig. 1J**).

Two nonmicroarray-based technologies are also finding applications in this area. In quantitative reverse-transcriptase polymerase chain reaction (qRT-PCR), RNA from the tumor is converted to cDNA and arrayed in different wells of a multiwell plate, each well containing specific PCR primers for a particular gene (see **Fig. 1F**). qRT-PCR analysis can then be used to rapidly and accurately quantify the expression level of each gene of interest within the sample. Unlike microarray analysis, which

Table 2
Commonly used methods for measuring gene expression

Method	Description	Advantages	Disadvantages
Spotted cDNA microarray (eg, Agilent)	Glass slides robotically spotted with purified cDNA clones, PCR products from clones, or oligonucleotides	Ability to design custom arrays	Operator dependent, labor intensive, not always reproducible, requires fresh or frozen tissue
Photolithography (eg, Affymetrix Gene Chips)	DNA probes directly synthesized on silicon chips	Ability to design custom arrays	Requires frozen tissue or placement in RNA preservative media
Real-time reverse transcriptase polymerase chain reaction (RT-PCR)	Generate DNA copies of RNA by reverse transcription, amplify DNA by PCR, quantify DNA product using specific fluorescent reagents	May be performed using RNA extracted from paraffin tissue	Requires development and validation of probes, technical limitations in number of genes that may be assayed
RNA sequencing	Massively parallel sequencing of all mRNAs in a sample	Can detect mutations, splice variants, and fusion genes in addition to changes in gene expression level	Expensive to run the experiments and time consuming to perform the analysis

interrogates tens of thousands of genes, the qRT-PCR technology is more appropriate when a limited group of genes is being investigated, although this method may still allow analysis of several hundred genes simultaneously.

The recent advent of high-throughput massively parallel sequencing machines has opened up an entirely new possibility for gene expression profiling, termed RNA sequencing. It is now feasible to profile samples by direct sequencing of cDNAs derived from many millions of RNA transcripts in a given sample. In addition to providing absolute expression levels (as the precise number of transcripts can be counted), this technology also allows the identification of alternatively spliced isoforms, mutations, and novel transcripts arising from fusion genes. In the example shown (see **Fig. 1**G), the blue gene is more highly expressed than the red gene, resulting in many more sequencing reads. Furthermore, mutations and fusion genes may be detected using this technology, which is not possible using the microarray platforms or qRT-PCR. In this example, the yellow gene has a mutation that is detected in the sequencing reactions, whereas the other transcript results from the fusion of 2 independent genes (green and purple) and is recognized from sequencing reads spanning the boundary between the 2 genes. Recent studies in breast, prostate, and leukemic cell lines show the potential of this approach.[27,28]

QUALITY CONTROL OF GENE EXPRESSION ANALYSIS METHODS

There are multiple sources of error in clinical application of multiparameter assays, including preanalytical, analytical, and postanalytical. Approval requires meeting specific technical requirements regarding performance, reliability, and reproducibility.

The Microarray Quality Control (MAQC) project was organized by the US Food and Drug Administration (FDA) to improve current and next-generation molecular profiling technologies and foster their proper applications in discovery, development, and review of FDA-regulated products (http://www.fda.gov/ScienceResearch/BioinformaticsTools/ MicroarrayQualityControlProject/default.htm). The effort includes multiple stakeholders, including multiple centers within the FDA and other federal agencies, major providers of microarray platforms and RNA samples, academic laboratories, and others. In MAQC-I, 2 human reference RNA samples were evaluated, and differential gene expression levels between the 2 samples were calibrated with microarrays and other technologies (eg, qRT-PCR). The resulting microarray data sets were used for assessing the precision and cross-platform/laboratory comparability of microarrays, and allowing individual laboratories to more easily identify and correct procedural failures.[29–34] In MAQC-II, teams developed classifiers for 13 end points from 6 relatively large training data sets, and produced more than 18,000 models that were tested by independent and blinded validation sets generated for MAQC-II. In MAQC-III, also called sequencing quality control, the technical performance of next-generation sequencing platforms is being evaluated by generating benchmark data sets with reference samples and evaluating advantages and limitations of various bioinformatics strategies in RNA and DNA analyses.

METHODS FOR BIOINFORMATICS ANALYSIS OF GENE EXPRESSION

The method by which gene expression data are analyzed depends on the objectives of the analysis, which may be broadly classified as class comparison, class prediction, or class discovery, as described by Simon and colleagues.[19] A description of the statistical analytical methods is beyond the scope of this article, but has been reviewed by others.[35] Class comparison involves determining differences in expression profiles associated with a specific known clinical characteristic (eg, BRCA mutation-associated cancer) or outcome (eg, recurrence or organ-specific recurrence). The primary goal of this type of analysis is to find an informative set of genes and to estimate corresponding population parameters, such as the individual effect of increased expression in each gene on the probability of recurrence. Given the multiplicity of testing at the gene level, gene importance is inferred by ranking all of the genes measured on the array by statistical significance, summarized by the magnitude of the test statistic, corresponding P-value or adjusted P-value.[36,37] Extending the univariate approach, modeling approaches such as linear or logistic regression may be used to adjust for other genes of interest or known clinical factors such as tumor stage, age, or treatment modality. Model building must take relationships between predictors (included in and omitted from the model) into account to produce precise estimates of effect as well as valid inferences. Statistical association does not confer predictive ability; in classification, for example, a marker exhibiting an odds ratio as high as 3.0 is a poor classification tool.[38] Similar to, but distinct from class comparison, class prediction involves developing a gene expression–based algorithm that accurately predicts group membership of a particular sample. It is well understood that high correlation between predictors in the model does not preclude a good fit; therefore less emphasis is placed on the interpretability of the final model in favor of highly accurate predictions. To this end, the error rate or mean squared error is of primary importance in assessing model performance. Predictive ability is first assessed through internal cross-validation approaches.[39] However, testing the model in independent and more heterogeneous data sets is vital to properly evaluate its true predictive value.

Class comparison and prediction fall into the category of top-down approaches, in which gene expression data from cohorts with known clinical outcomes are compared with genes that are associated with prognosis without any a priori biologic assumption. After this unbiased evaluation, it has become standard to test the subset of important genes from the ranked list or model for enrichment of specific molecular pathways using tools such as Ingenuity IPA (Ingenuity Systems, Redwood City, CA, USA).[40] Alternatively, a bottom-up approach may be used, in which gene expression patterns that are associated with a specific biologic phenotype or deregulated molecular pathway are first identified and then subsequently correlated with the clinical outcome.[26] Class discovery may also be based on unsupervised statistical clustering algorithms such as hierarchical or k-means clustering. An analysis of 4 validated gene expression signatures developed either by the class discovery or bottom-up approach (intrinsic gene set, wound-response signature) or class comparison or top-down approach (70-gene assay, 21-gene assay) showed significant agreement in their outcome predictions for individual patients, suggesting that they are tracking similar biologic phenomena despite being developed by differing methodologies.[41] Although proliferation is the strongest parameter predicting clinical outcome in the ER-positive/HER2-negative subtype and the common denominator of most currently available prognostic gene signatures, immune response and tumor invasion are predominant molecular processes associated with prognosis in the triple negative and HER2-positive subgroups, respectively.[42]

VALIDITY, REPRODUCIBILITY, AND REPORTING OF MICROARRAY STUDIES

Several steps are typically involved in properly developing a gene expression signature, including identifying the signature in a training set, and then validation of the signature in other data sets. There are methods for internally cross-validating the signature in the same data set, but external validation is always necessary in other data sets. Failure to properly adhere to these fundamental principles has led some to challenge the validity and reproducibility of microarray-based studies.[43] Dupuy and Simon[44] specifically evaluated the quality of 42 microarray-based breast cancer studies published in 2004 and found that at least 50% contained at least 1 fundamental methodological flaw. The most common design flaws included inadequate control for multiple testing, a spurious claim for class discovery using outcome-related genes, and biased estimation of predictive accuracy by improper cross-validation. All of these deficiencies could potentially contribute to false discovery. The investigators proposed guidelines including dos and don'ts that are essential reading for anyone engaged in the clinical development of gene expression signatures.

Criteria have been developed for assessing and reporting tumor markers, including multiparameter assays, called the REMARK guidelines (reporting recommendations for tumor marker prognostic studies). These guidelines were developed by an expert panel to address methodological deficiencies that were commonplace in most reports evaluating tumor markers, including multiparameter gene assays on recommendation of the first meeting held in 2000 of the National Cancer Institute-European Organization for Research and Treatment of Cancer (NCI-EORTC) First International Meeting on Cancer Diagnostics. The guidelines provide relevant information about the study design, preplanned hypotheses, patient and specimen characteristics, assay methods, and statistical analysis methods. The guidelines are intended to encourage transparent and complete reporting of the relevant information for the scientific community. Most peer-reviewed journals require that reports describing tumor markers, including multiparameter assays, follow the REMARK guidelines to be considered for publication. In addition, standards termed minimal information about a microarray experiment (MIAME) for reporting the data have been established by the Microarray Gene Expression Data Society,[45] and most journals require that the gene expression data described in the publication be deposited in a publicly available database (eg, Gene Expression Omnibus (http://www.ncbi.nlm.nih.gov/geo)).

REGULATORY APPROVAL OF MULTIPARAMETER ASSAYS

Approval of multiparameter breast cancer assays had been regulated in the past under the provisions of the Clinical Laboratory Improvement Act of 1988 (CLIA), which provided the basis for approval of the Oncotype DX assay.[46] The regulations apply to laboratories that examine human specimens for the diagnosis, prevention, or treatment of any disease or assessment of health. The FDA released a guidance document in 2007 indicating that approval of multiparameter assays falls under regulatory jurisdiction of the agency under regulations governing approval of medical devices (http://www.fda.gov/MedicalDevices/DeviceRegulationandGuidance/GuidanceDocuments/ucm079163.htm#1). A gene expression profiling test system for breast cancer prognosis was defined as a device that measures the RNA expression level of multiple genes and combines this information to yield a signature (pattern or classifier or index) to aid in prognosis. Approval provided by this mechanism is commonly known as 510(k) clearance. There are currently 4 approved multiparameter assays, which are summarized in **Table 3** and described in greater detail later.

CLASSIFIERS DEVELOPED BY SUPERVISED ANALYSIS

Several classifiers have been developed by comparing gene expression profiles from relapsing versus nonrelapsing cancers, including a 70-gene profile,[47,48] 76-gene profile,[49,50] 21-gene profile,[51,52] and 2-gene HOXB13/IL17BR ratio.[53–56] The characteristics of the populations used for the external validations studies and key results are shown in **Table 4**.

70-Gene Assay

A 70-gene assay associated with prognosis was first identified in a test set of breast tumors derived from 117 women treated at the Netherlands Cancer Institute in Amsterdam.[63] RNA extracted from frozen tumor specimens was analyzed using the Rosetta Hu25K microarrays for expression of nearly 25,000 genes, and supervised classification was applied to identify a gene expression signature strongly predictive of a short interval to distant metastases (poor prognosis signature) in patients with lymph node–negative disease, and a signature that identified tumors of BRCA1 carriers. The poor prognosis signature consisted of genes regulating cell cycle, invasion, metastasis, and angiogenesis. The signature was then prospectively validated in a separate cohort of 295 consecutive patients treated at the same institution less than 53 years of age with stage I to II primary breast carcinoma associated with negative (n = 151) or positive (N = 144) axillary lymph nodes, of whom 180 (61%) had a poor prognosis signature and 115 (39%) had a good-prognosis signature.[48] The probability of remaining free of distant metastases was 51% and 85% for the high- and low-risk signatures, respectively. The estimated hazard ratio (HR) for distant metastases 5.1 (95% confidence interval [CI] 2.9–9.0) for the high- compared with the low-risk signature, which remained significant when adjusted for clinical covariates in a multivariable Cox regression analysis. The 70-gene signature subsequently was externally validated in a separate validation set consisting of 307 patients 60 years of age or less with primary breast cancers measuring 5 cm or less associated with negative axillary lymph

Table 3
Multiparameter assays for breast cancer approved by regulatory agencies

Assay (Company)	Method	Tissue Type	Approval	Patient Population	Prognosis/Prediction
Mammaprint 70-gene assay (Agendia)	DNA microarray	Fresh or frozen	Europe and United States (FDA)	ER-positive/negative stage I–II breast cancer	Prognostic for distant recurrence
Oncotype DX 21-gene assay (Genomic Health)	qRT-PCR	FFPE	Europe and United States (CLIA)	ER-positive stage I–II breast cancer	Prognostic for distant recurrence Predictive of chemotherapy benefit if RS high
Theros 2-gene ratio (Biotheranotics)	qRT-PCR	FFPE	United States (CLIA)	ER-positive, lymph node–negative breast cancer	Prognostic for distant recurrence
MapQuantDX 5-gene molecular grade (Ipsogen)	DNA microarray	Fresh or frozen	Europe	ER-positive, grade 2 tumors	Prognosis: reclassification of tumors from grade 2 to grade 1 or 3

Abbreviation: FFPE, formalin-fixed paraffin-embedded.

nodes who received no adjuvant systemic therapy, including endocrine therapy (71% had ER-positive disease).[47]

76-Gene Assay

A 76-gene assay associated with prognosis was first identified in a test set derived from 286 patients with lymph node–negative breast cancer who received no adjuvant systemic therapy treated at the Erasmus Cancer Institute in Rotterdam, the Netherlands, of whom 73% had ER-positive disease.[50] In contrast to the populations in which the 70-gene assay was validated, this analysis did include patients 60 years or older, or who had T3 to T4 tumors (only 3% for the latter). RNA extracted from frozen tumor specimens was analyzed using the Affymetrix Human U133a GeneChips for expression of 22,000 transcripts. In a training set of 115 tumors, a 76-gene signature consisting of 60 genes for ER-positive tumors and 16 genes for ER-negative tumors was identified. An external validation study was subsequently performed in 180 patients of any age with tumors less than 5 cm in diameter and negative axillary nodes who received no systemic adjuvant therapy, including endocrine therapy.[49] The HR for distant metastasis within 5 years was 7.4 (95% CI 2.6–20.9), and was 11.4 (95% CI 2.67–48.4) when adjusted for clinical covariates. For distant metastases at 5 years, the sensitivity was 90% and specificity was 50%. The positive and negative predictive values were 38% (95% CI 29%–47%) and 94% (95% CI 86%–97%), respectively.

2-Gene HOXB13/IL17BR Ratio

Ma and colleagues developed a 2-gene ratio training set which included 60 women with ER-positive breast cancer. An expression signature predictive of disease-free survival was reduced to a 2-gene ratio, HOXB13/IL17BR.[61] The investigators also evaluated the biologic function by ectopic expression of HOXB13 in MCF10A breast epithelial cells, and showed that transfection enhanced motility and invasion in vitro. High HOXB13/IL17BR ratio was subsequently evaluated in a separate validation set including 206 women with ER-positive breast cancer and was significantly associated with inferior disease-free survival (HR 2.38, 95% CI 1.30–4.36) and overall survival (HR, 2.48, 95% CI 1.22–5.06) in 130 patients with axillary lymph node–negative disease, but not in the 76 patients with lymph node–positive disease. A separate validation study was performed in 619 patients with operable ER-positive breast cancer treated with adjuvant tamoxifen, and 193 patients with metastatic breast cancer receiving first-line tamoxifen therapy for metastatic disease. An increased HOXB13/IL17BR ratio was inferior disease-free survival for node-negative patients only. For patients with metastatic disease when adjusted for clinical covariates, a high ratio was the strongest predictor in multivariate analysis for a poor response to tamoxifen therapy (odds ratio = 0.16; 95% CI 0.06–0.45) and a shorter progression-free survival (HR 2.97; 95% CI 1.82–4.86).

Genomic Grade Index

Sotiriou and colleagues[64] compared the gene expression profile of tumors associated with poor and good histologic grade, and applied the grade signature to those with intermediate grade to predict outcomes in those with an intermediate grade. Microarray data from 64 ER-positive breast cancers derived from 3 published gene expression data sets were analyzed for differential gene expression in tumors associated with a poor versus good histologic grade, which identified 97 genes that were differentially expressed, most involved in cell cycle regulation and proliferation. In an independent validation data set including 597 tumors, the gene expression grade index was strongly associated with histologic grade. However, among tumors with

Table 4
Results of pivotal validation studies for selected multiparameter markers developed by class comparison/prediction or top-down approaches

Assay and Reference	Patient Population	Treatment	No. of Patients	Key Findings
70-Gene Assay (Mammaprint)				
Van de Vijver et al[48]	Stage I–II breast cancer < 53 years	Chemo (38%), endocrine therapy (14%), or no adjuvant therapy	295	70-gene signature (good vs poor risk) prognostic for distant recurrence
Buyse et al[47]	Stage I–II breast cancer < 61 years	No adjuvant therapy	302	70-gene signature adds independent prognostic information to clinicopathologic risk assessment
76-Gene Assay				
Foekens et al[49]	Lymph node–negative	None	180	76-gene signature (good vs poor risk) prognostic for distant recurrence
21-Gene Assay (Oncotype DX)				
Paik et al[52]	ER-positive, lymph node–negative breast cancer	Tamoxifen	668	RS is prognostic for risk of distant recurrence as a categorical (low, intermediate, or high) or continuous variable
Habel et al[51]	ER-positive, lymph node–negative	Tamoxifen	790	External population-based validation study shows RS predictive of breast cancer death in tamoxifen-treated patients with ER-positive, lymph node–negative breast cancer

Paik et al[57]	ER-positive, lymph-node negative	Tamoxifen ± CMF	651	RS is predictive of benefit from adjuvant CMF chemotherapy (beneficial only if RS ≥ 31)
Goldstein et al[58]	ER-positive, 0–3 positive lymph nodes	Tamoxifen + doxorubicin and cyclophosphamide or docetaxel	465	RS is prognostic in patients treated with adjuvant endocrine therapy plus chemotherapy and provides information complementary to classic clinicopathologic features
Albain et al[59]	ER-positive, lymph node-positive and postmenopausal	Tamoxifen ± CAF	367	RS is predictive of benefit from adjuvant CAF chemotherapy (beneficial only if RS ≥ 31)
Dowsett et al[60]	ER-positive, lymph node-negative or -positive	Anastrozole versus tamoxifen ± chemotherapy	1308	RS is prognostic in anastrozole treated patients
2-Gene Ratio				
Goetz et al[61]	ER-positive, lymph node-negative or -positive	Tamoxifen	211	2-gene $HOX13/IL17B$ ratio prognostic in node-negative but not node-positive disease
Jansen et al[62]	ER-positive lymph node-negative or -positive	No adjuvant therapy	468	2-gene $HOX13/IL17B$ ratio prognostic in node-negative disease
	ER-positive metastatic disease	Tamoxifen	193	2-gene $HOX13/IL17B$ ratio associated with progression-free survival

intermediate histologic grade, the index spanned the values for histologic grade 1 to 3 tumors, and a high molecular grade gene expression grade index was associated with a higher risk of recurrence (HR 3.61, 95% CI 2.25–5.78). The 97-gene genomic grade index (GGI) was subsequently reduced to a 5-cell cycle-related genes to molecular grade index (MGI) and evaluated in 2 publicly available microarray data sets including 410 patients, followed by development of a real-time RT-PCR assay that was tested in 2 additional cohorts including 323 patients. MGI performed as consistently as the more complex 97-gene GGI.[55] In addition, the analysis showed that in patients treated with endocrine therapy, MGI and HOXB13/IL17BR modified each other's prognostic performance; high MGI was associated with significantly worse outcome only in combination with high HOXB13/IL17BR ratio, and likewise, high HOXB13/IL17BR was significantly associated with poor outcome only in combination with high MGI.

21-Gene Assay (Oncotype DX Recurrence Score)

The 21-gene assay was developed using different methods from those previously described. The assay includes 16 tumor-associated genes and 5 reference genes, with the result expressed as a computed recurrence score (RS).[52] The genes selected for incorporation in the model were derived from a panel of 250 candidate genes that was assembled by searching the published literature, genomic databases, pathway analysis, and microarray-based gene expression profiling experiments performed in fresh frozen tissue to identify genes likely to be associated with prognosis. The gene panel was tested in formalin-fixed paraffin-embedded primary tumor samples from 447 patients with breast cancer.[52,65] Genes were tested in a heterogenous group because it was hypothesized that the genes most highly correlated with recurrence would survive evaluation across diverse patients and treatments. Genes that were consistently significant across multiple studies provided the basis for developing of the RS model. The tumor-related genes included in the algorithm include genes involved in ER signaling (ESR1, PGR, BCL2, SCUBE2), proliferation (Ki67, STK15, Survivin, CCNB1, MYLB2), Her2 signaling (HER2, GRB7), invasion (MMP-11, CTSL2), and other genes involved in immune function (CD68), drug metabolism (GSTM1), and apoptosis (BAG1). Relative expression levels of the 16 genes are measured in relation to average expression levels of 5 reference genes (the latter are not included in the RS calculation). A score is generated for each gene ranging from 0 to 15, with each integer of 1 corresponding to a 2-fold increase in RNA expression level. For each of the gene groups, the mean of the values from each gene group is obtained. The mean expression value for each of the 4 gene groups plus the expression level for each of the 3 individual genes are each multiplied by a coefficient. RS is calculated using the sum of the adjusted RNA expression values for each gene group or gene. Greater relative weight is reflected by the higher coefficient values derived for the proliferation, HER2, and ER-related genes. Higher expression levels for favorable genes (ER group, GSTM1, BAG1) result in a lower RS (as a result of a negative coefficient in the algorithm), whereas higher expression of unfavorable genes (proliferation group, HER2 group, invasion group, and CD68) contribute to a higher RS (as a result of a positive coefficient in the algorithm). The analytical and operational performance specifications defined for the Oncotype DX assay allow the reporting of quantitative RS values for individual patients with a standard deviation of within 2 RS units on a 100-unit scale.[66]

Several pivotal studies have been performed evaluating the 21-gene assay, which are summarized in **Table 4**. The assay was first tested in a prospective validation study that was performed in patients with ER-positive, node-negative breast cancer who received a 5-year course of tamoxifen in the National Surgical Adjuvant Breast and Bowel Project (NSABP) trial B-14.[52,67–69] The study included 668 of 675 patients for whom tumor blocks were available and who had sufficient tumor for analysis. When evaluated as a categorical variable, the proportions of patients categorized as having an RS defined as low (<18), intermediate (18–30), or high (>31) risk by the RT-PCR assay were 51%, 22%, and 27%, respectively. The Kaplan-Meier estimates of the rates of distant recurrence at 10 years in the low-, intermediate-, and high-risk groups were 7%, 14%, and 31%, respectively. In a multivariate Cox model, RS predicted distant recurrence independent of age and tumor size, and was also predictive of overall survival. The prognostic usefulness of the 21-gene assay was subsequently validated in other data sets including patients with ER-positive disease, including a population-based study including lymph node–negative patients treated with tamoxifen,[51] lymph node–positive or –negative patients treated with adjuvant anastrozole,[60] or patients with up to 3 positive axillary nodes treated with adjuvant tamoxifen plus doxorubicin-containing chemotherapy.[58] Subsequent evaluation in other data sets indicated that high RS was associated with benefit from adjuvant cyclophosphamide, methotrexate, and 5-fluorouracil (CMF) chemotherapy in patients with ER-positive, lymph node–negative breast cancer, and from cyclophosphamide, doxorubicin, and 5-fluoroucacil (CAF) in postmenopausal patients with node-positive breast cancer.[59]

MULTIPARAMETER ASSAYS COMPARED WITH INTEGRATED CLINICAL INFORMATION

Most studies evaluating multiparameter assays have evaluated the assay in models adjusted for clinical covariates to show that the assay provides additional information beyond that provided by clinical features.[26] Some reports have described models integrating molecular and clinical data into an algorithm that is more accurate in predicting clinical outcomes than either alone.[70] Some reports have described a comparison of risk stratification predicted by the assay compared with treatment guidelines (eg, St Gallen critieria[20]), indices based on clinical factors (eg, Nottingham Prognostic Index [NPI][71]), or Adjuvant! Online (http://www.adjuvantonline.com), a web-based tool that predicts 10-year breast cancer outcomes with and without adjuvant systemic therapy that has been validated in a population-based study.[72] Patients were also assigned to the clinicopathologic low-risk group if their 10-year survival probability, as estimated by Adjuvant! software,[72] was greater than 88% for ER-positive tumors or 92% for ER-negative tumors.

Buyse and colleagues[47] evaluated the 70-gene profile in 307 patients who received no adjuvant systemic therapy. The prognostic information provided with the 70-gene profile was compared with risk categories assigned by the St Gallen criteria, NPI, or Adjuvant!. Ten-year survival estimated by Adjuvant! was defined as low risk if 92% or higher for ER-positive disease, and 88% for ER-negative disease; a lower threshold was used for ER-positive disease because it was estimated that the use of endocrine therapy would result in a 4% absolute improvement in survival at 10 years. The gene signature exhibited comparable sensitivity for distant recurrence when compared with clinical features as assessed by Adjuvant! Online (87%), NPI (79%), or St Gallen criteria (96%). On the other hand, the specificity of the high-risk signature for distant metastases (42%) appeared better than some clinical predictors, such as the St Gallen criteria (10%) or Adjuvant! Online (29%), but not others such as the NPI (48%). Other studies have shown that the 21-gene assay does not correlate with Adjuvant! Online, suggesting that the assay provides complementary information.[58,73]

CLASSIFIERS DEVELOPED BY OTHER METHODS

Several markers that have been developed by other methods are summarized in **Table 5**, including the intrinsic gene set or PAM50 developed using what would be

Table 5
Results of pivotal validation studies for selected multiparameter markers developed by other methods

Assay and Reference	Patient Population	No. of Patients	Key Findings
Intrinsic Gene Set			
Sorlie et al[74,75]	Locally advanced breast cancer (publicly available data sets previously reported by Perou and Geisler)	115	Expression pattern of 535 intrinsic genes analyzed by hierarchical clustering confirmed identification of distinct subtypes including basal-like, HER2-overexpressing, and 2 luminallike, and 1 normal breast cancer subtypes with differing response to chemotherapy and prognosis
Parker et al[70]	Stage I–II breast cancer (publicly available data sets including data sets previously reported by Loi, Wang, and Ivshima)	761	PAM50 developed in training set using panel of 10 genes to define 4 distinct breast cancer subtypes, including basal-like, HER2-enriched, luminal A, and luminal B subtypes; normal expression pattern indicative not of distinct subtype but rather insufficient tumor tissue in specimen / Breast cancer subtypes identified by PAM 50 associated with distant prognosis
Wound Expression			
Chang et al[76]	Stage I–II breast cancer (publicly available data set reported by van de Vijver)	295	Wound-response signature identified by evaluating transcriptional response to normal serum / Wound-response signature associated with an adverse prognosis
Invasive Gene Signature			
Liu et al[77]	Stage I–II breast cancer (publicly available data sets reported by van de Vijver and Wang)	581	Differential gene expression profile of CD44+CD24 −/low tumorigenic breast cancer cells compared with normal breast epithelium used to identify a 186 IGS / IGS associated with recurrence and survival

best characterized as an unsupervised method, and the wound-response signature and invasive signature developed using a bottom-up approach.

Intrinsic Breast Cancer Subtypes and PAM50

Perou and colleagues[12] first reported the intrinsic breast cancer subtypes by evaluating variation in gene expression patterns using hierarchical clustering in a set of 65 breast cancers from 42 individuals using complementary DNA microarrays representing 8102 human genes. When a panel of 534 intrinsic genes selected from the microarray were tested in other data sets, the findings were recapitulated.[74,75] It was hypothesized that these subtypes had distinctive gene expression profiles because they originated from different cell types, including luminal epithelial cells (the cells that line the duct and give rise to most breast cancers) and basal epithelial cells of the normal mammary gland (characterized by expression of cytokeratins 5/6 and 17). The intrinsic gene panel was subsequently reduced to a panel of 50 genes, using microarray and qRT-PCR, with 10 genes selected for each centroid used to define each of 4 intrinsic subtypes, including luminal A, luminal B, basal, and HER2-enriched, plus a fifth category defined as normal, which indicates a sample that had insufficient tumor material to permit accurate classification.[70,78] This assay has been referred to as the PAM50, because it was developed using the prediction analysis of microarray method, and because it include 50 genes; each tumor analyzed by this method is assigned to gene expression centroid representing the specific subtype it is most similar to. After development of the assay in a training set including 189 prototype samples, its prognostic usefulness was subsequently validated in test sets from 761 patients who received no systemic adjuvant therapy, and its predictive usefulness was validated in 133 patients for prediction of pathologic complete response (pCR) to a neoadjuvant taxane and anthracycline regimen. With regard to prognosis, the intrinsic subtypes showed prognostic significance and remained significant in multivariable analyses that incorporated clinical covariates. In addition, a prognostic model for node-negative breast cancer was developed using intrinsic subtype and clinical information; the C-index estimate for the combined model (subtype and tumor size) was significantly better than either clinicopathologic model or subtype model alone. The intrinsic subtype model predicted neoadjuvant chemotherapy efficacy with a negative predictive value for pCR of 97%.

WOUND-RESPONSE SIGNATURE

Chang and colleagues[76] hypothesized that features of the molecular program of normal wound healing might play an important role in cancer metastasis and identified consistent features in the transcriptional response of normal fibroblasts to serum, which they characterized as the wound-response signature. This signature was found to be associated with distant metastases-free survival and overall survival in a data set including 295 patients with early breast cancer. The signature was subsequently validated in separate data set and found to reliably differentiate normal and malignant breast tissue,[79] and to be significantly associated with local recurrence.[80]

INVASIVE GENE SIGNATURE

Liu and colleagues[77] hypothesized that a subpopulation of breast cancer cells exhibited greater tumorigenic capacity that could be identified by expression of high expression of CD44 with low or undetectable expression of CD24 (CD44+CD24-/low), they developed a 186-gene invasive gene signature (IGS) by comparing the gene expression profile of CD44+CD24−/low tumorigenic breast cancer cells with that of normal breast epithelium. There was a significant association between the IGS and overall and metastasis-free survival that was independent of established clinical and pathologic variables, and was more significant when combined with the wound-response signature. The IGS was also associated with the prognosis in other cancer types, including medulloblastoma and carcinoma of the lung and prostate.

PROSPECTIVE CLINICAL TRIALS EVALUATING MULTIPARAMETER ASSAYS

Two clinical trials are prospectively evaluating multiparameter assays in clinical practice.[26] In the TAILORx trial (Trial Assigning Individualized Options for Treatment), patients 75 years of age or younger with ER-positive, HER2-negative, axillary node–negative breast cancer who meet established National Comprehensive Cancer Network (NCCN) guidelines for adjuvant chemotherapy have the treatment assigned or randomized from the 21-gene assay results (NCT00310180). Patients with a low RS are directed to endocrine therapy and those with high RS are directed to chemo-endocrine therapy, whereas those with an indeterminate midrange RS (11–25) are randomized to receive chemoendocrine therapy (the standard treatment arm) or endocrine therapy alone (the experimental arm).[81] In the MINDACT trial (Microarray in Node-Negative Disease May Avoid Chemotherapy) trial (NCT00433589), patients with stage I to II breast cancer undergo risk assessment by the 70-gene assay and Adjuvant! Online and are assigned to endocrine therapy alone if genomic and clinical criteria are concordant for low-risk disease and chemoendocrine if concordant for high-risk disease; patients whose risk is discordant by genomic and clinical features are randomized to treatment assigned by clinical or genomic criteria.

Several gene expression signatures have been identified that are predictive of response to neoadjuvant chemotherapy.[23,82–84] An ongoing prospective clinical trial is evaluating whether a multiparameter is more accurate in predicting response to therapy than clinical criteria (NCT00336791).

CLINICAL USEFULNESS OF MULTIPARAMETER ASSAYS AND CONCLUSIONS

Clinical usefulness is defined by whether a marker informs clinical decision making, and whether patients benefit from that information. Two expert reviews have indicated that evidence supporting the clinical usefulness of gene expression profiles for breast cancer is insufficient.[85,86] On the other hand, expert panels convened by the American Society of Clinical Oncology (ASCO) and NCCN concluded that certain multiparameter assays such as the 21-gene assay show clinical usefulness and recommend their use in specific clinical scenarios.[14,87] These recommendations are based largely on validation studies reporting a benefit from chemotherapy in high-risk subjects as identified by multiparameter gene expression assay.[57] It is biologically plausible that high-risk populations identified by other assays might also benefit from chemotherapy, because poor-risk signatures are driven by high expression of proliferation-associated genes that predict response to chemotherapy (particularly in ER-positive, HER2-negative disease).[42]

Information provided by markers may influence clinical decision making in several ways summarized in **Table 6**, including treatment sparing, selection, direction, and confirmation. Markers have been used thus far predominantly in patients with ER-positive disease; in this clinical scenario, although the risk of recurrence is reduced by adjuvant endocrine therapy, there may be a considerable residual risk of recurrence that typically results in a recommendation for adjuvant chemotherapy according to expert-based guidelines to further reduce the risk of recurrence.[14,20] The residual risk of recurrence after endocrine therapy, and the potential benefits of adding

Influence of Marker on Treatment	Therapeutic Recommendation Based on Clinical Features	Therapeutic Recommendation Based on Molecular Markers	Clinical Usefulness/ Benefit
Table 6 Potential influence of multiparameter assay in clinical decision making			
Sparing	Yes	No	Reduce unnecessary therapy
Selection	No	Yes	Reduce recurrence risk
Direction	Uncertain	Yes or no	Provide therapeutic recommendation
Confirmation	Yes or no	Same as recommendation based on clinical features	Reinforce therapeutic recommendation
No influence	Uncertain	Uncertain	None

chemotherapy, may be estimated by using validated algorithms such as Adjuvant! Online that integrate clinicopathologic and treatment information.[72] Although adding chemotherapy reduces the risk of recurrence on average by about 25% to 30%, the absolute benefit for an individual patient is small, ranging from 1% to 5%.[69] However, many patients are willing to accept adjuvant chemotherapy even if the likelihood of benefit is small.[88] Therefore, many subjects with low-risk disease (eg, ER-positive, node-negative) are overtreated with chemotherapy, because most would have been cured with endocrine therapy alone. In treatment sparing, the clinical features indicate a need for chemotherapy, but the molecular marker is discordant by indicating a favorable prognosis without therapy, thereby resulting in sparing of adjuvant chemotherapy. In treatment selection, the clinical features indicate a favorable prognosis, but the molecular marker is discordant by indicating an unfavorable prognosis with endocrine therapy alone, thereby resulting in selection of chemotherapy in an individual for whom it otherwise would not have been recommended. In treatment direction, there is a position of therapeutic equipoise regarding a recommendation for adjuvant chemotherapy based on clinical criteria, and the marker provides direction toward a clear treatment path. Treatment confirmation occurs when a marker confirms a therapeutic recommendation that was made on clinical features alone, which may be of intangible value to the patient and the clinician. However, only treatment sparing and selection, and arguably treatment direction, seem to meet the definition of demonstrable clinical usefulness. It has also been clearly established that equipoise or uncertainty may remain even after the results of a molecular marker are available. Several reports have indicated that application of the 21-gene assay or the 70-gene assay results in a change in therapeutic recommendations in approximately 20% to 25% of patients, usually in the direction of treatment sparing.[89–91]

Although these principles currently apply primarily to the use of multiparameter markers for providing a recommendation for adjuvant chemotherapy recommendation, particularly in ER-positive disease, these same principles could be applied to in other scenarios. For example, specific signatures have been identified for organ-specific recurrence, including recurrence in bones,[92] lungs,[93] and brain[94] These signatures may be useful for selecting individuals most likely to benefit from organ-specific therapies, such as bisphosphonates to prevent bone metastases,[95] or for specific therapies more likely to penetrate the blood-brain barrier.[96] Other potential applications include identification of cancers that may need no additional local or systemic therapy after diagnostic biopsy, locally therapeutic excision, or ablation.[97]

REFERENCES

1. Hede K. Superhighway or blind alley? The cancer genome atlas releases first results. J Natl Cancer Inst 2008;100:1566.
2. Wood LD, Parsons DW, Jones S, et al. The genomic landscapes of human breast and colorectal cancers. Science 2007;318:1108.
3. Stephens PJ, McBride DJ, Lin ML, et al. Complex landscapes of somatic rearrangement in human breast cancer genomes. Nature 2009;462:1005.
4. Joensuu H, Roberts PJ, Sarlomo-Rikala M, et al. Effect of the tyrosine kinase inhibitor STI571 in a patient with a metastatic gastrointestinal stromal tumor. N Engl J Med 2001;344:1052.
5. Hatchwell E, Greally JM. The potential role of epigenomic dysregulation in complex human disease. Trends Genet 2007;23:588.
6. Thompson RF, Suzuki M, Lau KW, et al. A pipeline for the quantitative analysis of CG dinucleotide methylation using mass spectrometry. Bioinformatics 2009;25:2164.
7. Iorio MV, Casalini P, Tagliabue E, et al. MicroRNA profiling as a tool to understand prognosis, therapy response and resistance in breast cancer. Eur J Cancer 2008;44:2753.
8. Gast MC, Schellens JH, Beijnen JH. Clinical proteomics in breast cancer: a review. Breast Cancer Res Treat 2009;116:17.
9. Figueroa ME, Reimers M, Thompson RF, et al. An integrative genomic and epigenomic approach for the study of transcriptional regulation. PLoS One 2008;3:e1882.
10. Hanash S. Integrated global profiling of cancer. Nat Rev Cancer 2004;4:638.
11. Simon R. Diagnostic and prognostic prediction using gene expression profiles in high-dimensional microarray data. Br J Cancer 2003;89:1599.
12. Perou CM, Sorlie T, Eisen MB, et al. Molecular portraits of human breast tumours. Nature 2000;406:747.
13. Freidlin B, Jiang W, Simon R. The cross-validated adaptive signature design. Clin Cancer Res 2010;16:691-8.
14. Harris L, Fritsche H, Mennel R, et al. American Society of Clinical Oncology 2007 update of recommendations for the use of tumor markers in breast cancer. J Clin Oncol 2007;25:5287.
15. Hayes DF, Bast RC, Desch CE, et al. Tumor marker utility grading system: a framework to evaluate clinical utility of tumor markers. J Natl Cancer Inst 1996;88:1456.
16. Dobbin K, Simon R. Sample size determination in microarray experiments for class comparison and prognostic classification. Biostatistics 2005;6:27.
17. Dobbin KK, Simon RM. Sample size planning for developing classifiers using high dimensional DNA microarray data. Biostatistics 2007;8:101-7.
18. Ransohoff DF. Rules of evidence for cancer molecular-marker discovery and validation. Nat Rev Cancer 2004;4:309.
19. Simon R, Radmacher MD, Dobbin K, et al. Pitfalls in the use of DNA microarray data for diagnostic and prognostic classification. J Natl Cancer Inst 2003;95:14.
20. Goldhirsch A, Ingle JN, Gelber RD, et al. Thresholds for therapies: highlights of the St Gallen International Expert Consensus on the primary therapy of early breast cancer 2009. Ann Oncol 2009;20:1319.

21. Sargent DJ, Conley BA, Allegra C, et al. Clinical trial designs for predictive marker validation in cancer treatment trials. J Clin Oncol 2005;23:2020.

22. Popovici V, Chen W, Gallas BG, et al. Effect of training sample size and classification difficulty on the accuracy of genomic predictors. Breast Cancer Res 2010; 112:R5.

23. Hess KR, Anderson K, Symmans WF, et al. Pharmacogenomic predictor of sensitivity to preoperative chemotherapy with paclitaxel and fluorouracil, doxorubicin, and cyclophosphamide in breast cancer. J Clin Oncol 2006;24:4236.

24. Shak S, Baehner FL, Palmer G, et al. Relationship between proliferation genes and expression of hormone and growth factor receptors: quantitative RT-PCR in 10,618 breast cancers [abstract 6111]. Breast Cancer Res Treat 2006;100(Suppl 1).

25. Quackenbush J. Microarray analysis and tumor classification. N Engl J Med 2006;354:2463.

26. Sotiriou C, Pusztai L. Gene-expression signatures in breast cancer. N Engl J Med 2009;360:790.

27. Levin JZ, Berger MF, Adiconis X, et al. Targeted next-generation sequencing of a cancer transcriptome enhances detection of sequence variants and novel fusion transcripts. Genome Biol 2009;10:R115.

28. Maher CA, Palanisamy N, Brenner JC, et al. Chimeric transcript discovery by paired-end transcriptome sequencing. Proc Natl Acad Sci U S A 2009;106: 12353.

29. Canales RD, Luo Y, Willey JC, et al. Evaluation of DNA microarray results with quantitative gene expression platforms. Nat Biotechnol 2006;24:1115.

30. Guo L, Lobenhofer EK, Wang C, et al. Rat toxicogenomic study reveals analytical consistency across microarray platforms. Nat Biotechnol 2006;24:1162.

31. Patterson TA, Lobenhofer EK, Fulmer-Smentek SB, et al. Performance comparison of one-color and two-color platforms within the MicroArray Quality Control (MAQC) project. Nat Biotechnol 2006;24:1140.

32. Shi L, Reid LH, Jones WD, et al. The microarray quality control (MAQC) project shows inter- and intraplatform reproducibility of gene expression measurements. Nat Biotechnol 2006;24:1151.

33. Shippy R, Fulmer-Smentek S, Jensen RV, et al. Using RNA sample titrations to assess microarray platform performance and normalization techniques. Nat Biotechnol 2006;24:1123.

34. Tong W, Lucas AB, Shippy R, et al. Evaluation of external RNA controls for the assessment of microarray performance. Nat Biotechnol 2006;24:1132.

35. Asyali MH, Colak D, Demirkaya O, et al. Gene expression profile cllassification: a review. Curr Bioinform 2006;1:55.

36. Benjamini Y, Hochberg Y. Controlling the false discovery rate: a practical and powerful approach to multiple testing. J R Stat Soc Ser A 1995;B57:289.

37. Storey JD, Tibshirani R. Statistical significance for genomewide studies. Proc Natl Acad Sci U S A 2003;100:9440.

38. Pepe MS, Janes H, Longton G, et al. Limitations of the odds ratio in gauging the performance of a diagnostic, prognostic, or screening marker. Am J Epidemiol 2004;159:882.

39. Molinaro AM, Simon R, Pfeiffer RM. Prediction error estimation: a comparison of resampling methods. Bioinformatics 2005;21:3301.

40. Ingenuity® Systems, Redwood City, CA, USA. Available at: http://www.ingenuity.com. Accessed March 27, 2010.

41. Fan C, Oh DS, Wessels L, et al. Concordance among gene-expression-based predictors for breast cancer. N Engl J Med 2006;355:560.

42. Desmedt C, Haibe-Kains B, Wirapati P, et al. Biological processes associated with breast cancer clinical outcome depend on the molecular subtypes. Clin Cancer Res 2008;14:5158.
43. Marshall E. Getting the noise out of gene arrays. Science 2004;306:630.
44. Dupuy A, Simon RM. Critical review of published microarray studies for cancer outcome and guidelines on statistical analysis and reporting. J Natl Cancer Inst 2007;99:147–57.
45. Ball CA, Sherlock G, Parkinson H, et al. Standards for microarray data. Science 2002;298:539.
46. Medicare, Medicaid and CLIA programs; regulations implementing the Clinical Laboratory Improvement Amendments of 1988 (CLIA)–HCFA. Final rule with comment period. Fed Regist 1992;57:7002.
47. Buyse M, Loi S, van't Veer L, et al. Validation and clinical utility of a 70-gene prognostic signature for women with node-negative breast cancer. J Natl Cancer Inst 2006;98:1183.
48. van de Vijver MJ, He YD, van't Veer LJ, et al. A gene-expression signature as a predictor of survival in breast cancer. N Engl J Med 2002;347:1999.
49. Foekens JA, Atkins D, Zhang Y, et al. Multicenter validation of a gene expression-based prognostic signature in lymph node-negative primary breast cancer. J Clin Oncol 2006;24:1665.
50. Wang Y, Klijn JG, Zhang Y, et al. Gene-expression profiles to predict distant metastasis of lymph-node-negative primary breast cancer. Lancet 2005;365:671.
51. Habel LA, Shak S, Jacobs MK, et al. A population-based study of tumor gene expression and risk of breast cancer death among lymph node-negative patients. Breast Cancer Res 2006;8:R25.
52. Paik S, Shak S, Tang G, et al. A multigene assay to predict recurrence of tamoxifen-treated, node-negative breast cancer. N Engl J Med 2004;351:2817.
53. Jerevall PL, Brommesson S, Strand C, et al. Exploring the two-gene ratio in breast cancer–independent roles for HOXB13 and IL17BR in prediction of clinical outcome. Breast Cancer Res Treat 2008;107:225.
54. Ma XJ, Hilsenbeck SG, Wang W, et al. The HOXB13:IL17BR expression index is a prognostic factor in early-stage breast cancer. J Clin Oncol 2006;24:4611.
55. Ma XJ, Salunga R, Dahiya S, et al. A five-gene molecular grade index and HOXB13:IL17BR are complementary prognostic factors in early stage breast cancer. Clin Cancer Res 2008;14:2601.
56. Ma XJ, Wang Z, Ryan PD, et al. A two-gene expression ratio predicts clinical outcome in breast cancer patients treated with tamoxifen. Cancer Cell 2004;5:607.
57. Paik S, Tang G, Shak S, et al. Gene expression and benefit of chemotherapy in women with node-negative, estrogen receptor-positive breast cancer. J Clin Oncol 2006;24:3726.
58. Goldstein LJ, Gray R, Badve S, et al. Prognostic utility of the 21-gene assay in hormone receptor-positive operable breast cancer compared with classical clinicopathologic features. J Clin Oncol 2008;26:4063.
59. Albain KS, Barlow WE, Shak S, et al. Prognostic and predictive value of the 21-gene recurrence score assay in postmenopausal women with node-positive, oestrogen-receptor-positive breast cancer on chemotherapy: a retrospective analysis of a randomised trial. Lancet Oncol 2010;11:55–65.
60. Dowsett M, Cuzick J, Wales C, et al. Prediction of risk of distant recurrence using the 21-gene recurrence score in node-negative and node-positive postmenopausal patients with breast cancer treated with anastrozole or tamoxifen: a TransATAC study. J Clin Oncol 2010;28:1829–34.

61. Goetz MP, Suman VJ, Ingle JN, et al. A two-gene expression ratio of homeobox 13 and interleukin-17B receptor for prediction of recurrence and survival in women receiving adjuvant tamoxifen. Clin Cancer Res 2006;12:2080.
62. Jansen MP, Sieuwerts AM, Look MP, et al. HOXB13-to-IL17BR expression ratio is related with tumor aggressiveness and response to tamoxifen of recurrent breast cancer: a retrospective study. J Clin Oncol 2007;25:662.
63. van't Veer LJ, Dai H, van de Vijver MJ, et al. Gene expression profiling predicts clinical outcome of breast cancer. Nature 2002;415:530.
64. Sotiriou C, Wirapati P, Loi S, et al. Gene expression profiling in breast cancer: understanding the molecular basis of histologic grade to improve prognosis. J Natl Cancer Inst 2006;98:262.
65. Cobleigh MA, Tabesh B, Bitterman P, et al. Tumor gene expression and prognosis in breast cancer patients with 10 or more positive lymph nodes. Clin Cancer Res 2005;11:8623.
66. Cronin M, Sangli C, Liu ML, et al. Analytical validation of the oncotype DX genomic diagnostic test for recurrence prognosis and therapeutic response prediction in node-negative, estrogen receptor-positive breast cancer. Clin Chem 2007;53:1084.
67. Fisher B, Costantino J, Redmond C, et al. A randomized clinical trial evaluating tamoxifen in the treatment of patients with node-negative breast cancer who have estrogen-receptor-positive tumors. N Engl J Med 1989;320:479.
68. Fisher B, Jeong JH, Bryant J, et al. Treatment of lymph-node-negative, oestrogen-receptor-positive breast cancer: long-term findings from National Surgical Adjuvant Breast and Bowel Project randomised clinical trials. Lancet 2004;364:858.
69. Fisher B, Jeong JH, Dignam J, et al. Findings from recent National Surgical Adjuvant Breast and Bowel Project adjuvant studies in stage I breast cancer. J Natl Cancer Inst Monogr 2001;30:62–6.
70. Parker JS, Mullins M, Cheang MC, et al. Supervised risk predictor of breast cancer based on intrinsic subtypes. J Clin Oncol 2009;27:1160.
71. Balslev I, Axelsson CK, Zedeler K, et al. The Nottingham prognostic index applied to 9,149 patients from the studies of the Danish Breast Cancer Cooperative Group (DBCG). Breast Cancer Res Treat 1994;32:281.
72. Olivotto IA, Bajdik CD, Ravdin PM, et al. Population-based validation of the prognostic model ADJUVANT! for early breast cancer. J Clin Oncol 2005;23:2716.
73. Bryant J. Oncotype DX correlates more closely with prognosis than adjuvant online. 9th International Conference: Primary therapy of early breast cancer. St Gallen (Switzerland), January 25–28, 2005.
74. Sorlie T, Perou CM, Tibshirani R, et al. Gene expression patterns of breast carcinomas distinguish tumor subclasses with clinical implications. Proc Natl Acad Sci U S A 2001;98:10869.
75. Sorlie T, Tibshirani R, Parker J, et al. Repeated observation of breast tumor subtypes in independent gene expression data sets. Proc Natl Acad Sci U S A 2003;100:8418.
76. Chang HY, Nuyten DS, Sneddon JB, et al. Robustness, scalability, and integration of a wound-response gene expression signature in predicting breast cancer survival. Proc Natl Acad Sci U S A 2005;102:3738.
77. Liu R, Wang X, Chen GY, et al. The prognostic role of a gene signature from tumorigenic breast-cancer cells. N Engl J Med 2007;356:217.
78. Cheang MC, Voduc D, Bajdik C, et al. Basal-like breast cancer defined by five biomarkers has superior prognostic value than triple-negative phenotype. Clin Cancer Res 2008;14:1368.

79. Troester MA, Lee MH, Carter M, et al. Activation of host wound responses in breast cancer microenvironment. Clin Cancer Res 2009;15:7020.
80. Nuyten DS, Kreike B, Hart AA, et al. Predicting a local recurrence after breast-conserving therapy by gene expression profiling. Breast Cancer Res 2006;8:R62.
81. Sparano JA. TAILORx: trial assigning individualized options for treatment (Rx). Clin Breast Cancer 2006;7:347.
82. Chang JC, Wooten EC, Tsimelzon A, et al. Gene expression profiling for the prediction of therapeutic response to docetaxel in patients with breast cancer. Lancet 2003;362:362.
83. Cleator S, Tsimelzon A, Ashworth A, et al. Gene expression patterns for doxorubicin (adriamycin) and cyclophosphamide (cytoxan) (AC) response and resistance. Breast Cancer Res Treat 2006;95:229.
84. Gianni L, Zambetti M, Clark K, et al. Gene expression profiles in paraffin-embedded core biopsy tissue predict response to chemotherapy in women with locally advanced breast cancer. J Clin Oncol 2005;23:7265.
85. Recommendations from the EGAPP Working Group: can tumor gene expression profiling improve outcomes in patients with breast cancer? Genet Med 2009;11:66.
86. Marchionni L, Wilson RF, Wolff AC, et al. Systematic review: gene expression profiling assays in early-stage breast cancer. Ann Intern Med 2008;148:358.
87. Carlson RW, Allred DC, Anderson BO, et al. Breast cancer. Clinical practice guidelines in oncology. J Natl Compr Canc Netw 2009;7:122.
88. Simes RJ, Coates AS. Patient preferences for adjuvant chemotherapy of early breast cancer: how much benefit is needed? J Natl Cancer Inst Monogr 2001;30:146–52.
89. Bueno-de-Mesquita JM, van Harten WH, Retel VP, et al. Use of 70-gene signature to predict prognosis of patients with node-negative breast cancer: a prospective community-based feasibility study (RASTER). Lancet Oncol 2007;8:1079.
90. Lo SS, Mumby PB, Norton J. Prospective multicenter study of the impact of the 21-gene recurrence score assay on medical oncologist and patient adjuvant breast cancer treatment selection. Biostatistics 2010;28:1671–6.
91. Sparano JA, Solin LJ. Defining the clinical utility of gene expression assays in breast cancer: the intersection of science and art in clinical decision making. J Clin Oncol 2010;10:1625–7.
92. Smid M, Wang Y, Klijn JG, et al. Genes associated with breast cancer metastatic to bone. J Clin Oncol 2006;24:2261.
93. Landemaine T, Jackson A, Bellahcene A, et al. A six-gene signature predicting breast cancer lung metastasis. Cancer Res 2008;68:6092.
94. Bos PD, Zhang XH, Nadal C, et al. Genes that mediate breast cancer metastasis to the brain. Nature 2009;459:1005.
95. Gnant M, Mlineritsch B, Schippinger W, et al. Endocrine therapy plus zoledronic acid in premenopausal breast cancer. N Engl J Med 2009;360:679.
96. Geyer CE, Forster J, Lindquist D, et al. Lapatinib plus capecitabine for HER2-positive advanced breast cancer. N Engl J Med 2006;355:2733.
97. Zahl PH, Maehlen J, Welch HG. The natural history of invasive breast cancers detected by screening mammography. Arch Intern Med 2008;168:2311.

Neoadjuvant Chemotherapy for Operable Breast Cancer: Individualizing Locoregional and Systemic Therapy

Harry D. Bear, MD, PhD

KEYWORDS

- Breast cancer • Neoadjuvant • Chemotherapy
- Breast conservation surgery • Sentinel lymph nodes

POTENTIAL BENEFITS OF NEOADJUVANT CHEMOTHERAPY FOR BREAST CANCER

Classically, neoadjuvant chemotherapy (NAC) was used only for patients with locally advanced breast cancer (LABC), corresponding approximately to American Joint Commission on Cancer stage III.[1] Once the success of downstaging those patients with chemotherapy was appreciated, similar strategies began to be used for patients with operable breast cancer but who were not ideal candidates for breast-conserving surgery (BCS). Initially, this approach was tested to determine whether primary or neoadjuvant chemotherapy might prove superior to postoperative or adjuvant therapy, but it was hoped that this also might allow BCS for women who would otherwise require mastectomy. As shown in the National Surgical Adjuvant Breast and Bowel Project's (NSABP) Protocol B-18, the former was not the case, but the latter was feasible.[2,3] In this trial, women with palpable operable breast cancer (median tumor size = 3.5 cm) diagnosed by needle biopsy were randomized to receive 4 cycles of doxorubicin (Adriamycin) + cyclophosphamide (AC) preoperatively or the same regimen postoperatively in the adjuvant setting. The breast conservation rates were 68% and 60% for the 2 groups, respectively, and the overall outcomes (disease-free survival [DFS] and overall survival [OS]) for both groups of patients were identical. These data showed that NAC could be used to increase the likelihood of BCS without

Division of Surgical Oncology, Department of Surgery, Massey Cancer Center, Virginia Commonwealth University, Box 980011, Richmond, VA 23298-0011, USA
E-mail address: hdbear@vcu.edu

Surg Oncol Clin N Am 19 (2010) 607–626
doi:10.1016/j.soc.2010.04.001
1055-3207/10/$ – see front matter © 2010 Elsevier Inc. All rights reserved.

surgonc.theclinics.com

compromising survival. The increase in BCS was even more striking in the European Cooperative Trial in Operable Breast Cancer (ECTO) trial, as shown in **Fig. 1.**[4] The BCS rate for primary surgery patients in the European study was lower than in B-18, which may reflect a greater frequency of larger tumors (80% >4 cm), as well as possible systematic differences in surgical practice. Nevertheless, other studies have confirmed the potential to increase BCS, as well as the potential to decrease the volume of tissue that needs to be removed and the need for re-excision.[5,6] The NSABP B-18 study also demonstrated a strong relationship between pathologic complete response (pCR, defined in B-18 as no invasive breast cancer cells in the breast) with NAC and patient outcomes (**Fig. 2**), which has been observed repeatedly in other series as well.[4,7–10] It has been suggested that the ability to observe responses during neoadjuvant chemotherapy treatment constitutes another potential advantage to this approach, but it is not clear how this information should be used to modify the treatment of each patient in real time. A German study designed to determine whether an early change in chemotherapy drugs would benefit patients who do not respond well to the initial regimen showed that nonresponders are unlikely to experience a pCR with either more of the same or a different cytotoxic regimen.[11] Nevertheless, even without a pCR, continuing chemotherapy may reduce tumor burden sufficiently to make inoperable cancers operable or to allow BCS. Moreover, it may be beneficial for patients to see the effects of treatment as the tumors regress, in contrast to the adjuvant setting where the benefits are hypothetical and the toxicities extremely concrete. Another advantage, albeit controversial, to neoadjuvant chemotherapy is the potential to downstage the axillary nodes and decrease the need for axillary node dissection and the risk of lymphedema. This aspect of surgical management after NAC is discussed in more detail later. The potential clinical advantages of NAC for breast cancer are

1. Increased chance for BCT
2. Improved cosmesis by removal of less tissue and fewer re-excisions
3. Decreased need for axillary node dissection
4. Time for genetic testing before surgery
5. Observation of response to treatment
6. Opportunity for discovery.

Because of the strong relationship of response (especially pCR) to patient outcomes, NAC offers a valuable research platform to test new treatment regimens

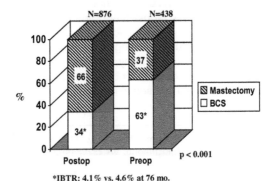

Fig. 1. BCS and mastectomy rates in women receiving postoperative adjuvant versus preoperative chemotherapy in the ECTO trial.

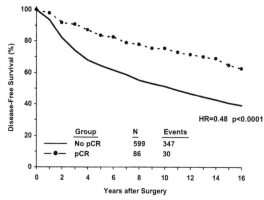

Fig. 2. Disease-free survival for patients receiving preoperative chemotherapy in NSABP Protocol B-18 who did or did not achieve a pathologic complete response (pCR) in the breast.

and agents, and to increase our understanding of breast cancer biology; these in turn will lead to truly individualized therapy based on biologic and molecular parameters.

PREDICTING RESPONSE TO NEOADJUVANT CHEMOTHERAPY

Based on these advantages, it has been suggested that anyone with a T2 or larger tumor or clinically evident or ultrasound (US)-detected lymph node involvement at presentation is a potential candidate for NAC. A less well-defined, but perhaps more practical, guideline might be that NAC should be considered for any patient in whom it is clear that adjuvant chemotherapy would be indicated. As more is learnt about breast cancer biology, this decision will be based only partly on the anatomic clinical stage and more on the pathologic and molecular features of each cancer.

Indeed, as NAC has become more widely applied, it has become evident that some patients may benefit more from NAC than others. At the simplest level, multiple studies, including the NSABP B-27 and ECTO trials, have shown that hormone-responsive breast cancers are less likely to achieve pCR than hormone receptor negative cancers.[10,12–16] In the B-27 trial, for example, estrogen receptor (ER)-positive cancers had a pCR rate of 8.3% versus 16.7% for ER-negative tumors.[12] However, both subsets of patients appeared to benefit, in terms of pCR, from the addition of a taxane to the neoadjuvant regimen. In the ECTO trial, ER was a highly significant predictor of pCR (12% for ER+ vs 42% for ER−).[17] Despite the emphasis on pCR in the literature, many patients with ER+ cancers may still benefit substantially from NAC.[18] In the B-18 trial, 80% of all patients experienced an objective clinical response to AC, and in B-27 more than 90% of patients treated with AC + docetaxel had an objective response.[2,12] In the ECTO trial, 42% of patients with ER+ tumors had a clinical complete response (cCR) compared with 60% in the ER− subset.[17] The MD Anderson experience shows that pCR is strongly predictive for outcomes in the ER+ subset.[19] Thus, a predictably low likelihood of a pCR does not mean that NAC would not be clinically useful, perhaps allowing BCS in many ER− and ER+ patients who would otherwise require a mastectomy. What might be more helpful, and could perhaps be provided by the more detailed molecular characterizations to be discussed later, would be the ability to predict which patients are unlikely to have an objective and clinically useful response to chemotherapy. These patients would then be candidates for immediate surgery, neoadjuvant hormonal therapy, or neoadjuvant treatment with novel agents.

Patients with invasive lobular cancers (ILC) have also been singled out in multiple studies as a subset who are less likely to achieve a pCR. In some studies, the pCR rate for these patients has been less than 5%, but in the in B-27 trial 10.2% of ILC patients (vs 17.5% for IDC) had a pCR.[20–25] Moreover, it has recently been suggested that NAC may not dramatically increase the likelihood of BCS in patients with lobular cancers, making this approach less advantageous.[23] Despite the low response rates compared with IDC, patients with ILC generally have better long-term outcomes.[20,21,24,26] The low chemosensitivity of ILC likely reflects the strong hormone responsiveness for most of these tumors, and the better outcomes reflect a less aggressive biology. This group of patients may benefit more from hormonal neoadjuvant therapy than from cytotoxic chemotherapy.

A clinical and histopathologic scoring system to predict the likelihood of responding well to NAC has been described.[27] Recently, molecular/genetic profiles of tumors have been shown to be potentially more precise predictors of who will or will not respond to NAC for breast cancer. Gianni and colleagues[28] showed that the 21-gene expression profile originally developed to predict outcomes for patients with node-negative ER+ cancers was highly predictive of pCR to NAC. Only patients with high recurrence scores exhibited pCR to polychemotherapy. Using clinical response as an end point, it has also been shown that recurrence score could identify patients who were most likely to have a clinical complete response to single-agent taxane therapy.[29] Many other studies have shown that some gene expression profiles that correlate with a poor prognosis (eg, HER-2 enriched and basal-like) also correlate with a high likelihood of a good response to NAC (**Fig. 3**; **Table 1**).[28–35] Conversely, these data show that tumors with profiles indicating less aggressive behavior are also less likely to respond to chemotherapy, which is probably the major reason for the imperfect relationship between pCR and patient outcomes and may also explain why doubling the pCR rate with the addition of a taxane to AC in B-27 did not lead to a significant increase in survival.[7,15] Because patients who do not have a pCR with NAC are a mixture of patients with nonaggressive tumors with a good prognosis (eg, the luminal A subset) and more aggressive tumors with a poor prognosis that are also chemoresistant, these patients have intermediate outcomes. If both subsets of chemoresistant patients could be clearly identified, the patients with good prognosis could avoid toxic therapies and the subset with poor prognosis would be candidates for trials of novel agents. A recent report combining patients from the B-27 trial, the I-SPY trial, and patients from MD Anderson, all of whom received anthracycline

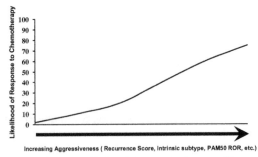

Fig. 3. Generalized graph of the correlation between various profiles or signatures of tumor aggressiveness and the likelihood of response (especially pCR) to cytotoxic chemotherapy.

Table 1
Correlations of genomic expression profiles with likelihood of pathologic complete response (pCR) with neoadjuvant chemotherapy for breast cancer

Study	(Method)/Subsets	% pCR
Esserman, ASCO 2009[33]	(21-gene score)	
	Low RS	3
	Intermediate RS	0
	High RS	36
Parker, SABCS 2009[35]	(PAM 50)	
	Luminal A	7
	Luminal B	17
	HER-2	36
	Basal-like	43
	Normal-like	19
Straver[34]	(70-gene signature [Mammaprint])	
	Good signature	0
	Poor signature	20
Chang, 2008[29]	21-gene score	
	Low RS	0[a]
	High RS	21[a]
Liedtke, 2009[32]	97-gene genomic grade index	
	High risk	12[b]
	Low risk	40[b]

Abbreviation: RS, recurrence score.
[a] Clinical complete responses.
[b] pCR + Residual Cancer Burden Class 1.
Data from Symmans WF, Peintinger F, Hatzis C, et al. Measurement of residual breast cancer burden to predict survival after neoadjuvant chemotherapy. J Clin Oncol 2007;25(28):4414–22.

+ taxane NAC, suggests that the luminal B subset responds poorly to chemotherapy and has a poor prognosis.[35] As suggested earlier, rather than focusing on pCR, it may be more important to understand which patients may not benefit clinically from NAC (eg, by increasing the chance for BCS) or from adjuvant chemotherapy. Such patients may benefit more from hormonal therapy or new biologic agents and might avoid chemotherapy altogether. Although it is not yet standard to perform a molecular/genetic assessment of breast cancers from core needle biopsy material before making a decision about neoadjuvant treatment, we are certainly heading in that direction. One of the major goals of the current NSABP B-40 trial is to gather data that will inform that course.

CHEMOTHERAPY VERSUS HORMONAL THERAPY

As noted earlier, there are emerging data suggesting that certain subsets of tumors, especially among those that are ER+ and/or PR+, may not respond well or in a clinically useful way to chemotherapy. For example, in the I-SPY trial, only 5% of luminal A tumors had a pCR to chemotherapy.[33] As recently reviewed, aromatase inhibitors seem to be superior to tamoxifen as neoadjuvant therapy for postmenopausal women with hormone-responsive tumors.[36–40] Aromatase inhibitors as neoajduvant treatment of such women have been shown to be at least as effective as, if not superior to, chemotherapy in terms of clinical responses and conversion to BCS.[41,42] However, pCR rates are consistently low for hormonal neoadjuvant therapy. As increasingly sophisticated molecular predictors of response to neoadjuvant chemotherapy or hormonal therapy are developed, we will be better able to choose among these alternative approaches for individual patients. Recently it has been proposed that early molecular assessments of response to hormonal therapy based on re-biopsy after 2 to 4 weeks of treatment may be a useful tool for deciding whether to continue hormonal therapy or switch to chemotherapy.[43] This concept is being tested directly in the ongoing American College of Surgeons Oncology Group (ACOSOG) Z1031B trial (**Fig. 4**). There are also subsets of patients, based on age and comorbidities, who may not be appropriate candidates for cytotoxic chemotherapy, but who may benefit from neoadjuvant hormonal therapy.

PRE-THERAPY ASSESSMENT AND STAGING

Once the decision has been made to treat a patient with breast cancer with NAC, several studies in addition to those that are routine (mammograms, routine laboratory tests, and so forth) should be performed. Although controversial as a standard study for all breast cancers, magnetic resonance imaging (MRI) of the breasts is particularly valuable for NAC patients.[44–48] MRI provides information about the extent of the known cancer, possible multicentric disease, axillary and internal mammary nodes, and serves as a baseline for evaluation of the primary tumor and nodal response to treatment. It has also been suggested that the appearance of the breast primary on MRI may be predictive of the likelihood of response to NAC.[49,50] For patients with LABC (stage III), evaluation for metastatic disease would be appropriate. It is also valuable to examine the axilla by US and to perform a biopsy on any suspicious-appearing nodes before starting treatment. This will provide important information that may influence lymph node surgery and/or radiation decisions later.

If the patient is being considered for BCS, it is critically important that the primary tumor site be tagged so that the appropriate area is excised at definitive surgery. At the completion of therapy, many palpable tumors will no longer be clinically or even mammographically detectable (**Fig. 5**), and the clip can be targeted preoperatively

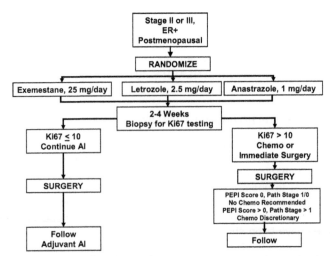

Fig. 4. The ACOSOG Protocol Z1031, Cohort B. PEPI, preoperative endocrine prognostic index, reflecting pT stage, pN stage, Ki67 level, and estrogen receptor status (Allred score).

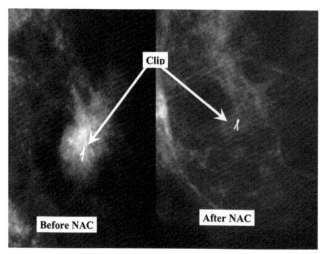

Fig. 5. Mammographic images of a breast cancer before and after NAC, showing the clip placed before the start of treatment on the left and the disappearance of all evidence of tumor, other than the clip, after treatment on the right.

with a localizing wire or by intraoperative US. In some centers, a radiographically guided clip is placed only if the tumor shows evidence of rapid regression, but it is our routine to place a clip in all of these tumors before starting therapy to avoid missing the opportunity to do so mid-therapy.[51] Placement of clips in patients receiving NAC has even been shown to improve local control after BCS.[51] Even if a total mastectomy is planned at the time of presentation, the clip can be helpful to the pathologist who examines the resection specimen, because the primary tumor site may become difficult to identify grossly. Moreover, some patients and/or their surgeons may change their minds about the surgical plan. In addition, we routinely tattoo the skin overlying the margins of the palpable tumor mass in the breast (usually at the time of venous access placement in the operating room), even if the patient has had a clip placed in the tumor (**Fig. 6**). This marking is a valuable aid to the ongoing clinical evaluation of the tumor response during therapy and helps to plan surgery, often making wire localization of the tumor site unnecessary.[52]

OPTIMAL CHEMOTHERAPY REGIMEN

Space does not allow a detailed review of the different chemotherapy regimens that can be used in the neoadjuvant setting for operable breast cancers. A recent expert consensus panel concluded that for most patients, regimens that combine anthracycline and taxane therapy, either concurrently or sequentially, have the greatest likelihood of a good clinical and pathologic response, and that the duration of therapy should extend to 4 to 6 months.[15,53–57] Indeed, recent trials have demonstrated that a longer duration of therapy is superior to a shorter duration with the same drugs.[58,59] However, this does not extend indefinitely, as demonstrated in the GeparTrio trial, which showed that 8 cycles of TAC were not better than 6 in patients who responded to the initial 2 cycles.[60] This trial also demonstrated that switching chemotherapy to a different combination of cytotoxic drugs did not improve the chances of a pCR in patients who did not respond to the first 2 cycles of TAC.[11] In other words, chemotherapy nonresponders are not likely to respond to different chemotherapy; some other novel form of therapy is needed. As noted recently at the 2009 San Antonio

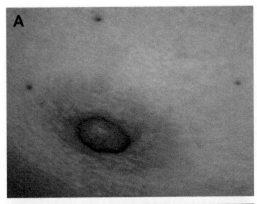

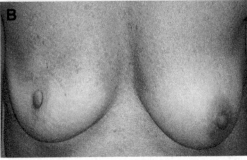

Fig. 6. (*A*) A patient with a large upper central breast cancer before NAC, with tattoos marking the upper, medial, and lateral extent of the palpable tumor; the lower edge of the tumor extended to the nipple. (*B*) The same patient 5 years after completion of NAC, surgery, and radiation. (*Adapted from* Bear HD, Preoperative chemotherapy for operable breast cancer: lessons from a patient and a randomized trial. Am J Oncol Rev 2004;3(4):194; with permission.)

Breast Symposium, the choice of regimens to be used in the neoadjuvant setting should be based on data from that setting and it is not an appropriate venue to practice creative oncology.[61]

Tumors that over express HER-2 are more likely to respond to cytotoxic chemotherapy and the addition of taxanes than HER-2-normal tumors.[13,62–65] Beyond this, however, the available data, albeit from a limited number of randomized patients, suggest that the addition of trastuzumab to chemotherapy significantly increases the likelihood of a pCR for tumors that have amplified HER-2.[66–68] Ongoing trials (NSABP B-41 and Neo-ALLTO) seek to determine whether the tyrosine kinase inhibitor lapatanib or lapatanib + trastuzumab combined with neoadjuvant chemotherapy will be superior to trastuzumab. Recently, it has been suggested that breast cancers arising in women with inherited BRCA1 mutations may have high rates of pCR with platinum-based regimens.[69]

ASSESSING RESPONSE TO NEOADJUVANT CHEMOTHERAPY

One of the more difficult tasks associated with the use of NAC for breast cancer is the assessment of the tumor response during and at the completion of treatment. Clinical examination has been used in several studies, but suffers from a lack of reproducibility, especially when different examiners are involved. The German neoadjuvant trials have depended on US examination of the breast to assess changes in tumor size more accurately.[60] Recently, there has been a great deal of interest in the use of MRI or positron emission tomography (PET) scans early in the planned treatment course to determine whether the tumor is responding and to predict the ultimate response to therapy.[44,47,48,70–72] We have started evaluating the use of PET scanning based on uptake of ^{18}F-labeled thymidine as a measure of breast tumor responses to NAC, and this trial has been expanded to multiple centers. Scans are being obtained at baseline, soon after the first dose of chemotherapy, and at the end of treatment before surgery. The results of these scans will be correlated with measures of tumor cell proliferation, such as Ki67, and with pCR. As noted earlier for hormonal therapy, re-biopsy of the primary tumor and molecular characterization of the tumor may also be a useful way to assess responses. The value of being able to identify responders and nonresponders early after the initiation of treatment rests on the potential to cease treatment that is likely to be futile in favor of other forms of therapy.

Assessment of the final tumor response by imaging may not be as valuable for determining whether the therapy has been successful, because all the treatment has been given already, and pathologic analysis will be more accurate. Nevertheless, accurate imaging evaluation of residual tumor at the end of NAC could be useful for surgical planning. Assuming that chemotherapy has resulted in an objective clinical response, which should occur in 90% or more of all patients with initially operable breast cancer, it may then be quite challenging to determine the appropriate extent of resection to remove the residual cancer and minimize the risk of local recurrence.[12] The patterns of regression can be variable, ranging from no residual tumor to concentric shrinkage or multifocal residual cancer occupying the original tumor volume (so-called cookie-crumble pattern), as illustrated in **Fig. 7**. At present, MRI seems to be the most accurate method for measuring residual disease before surgery and for planning BCS.[44,47,48] Nevertheless, because contrast-enhanced MRI depends to a large extent on vascularity, interpretation can be difficult. Nonvascularized tumor masses may or may not be viable (**Fig. 8**), and MRI imaging may miss the presence of microscopic foci of cancer, especially after a cookie-crumble pattern of response.[71] Currently there is no method reliable enough for determining the absence of cancer (invasive and noninvasive) on which to base omission of surgery after NAC.

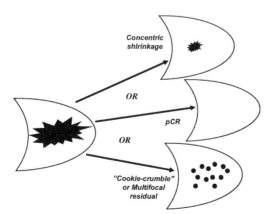

Fig. 7. Cartoon depicting different potential patterns of response of a breast cancer to NAC. *Abbreviation:* pCR, pathologic complete response. (*Adapted from* Bear HD. Preoperative chemotherapy for operable breast cancer: lessons from a patient and a randomized trial. Am J Oncol Rev 2004;3(4):196; with permission.)

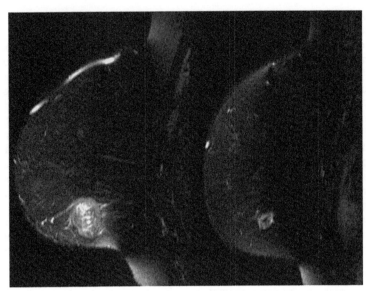

Fig. 8. MRI of a triple-negative breast cancer before (*left*) and after (*right*) neoadjuvant chemotherapy. After treatment, the residual tumor mass had minimal contrast enhancement, and pathology on the excision specimen showed a necrotic tumor with no viable cancer cells seen.

Even the pathologic assessment of residual disease can be based on variable criteria, and several different grading schema have been proposed. Perhaps the most widely used criteria for pCR are the absence of invasive tumor in the breast, either as a stand-alone end point or combined with the absence of cancer in the regional lymph nodes.[10,54,73] An index of residual cancer burden was recently described by Symmans and colleagues[8] based on features of the primary tumor site and lymph nodes. This index categorizes patients into 5 groups (0–4) that correlate with the long-term risk of metastatic disease. Aside from its potential for prognostic classification of patients, it also demonstrates that the relationship of pathologic response to outcomes is not all or none, with only pCR patients having a relatively good prognosis.

RESECTION OF THE PRIMARY TUMOR: BREAST CONSERVATION VERSUS MASTECTOMY

It is easy to appreciate that the type of response can profoundly influence the likelihood of obtaining a negative margin with BCS and the risk of ipsilateral breast tumor recurrence (IBTR). Unfortunately, as noted earlier, there are no highly reliable clinical or radiographic methods for assessing the extent and type of response accurately. A scoring system, based on clinical nodal stage, residual pathologic tumor size, lymphovascular invasion, and multifocal pattern of residual cancer has been proposed to categorize NAC patients's risk of local recurrence.[18] Patients with a score of 3 to 4 on this scale had a high risk of locoregional recurrence. Fortunately, only a small minority of patients were in this subset. However, 3 of the 4 parameters in this suggested scoring system are not available until after definitive surgery, making it of questionable value for deciding which patients are candidates for BCS. The surgeon should not resect the volume of tissue that would originally have been required before NAC, as this would defeat the purpose of treatment. Although it may someday be possible to omit surgery in a subset of patients who respond well to NAC, there is no reliable method for determining which patients have had a pCR before surgery. At present, surgical resection should not be omitted, because this may lead to unacceptably high rates of local recurrence.[74,75] It has been suggested that resection should extend to the original margins of the pretreatment tumor.[52] The simplest practical guide is that as much tissue around the original tumor site should be excised as is consistent with good cosmesis and a negative margin. This, combined with oncoplastic techniques when appropriate, will minimize the risk of IBTR and optimize the cosmetic outcomes.

MANAGEMENT OF REGIONAL LYMPH NODES IN PATIENTS TREATED WITH NCT

Although sentinel lymph node biopsy (SLNB) has largely replaced complete axillary node dissection for women with clinically negative lymph nodes undergoing primary surgery for breast cancer, the role and timing of SLNB in women who are treated with primary systemic therapy is highly controversial. Widely consulted guidelines suggest that NAC is a contraindication to the use of SLNB for staging of the regional lymph nodes.[76,77] Some have advocated pretreatment SLNB for patients with clinically and US-negative nodes.[76,78–87] If positive nodes are identified by any method before treatment, then most of these same investigators recommend completion axillary lymph node dissection (ALND) as part of definitive surgery after systemic treatment.[47,79,83,88] The arguments in favor of this approach are based on several concerns. First, there is a perceived need to determine the initial pathologic nodal stage of each patient before treatment. Second, there is concern that changes in the axillary nodes and lymphatics induced by chemotherapy will make SLNB either unsuccessful or inaccurate. Of particular concern has been the possibility of uneven regression of tumor in lymph nodes, with sentinel nodes becoming negative and other nodes remaining positive. These might lead to false-negative results, resulting in under staging of the patient after chemotherapy, increasing the risk of regional recurrence, and omission of beneficial regional irradiation.

However, one of the potential advantages to the use of NAC is that the morbidity of ALND may be avoided in a significant fraction of patients. By extrapolation from the NSABP B-18 and B-27 trials, it is likely that chemotherapy with anthracycline + taxane regimens could eliminate the need for ALND in more than 40% of initially node-positive patients.[2,12] As pathologic response rates increase further with the addition of targeted agents, the potential number of patients who might avoid ALND may increase. For example, in a group of 109 patients with HER-2+ cancers and biopsy-proven node metastases who received trastuzumab + chemotherapy preoperatively, 74% had negative nodes at the time of surgery.[89] Available clinical data suggest that SLNB after NAC is likely to be successful and accurate.[90–93] In the NSABP B-27 trial, SLNB was attempted in 428 patients and was successful in 343 (85%).[90] Although this seems low, it must be remembered that these patients had sentinel lymph node mapping performed ad hoc, with no mandated method (many with blue dye alone) and many were early on the learning curves for the surgeons involved. Furthermore, failure to map should not really be an issue of major concern, because this should lead to a full ALND, which opponents of SLNB in this setting propose anyway. False-negatives, on the other hand, are more worrisome, as these would lead to under staging and potentially leaving tumor behind. The false-negative rate for the B-27 patients, however, was 10.7% and was not significantly different for patients with clinically node-negative or -positive disease.[90] Two subsequent meta-analyses have confirmed similar false-negative rates for multiple studies (8% and 12%).[94,95] These figures are similar to large single institutional and multi-institutional series of SLN biopsy done at the time of primary surgery, without NAC (**Table 2**). The group at MD Anderson has confirmed that the success rates and accuracy of SLN biopsy after NCT are similar to those for primary surgical patients if the nodes are negative by clinical and US examination before treatment.[92] Moreover, SLNB dramatically reduced the need for ALND in NAC patients with T2 or T3 tumors, without any increase in regional recurrences. Thus, it should be reasonably well accepted that SLN biopsy can be used after treatment in N0 patients, particularly if US examination of the nodes before chemotherapy is negative. What to do about patients with known N1 to N3 disease is more controversial. Some small series have shown false-negative rates of 25% or higher for SLNB after NAC in patients with proven node spread.[88,91] Two recent European studies, on the other hand, did not find any significant difference in accuracy of SLN biopsy after chemotherapy between N0 and N1 patients.[96,97] Although it might be argued that significant prognostic information would be lost if nodal status is not determined at the time of diagnosis, the prognostic effect of residual cancer in lymph nodes after chemotherapy has been shown to be profound, and perhaps more important than initial nodal status. It might be argued, therefore, that SLNB before treatment, by potentially removing the only positive nodes, negates obtaining even more important prognostic information after treatment, and exposes the patient to 2 operations on the axilla and to potentially unnecessary radical surgery. The question of SLN accuracy after treatment of patients with known node spread may be answered definitively by an ongoing ACOSOG trial (Z-1071), illustrated in **Fig. 9**. Systemic treatment decisions, at least for now, are unlikely to be affected for the few patients whose nodes may be under staged by SLNB, because most of these patients receive a full course of chemotherapy preoperatively and there is no evidence that additional chemotherapy after surgery benefits those with residual disease.

POSTMASTECTOMY REGIONAL/CHEST WALL IRRADIATION AFTER NEOADJUVANT CHEMOTHERAPY

One remaining concern about these patients is whether to treat with regional and/or chest wall irradiation. Data from NSABP trials and from MD Anderson indicate a high risk for locoregional recurrence in patients with residual cancer after chemotherapy who do not receive regional irradiation.[98–100] Conversely, patients who were not stage IIIB or C and who have negative nodes after chemotherapy seem to be at low risk for locoregional recurrence.[98,101,102] However, until definitive data from

Table 2
Success rates and accuracy of sentinel lymph node biopsy with primary surgery or with surgery following neoadjuvant chemotherapy

Study	References	Timing	False-Negative Rate (%)
Multicenter SLN Trial	Krag et al[103]	Primary	11
Italian Randomized Trial	Veronesi et al[104]	Primary	9
University of Louisville	McMasters et al[105]	Primary	7
Ann Arundel, Multicenter	Tafra et al[106]	Primary	13
NSABP B-32	Krag et al[107]	Primary	10
NSABP B-27	Mamounas et al[90]	Post-NAC	11
Meta-analysis, 2006	Xing et al[94]	Post-NAC	12
Meta-analysis, 2009	Kelly et al[95]	Post-NAC	8

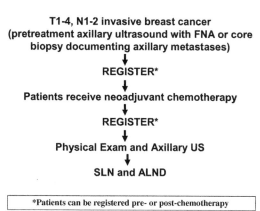

Fig. 9. ACOSOG Protocol Z1071. ALND, axillary lymph node dissection; FNA, fine-needle aspiration; SLN, sentinel lymph node.

a prospective trial demonstrate that these patients do not need regional or chest wall irradiation, it seems prudent to base this decision on a combination of the clinical stage at presentation and the pathologic stage after NAC.

SUMMARY

Neoadjuvant chemotherapy has many practical advantages for women with operable breast cancer, including increased chance for breast conservation. The potential to decrease the need for ALND is promising, but controversial. Hormonal neoadjuvant therapy may be more appropriate for some women. Perhaps most importantly, correlating responses to NAC with molecular profiles has the potential to increase our understanding of breast cancer biology and accelerate progress toward optimizing and individualizing therapy for women with breast cancer in the neoadjuvant and adjuvant settings.

REFERENCES

1. Singletary SE, Allred C, Ashley P, et al. Breast. In: Greene FL, Page DL, Fleming ID, et al, editors. AJCC cancer staging manual. 6th edition. New York: Springer; 2002. p. 221–40.
2. Fisher B, Brown A, Mamounas E, et al. Effect of preoperative chemotherapy on local-regional disease in women with operable breast cancer: findings from National Surgical Adjuvant Breast and Bowel Project B-18. J Clin Oncol 1997; 15(7):2483–93.
3. Fisher B, Bryant J, Wolmark N, et al. Effect of preoperative chemotherapy on the outcome of women with operable breast cancer. J Clin Oncol 1998;16(8): 2672–85.
4. Gianni L, Baselga J, Eiermann W, et al. Phase III trial evaluating the addition of paclitaxel to doxorubicin followed by cyclophosphamide, methotrexate, and fluorouracil, as adjuvant or primary systemic therapy: European Cooperative Trial in Operable Breast Cancer. J Clin Oncol 2009;27(15):2474–81.
5. Boughey JC, Peintinger F, Meric-Bernstam F, et al. Impact of preoperative versus postoperative chemotherapy on the extent and number of surgical

procedures in patients treated in randomized clinical trials for breast cancer. Ann Surg 2006;244(3):464–70.

6. Christy CJ, Thorsteinsson D, Grube BJ, et al. Preoperative chemotherapy decreases the need for re-excision of breast cancers between 2 and 4 cm diameter. Ann Surg Oncol 2009;16(3):697–702.

7. Rastogi P, Anderson SJ, Bear HD, et al. Preoperative chemotherapy: updates of National Surgical Adjuvant Breast and Bowel Project Protocols B-18 and B-27. J Clin Oncol 2008;26(5):778–85.

8. Symmans WF, Peintinger F, Hatzis C, et al. Measurement of residual breast cancer burden to predict survival after neoadjuvant chemotherapy. J Clin Oncol 2007;25(28):4414–22.

9. Hennessy BT, Hortobagyi GN, Rouzier R, et al. Outcome after pathologic complete eradication of cytologically proven breast cancer axillary node metastases following primary chemotherapy. J Clin Oncol 2005;23(36):9304–11.

10. Kuerer HM, Newman LA, Smith TL, et al. Clinical course of breast cancer patients with complete pathologic primary tumor and axillary lymph node response to doxorubicin-based neoadjuvant chemotherapy. J Clin Oncol 1999;17(2):460–9.

11. von Minckwitz G, Kummel S, Vogel P, et al. Neoadjuvant vinorelbine-capecitabine versus docetaxel-doxorubicin-cyclophosphamide in early nonresponsive breast cancer: phase III randomized GeparTrio trial. J Natl Cancer Inst 2008;100(8):542–51.

12. Bear HD, Anderson S, Brown A, et al. The effect on tumor response of adding sequential preoperative docetaxel (Taxotere) to preoperative doxorubicin and cyclophosphamide (AC): preliminary results from National Surgical Adjuvant Breast and Bowel Project (NSABP) Protocol B-27. J Clin Oncol 2003;21(22): 4165–74.

13. Tan MC, Al MF, Gao F, et al. Predictors of complete pathological response after neoadjuvant systemic therapy for breast cancer. Am J Surg 2009; 198(4):520–5.

14. Colleoni M, Viale G, Zahrieh D, et al. Chemotherapy is more effective in patients with breast cancer not expressing steroid hormone receptors: a study of preoperative treatment. Clin Cancer Res 2004;10(19):6622–8.

15. Bear HD, Anderson S, Smith RE, et al. Sequential preoperative or postoperative docetaxel added to preoperative doxorubicin plus cyclophosphamide for operable breast cancer: National Surgical Adjuvant Breast and Bowel Project Protocol B-27. J Clin Oncol 2006;24(13):2019–27.

16. Stearns V, Sing B, Tsangaris T, et al. A prospective randomized pilot study to evaluate predictors of response in serial core biopsies to single agent neoadjuvant doxorubicin or paclitaxel for patients with locally advanced breast cancer. Clin Cancer Res 2003;9:124–33.

17. Gianni L, Baselga J, Eiermann W, et al. Feasibility and tolerability of sequential doxorubicin/paclitaxel followed by cyclophosphamide, methotrexate, and fluorouracil and its effects on tumor response as preoperative therapy. Clin Cancer Res 2005;11(24 Pt 1):8715–21.

18. Chen AM, Meric-Bernstam F, Hunt KK, et al. Breast conservation after neoadjuvant chemotherapy. A prognostic index for clinical decision-making. Cancer 2005;103(4):689–95.

19. Guarneri V, Broglio K, Kau SW, et al. Prognostic value of pathologic complete response after primary chemotherapy in relation to hormone receptor status and other factors. J Clin Oncol 2006;24(7):1037–44.

20. Wenzel C, Bartsch R, Hussian D, et al. Invasive ductal carcinoma and invasive lobular carcinoma of breast differ in response following neoadjuvant therapy with epidoxorubicin and docetaxel + G-CSF. Breast Cancer Res Treat 2007; 104(1):109–14.

21. Cristofanilli M, Gonzalez-Angulo A, Sneige N, et al. Invasive lobular carcinoma classic type: response to primary chemotherapy and survival outcomes. J Clin Oncol 2005;23(1):41–8.

22. Mathieu MC, Rouzier R, Llombart-Cussac A, et al. The poor responsiveness of infiltrating lobular breast carcinomas to neoadjuvant chemotherapy can be explained by their biological profile. Eur J Cancer 2004;40(3):342–51.

23. Boughey JC, Wagner J, Garrett BJ, et al. Neoadjuvant chemotherapy in invasive lobular carcinoma may not improve rates of breast conservation. Ann Surg Oncol 2009;16(6):1606–11.

24. Julian TB, Anderson S, Fourchotte V, et al. Is invasive lobular cancer a prognostic factor for neoadjuvant chemotherapy response and long term outcomes? [abstract]. Ann Surg Oncol 2007;14(Suppl):17.

25. Sullivan PS, Apple SK. Should histologic type be taken into account when considering neoadjuvant chemotherapy in breast carcinoma? Breast J 2009; 15(2):146–54.

26. Bharat A, Gao F, Margenthaler JA. Tumor characteristics and patient outcomes are similar between invasive lobular and mixed invasive ductal/lobular breast cancers but differ from pure invasive ductal breast cancers. Am J Surg 2009; 198(4):516–9.

27. Rouzier R, Pusztai L, Delaloge S, et al. Nomograms to predict pathologic complete response and metastasis-free survival after preoperative chemotherapy for breast cancer. J Clin Oncol 2005;23(33):8331–9.

28. Gianni L, Zambetti M, Clark K, et al. Gene expression profiles in paraffin-embedded core biopsy tissue predict response to chemotherapy in women with locally advanced breast cancer. J Clin Oncol 2005;23(29):7265–77.

29. Chang JC, Makris A, Gutierrez MC, et al. Gene expression patterns in formalin-fixed, paraffin-embedded core biopsies predict docetaxel chemosensitivity in breast cancer patients. Breast Cancer Res Treat 2008;108(2):233–40.

30. Parker JS, Mullins M, Cheang MC, et al. Supervised risk predictor of breast cancer based on intrinsic subtypes. J Clin Oncol 2009;27(8):1160–7.

31. Iwao-Koizumi K, Matoba R, Ueno N, et al. Prediction of docetaxel response in human breast cancer by gene expression profiling. J Clin Oncol 2005;23(3):422–31.

32. Liedtke C, Hatzis C, Symmans WF, et al. Genomic grade index is associated with response to chemotherapy in patients with breast cancer. J Clin Oncol 2009;27(19):3185–91.

33. Esserman LJ, Perou C, Cheang M, et al. Breast cancer molecular profiles and tumor response of neoadjuvant doxorubicin and paclitaxel: the I-SPY TRIAL (CALGB 15007/150012, ACRIN 6657) [abstract]. J Clin Oncol 2009;27(18S, Part II):797s.

34. Straver ME, Glas AM, Hannemann J, et al. The 70-gene signature as a response predictor for neoadjuvant chemotherapy in breast cancer. Breast Cancer Res Treat 2009;119(3):551–8.

35. Parker JS, Prat A, Cheang MCU, et al. Breast cancer molecular subtypes predict response to anthracycline/taxane-based chemotherapy [abstract]. Cancer Res 2009;69(24):598s.

36. Mathew J, Asgeirsson KS, Jackson LR, et al. Neoadjuvant endocrine treatment in primary breast cancer - review of literature. Breast 2009;18(6):339–44.

37. Mamounas EP. Facilitating breast-conserving surgery and preventing recurrence: aromatase inhibitors in the neoadjuvant and adjuvant settings. Ann Surg Oncol 2008;15(3):691–703.

38. Ellis M, Ma C. Femara and the future: tailoring treatment and combination therapies with Femara. Breast Cancer Res Treat 2007;105(Suppl 1):105–15.

39. Smith IE, Dowsett M, Ebbs SR, et al. Neoadjuvant treatment of postmenopausal breast cancer with anastrozole, tamoxifen, or both in combination: the Immediate Preoperative Anastrozole, Tamoxifen, or Combined with Tamoxifen (IMPACT) multicenter double-blind randomized trial. J Clin Oncol 2005;23(22):5108–16.

40. Cataliotti L, Buzdar AU, Noguchi S, et al. Comparison of anastrozole versus tamoxifen as preoperative therapy in postmenopausal women with hormone receptor-positive breast cancer: the Pre-Operative "Arimidex" Compared to Tamoxifen (PROACT) trial. Cancer 2006;106(10):2095–103.

41. Semiglazov VF, Semiglazov VV, Dashyan GA, et al. Phase 2 randomized trial of primary endocrine therapy versus chemotherapy in postmenopausal patients with estrogen receptor-positive breast cancer. Cancer 2007;110(2):244–54.

42. Olson JA Jr, Budd GT, Carey LA, et al. Improved surgical outcomes for breast cancer patients receiving neoadjuvant aromatase inhibitor therapy: results from a multicenter phase II trial. J Am Coll Surg 2009;208(5):906–14.

43. Dowsett M, Smith IE, Ebbs SR, et al. Prognostic value of Ki67 expression after short-term presurgical endocrine therapy for primary breast cancer. J Natl Cancer Inst 2007;99(2):167–70.

44. Segara D, Krop IE, Garber JE, et al. Does MRI predict pathologic tumor response in women with breast cancer undergoing preoperative chemotherapy? J Surg Oncol 2007;96(6):474–80.

45. Martincich L, Montemurro F, De RG, et al. Monitoring response to primary chemotherapy in breast cancer using dynamic contrast-enhanced magnetic resonance imaging. Breast Cancer Res Treat 2004;83(1):67–76.

46. Martincich L, Montemurro F, Cirillo S, et al. Role of magnetic resonance imaging in the prediction of tumor response in patients with locally advanced breast cancer receiving neoadjuvant chemo-therapy. Radiol Med 2003; 106(1–2):51–8.

47. Hylton N. MR imaging for assessment of breast cancer response to neoadjuvant chemotherapy. Magn Reson Imaging Clin N Am 2006;14(3):383–9, vii.

48. Bodini M, Berruti A, Bottini A, et al. Magnetic resonance imaging in comparison to clinical palpation in assessing the response of breast cancer to epirubicin primary chemotherapy. Breast Cancer Res Treat 2004;85(3):211–8.

49. Esserman L, Kaplan E, Partridge S, et al. MRI phenotype is associated with response to doxorubicin and cyclophosphamide neoadjuvant chemotherapy in stage III breast cancer. Ann Surg Oncol 2001;8(6):549–59.

50. Craciunescu OI, Blackwell KL, Jones EL, et al. DCE-MRI parameters have potential to predict response of locally advanced breast cancer patients to neoadjuvant chemotherapy and hyperthermia: a pilot study. Int J Hyperthermia 2009;25(6):405–15.

51. Oh JL, Nguyen G, Whitman GJ, et al. Placement of radiopaque clips for tumor localization in patients undergoing neoadjuvant chemotherapy and breast conservation therapy. Cancer 2007;110(11):2420–7.

52. Lannin DR, Grube B, Black DS, et al. Breast tattoos for planning surgery following neoadjuvant chemotherapy. Am J Surg 2007;194(4):518–20.

53. Kaufmann M, von Minckwitz G, Bear HD, et al. Recommendations from an international expert panel on the use of neoadjuvant (primary) systemic treatment of

operable breast cancer: new perspectives 2006. Ann Oncol 2007;18(12): 1927–34.

54. Smith IC, Heys SD, Hutcheon AW, et al. Neoadjuvant chemotherapy in breast cancer: significantly enhanced response with docetaxel. J Clin Oncol 2002; 20(6):1456–66.

55. Nowak AK, Wilcken NR, Stockler MR, et al. Systematic review of taxane-containing versus non-taxane-containing regimens for adjuvant and neoadjuvant treatment of early breast cancer. Lancet Oncol 2004;5(6):372–80.

56. Cuppone F, Bria E, Carlini P, et al. Taxanes as primary chemotherapy for early breast cancer: meta-analysis of randomized trials. Cancer 2008;113(2):238–46.

57. Bria E, Nistico C, Cuppone F, et al. Benefit of taxanes as adjuvant chemotherapy for early breast cancer: pooled analysis of 15,500 patients. Cancer 2006; 106(11):2337–44.

58. Han S, Kim J, Lee J, et al. Comparison of 6 cycles versus 4 cycles of neoadjuvant epirubicin plus docetaxel chemotherapy in stages II and III breast cancer. Eur J Surg Oncol 2009;35(6):583–7.

59. Steger GG, Galid A, Gnant M, et al. Pathologic complete response with six compared with three cycles of neoadjuvant epirubicin plus docetaxel and granulocyte colony-stimulating factor in operable breast cancer: results of ABCSG-14. J Clin Oncol 2007;25(15):2012–8.

60. von Minckwitz G, Kummel S, Vogel P, et al. Intensified neoadjuvant chemotherapy in early-responding breast cancer: phase III randomized GeparTrio study. J Natl Cancer Inst 2008;100(8):552–62.

61. Winer EP. The evolving role of adjuvant chemotherapy [abstract]. Cancer Res 2009;69(24):484s.

62. Miglietta L, Vanella P, Canobbio L, et al. Clinical and pathological response to primary chemotherapy in patients with locally advanced breast cancer grouped according to hormonal receptors, Her2 status, grading and Ki-67 proliferation index. Anticancer Res 2009;29(5):1621–5.

63. Goldstein NS, Decker D, Severson D, et al. Molecular classification system identifies invasive breast carcinoma patients who are most likely and those who are least likely to achieve a complete pathologic response after neoadjuvant chemotherapy. Cancer 2007;110(8):1687–96.

64. Wang J, Buchholz TA, Middleton LP, et al. Assessment of histologic features and expression of biomarkers in predicting pathologic response to anthracycline-based neoadjuvant chemotherapy in patients with breast cancer. Cancer 2002;94(12):3107–14.

65. Hayes DF, Thor AD, Dressler LG, et al. HER2 and response to paclitaxel in node-positive breast cancer. N Engl J Med 2007;357(15):1496–506.

66. Buzdar AU, Ibrahim NK, Francis D, et al. Significantly higher pathologic complete remission rate after neoadjuvant therapy with trastuzumab, paclitaxel, and epirubicin chemotherapy: results of a randomized trial in human epidermal growth factor receptor 2-positive operable breast cancer. J Clin Oncol 2005;23(16):3676–85.

67. Buzdar AU, Valero V, Ibrahim NK, et al. Neoadjuvant therapy with paclitaxel followed by 5-fluorouracil, epirubicin, and cyclophosphamide chemotherapy and concurrent trastuzumab in human epidermal growth factor receptor 2-positive operable breast cancer: an update of the initial randomized study population and data of additional patients treated with the same regimen. Clin Cancer Res 2007;13(1):228–33.

68. Buzdar AU, Valero V, Ibrahim N, et al. Prospective data of additional patients treated with neoadjuvant therapy with paclitaxel followed by FEC chemotherapy

with trastuzumab in HER-2 positive operable breast cancer, and an update of initial study population [abstract]. Breast Cancer Res Treat 2005;94(S1):S223.

69. Byrski T, Gronwald J, Huzarski T, et al. Pathologic complete response rates in young women with BRCA1-positive breast cancers after neoadjuvant chemotherapy. J Clin Oncol 2010;28(3):375–9.

70. Johansen R, Jensen LR, Rydland J, et al. Predicting survival and early clinical response to primary chemotherapy for patients with locally advanced breast cancer using DCE-MRI. J Magn Reson Imaging 2009;29(6):1300–7.

71. Bahri S, Chen JH, Mehta RS, et al. Residual breast cancer diagnosed by MRI in patients receiving neoadjuvant chemotherapy with and without bevacizumab. Ann Surg Oncol 2009;16(6):1619–28.

72. Chen JH, Feig BA, Hsiang DJ, et al. Impact of MRI-evaluated neoadjuvant chemotherapy response on change of surgical recommendation in breast cancer. Ann Surg 2009;249(3):448–54.

73. Fisher B, Brown A, Mamounas E, et al. Effect of preoperative therapy for primary breast cancer (BC) on local-regional disease, disease-free survival (DFS) and survival (S): results from NSABP B-18 [abstract]. Proceedings of the American Society of Clinical Oncology 1997;16:127.

74. Mauri D, Pavlidis N, Ioannidis JP. Neoadjuvant versus adjuvant systemic treatment in breast cancer: a meta-analysis. J Natl Cancer Inst 2005;97(3):188–94.

75. Mauriac L, MacGrogan G, Avril A, et al. Neoadjuvant chemotherapy for operable breast carcinoma larger than 3 cm: a unicentre randomized trial with a 124-month median follow-up. Institut Bergonie Bordeaux Groupe Sein (IBBGS). Ann Oncol 1999;10(1):47–52.

76. Lyman GH, Giuliano AE, Somerfield MR, et al. American Society of Clinical Oncology guideline recommendations for sentinel lymph node biopsy in early-stage breast cancer. J Clin Oncol 2005;23(30):7703–20.

77. Carlson RW, Allred DC, Anderson BO, et al. Breast cancer. Clinical practice guidelines in oncology. J Natl Compr Canc Netw 2009;7(2):122–92.

78. Khan A, Sabel MS, Nees A, et al. Comprehensive axillary evaluation in neoadjuvant chemotherapy patients with ultrasonography and sentinel lymph node biopsy. Ann Surg Oncol 2005;12(9):697–704.

79. Kilbride KE, Lee MC, Nees AV, et al. Axillary staging prior to neoadjuvant chemotherapy for breast cancer: predictors of recurrence. Ann Surg Oncol 2008;15(11):3252–8.

80. Nason KS, Anderson BO, Byrd DR, et al. Increased false negative sentinel node biopsy rates after preoperative chemotherapy for invasive breast carcinoma. Cancer 2000;89(11):2187–94.

81. van Deurzen CH, Vriens BE, Tjan-Heijnen VC, et al. Accuracy of sentinel node biopsy after neoadjuvant chemotherapy in breast cancer patients: a systematic review. Eur J Cancer 2009;45(18):3124–30.

82. Menard JP, Extra JM, Jacquemier J, et al. Sentinel lymphadenectomy for the staging of clinical axillary node-negative breast cancer before neoadjuvant chemotherapy. Eur J Surg Oncol 2009;35(9):916–20.

83. Iwase H, Yamamoto Y, Kawasoe T, et al. Advantage of sentinel lymph node biopsy before neoadjuvant chemotherapy in breast cancer treatment. Surg Today 2009;39(5):374–80.

84. van Rijk MC, Nieweg OE, Rutgers EJ, et al. Sentinel node biopsy before neoadjuvant chemotherapy spares breast cancer patients axillary lymph node dissection. Ann Surg Oncol 2006;13(4):475–9.

85. Cox CE, Cox JM, White LB, et al. Sentinel node biopsy before neoadjuvant chemotherapy for determining axillary status and treatment prognosis in locally advanced breast cancer. Ann Surg Oncol 2006;13(4):483–90.
86. Jones JL, Zabicki K, Christian RL, et al. A comparison of sentinel node biopsy before and after neoadjuvant chemotherapy: timing is important. Am J Surg 2005;190(4):517–20.
87. Schrenk P, Hochreiner G, Fridrik M, et al. Sentinel node biopsy performed before preoperative chemotherapy for axillary lymph node staging in breast cancer. Breast J 2003;9(4):282–7.
88. Shen J, Gilcrease MZ, Babiera GV, et al. Feasibility and accuracy of sentinel lymph node biopsy after preoperative chemotherapy in breast cancer patients with documented axillary metastases. Cancer 2007;109(7):1255–63.
89. Dominici LS, Negron Gonzalez VM, Buzdar AU, et al. Eradication of axillary lymph node metastases occurs in 74% of patients receiving neoadjuvant chemotherapy with concurrent trastuzumab for HER2 positive breast cancer [abstract]. Cancer Res 2009;69(24):566s.
90. Mamounas EP, Brown A, Anderson S, et al. Sentinel node biopsy after neoadjuvant chemotherapy in breast cancer: results from National Surgical Adjuvant Breast and Bowel Project Protocol B-27. J Clin Oncol 2005;23(12):2694–702.
91. Gimbergues P, Abrial C, Durando X, et al. Sentinel lymph node biopsy after neoadjuvant chemotherapy is accurate in breast cancer patients with a clinically negative axillary nodal status at presentation. Ann Surg Oncol 2008;15(5):1316–21.
92. Hunt KK, Yi M, Mittendorf EA, et al. Sentinel lymph node surgery after neoadjuvant chemotherapy is accurate and reduces the need for axillary dissection in breast cancer patients. Ann Surg 2009;250(4):558–66.
93. Newman EA, Sabel MS, Nees AV, et al. Sentinel lymph node biopsy performed after neoadjuvant chemotherapy is accurate in patients with documented node-positive breast cancer at presentation. Ann Surg Oncol 2007;14(10):2946–52.
94. Xing Y, Foy M, Cox DD, et al. Meta-analysis of sentinel lymph node biopsy after preoperative chemotherapy in patients with breast cancer. Br J Surg 2006;93(5):539–46.
95. Kelly AM, Dwamena B, Cronin P, et al. Breast cancer sentinel node identification and classification after neoadjuvant chemotherapy-systematic review and meta analysis. Acad Radiol 2009;16(5):551–63.
96. Classe JM, Bordes V, Campion L, et al. Sentinel lymph node biopsy after neoadjuvant chemotherapy for advanced breast cancer: results of Ganglion Sentinelle et Chimiotherapie Neoadjuvante, a French prospective multicentric study. J Clin Oncol 2009;27(5):726–32.
97. Tausch C, Konstantiniuk P, Kugler F, et al. Sentinel lymph node biopsy after preoperative chemotherapy for breast cancer: findings from the Austrian Sentinel Node Study Group. Ann Surg Oncol 2008;15(12):3378–83.
98. Goldman B. Cancer vaccines: finding the best way to train the immune system. J Natl Cancer Inst 2002;94(20):1523–6.
99. Buchholz TA, Lehman CD, Harris JR, et al. Statement of the science concerning locoregional treatments after preoperative chemotherapy for breast cancer: a National Cancer Institute conference. J Clin Oncol 2008;26(5):791–7.
100. Huang EH, Strom EA, Perkins GH, et al. Comparison of risk of local-regional recurrence after mastectomy or breast conservation therapy for patients treated with neoadjuvant chemotherapy and radiation stratified according to a prognostic index score. Int J Radiat Oncol Biol Phys 2006;66(2):352–7.

101. McGuire SE, Gonzalez-Angulo AM, Huang EH, et al. Postmastectomy radiation improves the outcome of patients with locally advanced breast cancer who achieve a pathologic complete response to neoadjuvant chemotherapy. Int J Radiat Oncol Biol Phys 2007;68(4):1004–9.
102. Garg AK, Strom EA, McNeese MD, et al. T3 disease at presentation or pathologic involvement of four or more lymph nodes predict for locoregional recurrence in stage II breast cancer treated with neoadjuvant chemotherapy and mastectomy without radiotherapy. Int J Radiat Oncol Biol Phys 2004;59(1):138–45.
103. Krag D, Weaver D, Ashikaga T, et al. The sentinel node in breast cancer - a multicenter validation study. N Engl J Med 1998;339(14):941–6.
104. Veronesi U, Paganelli G, Viale G, et al. A randomized comparison of sentinel-node biopsy with routine axillary dissection in breast cancer. N Engl J Med 2003;349(6):546–53.
105. McMasters KM, Tuttle TM, Carlson DJ, et al. Sentinel lymph node biopsy for breast cancer: a suitable alternative to routine axillary dissection in multi-institutional practice when optimal technique is used. J Clin Oncol 2000;18(13):2560–6.
106. Tafra L, Lannin DR, Swanson MS, et al. Multicenter trial of sentinel node biopsy for breast cancer using both technetium sulfur colloid and isosulfan blue dye. Ann Surg 2001;233(1):51–9.
107. Krag DN, Anderson SJ, Julian TB, et al. Technical outcomes of sentinel-lymph-node resection and conventional axillary-lymph-node dissection in patients with clinically node-negative breast cancer: results from the NSABP B-32 randomised phase III trial. Lancet Oncol 2007;8(10):881–8.

Neoadjuvant Endocrine Therapy for Breast Cancer

Jane S. Chawla, MD[a], Cynthia X. Ma, MD, PhD[a,b],
Matthew J. Ellis, MB, BChir, PhD[a,b],*

KEYWORDS

- Breast cancer • Estrogen receptor
- Neoadjuvant endocrine therapy • Genomics • Relapse risk

The emergence of neoadjuvant systemic therapy has allowed surgically inoperable breast cancers to become operable and has increased the rate of breast-conserving surgery in those who would otherwise require a mastectomy. In premenopausal women, neoadjuvant chemotherapy is the current standard. However, in postmenopausal women with estrogen receptor (ER)-positive breast cancer, preoperative endocrine therapy with aromatase inhibitors (AIs) improves rates of breast conservation and minimizes treatment-related toxicities. In addition, the ability to obtain tumor specimens before and after neoadjuvant endocrine therapy has facilitated the development of biomarkers and gene profiles predictive of endocrine responsiveness and the evaluation of novel agents to improve the outcome of ER-positive breast cancer.

TAMOXIFEN VERSUS SURGERY

Early studies in the 1980s and 1990s focused on endocrine therapy use with tamoxifen as an alternative to surgery in patients aged 70 years and older who were poor surgical candidates. Although tumor shrinkage with tamoxifen was demonstrated, long-term disease control was poor.[1] A trial by the European Organization for Research and Treatment of Cancer (EORTC) randomized postmenopausal women aged 70 years and older to modified radical mastectomy versus tamoxifen 20 mg daily. They found that there was a higher rate of local progression or relapse in the tamoxifen-treated arm, but no difference in survival.[2] This and other studies paved the way for a shift

---

[a] Division of Oncology, Department of Medicine, Washington University, 660 South Euclid Avenue, Campus Box 8056, St Louis, MO 63110, USA
[b] Siteman Cancer Center, Washington University, 660 South Euclid Avenue, Campus Box 8056, St Louis, MO 63110, USA
* Corresponding author. Division of Oncology, Department of Medicine, Washington University, 660 South Euclid Avenue, Campus Box 8056, St Louis, MO 63110.
E-mail address: mellis@dom.wustl.edu

Surg Oncol Clin N Am 19 (2010) 627–638
doi:10.1016/j.soc.2010.04.004
1055-3207/10/$ – see front matter © 2010 Elsevier Inc. All rights reserved.

in treatment strategy to preoperative endocrine therapy before surgery, rather than in place of it.

AIS VERSUS TAMOXIFEN

AIs have been found to be superior to tamoxifen as endocrine therapy for postmenopausal women with hormone receptor–positive breast cancer in the settings of metastatic disease,[3–5] locally advanced disease,[6–8] and early-stage disease.[9,10] The molecular mechanism explaining the benefit of AIs compared with tamoxifen is still not clear, but may be related to the difference in the mechanism of action between the 2 classes of drugs or pharmacogenomic variables that differentially affect drug metabolism,[11–14] or both. For example, AIs block the conversion of androgens to estrogens in the peripheral tissues, thereby depriving the ER of its agonist. On the other hand, tamoxifen directly binds to the ER and acts as an agonist or antagonist in various tissues. Although the CYP2D6 genotype may be implicated in the efficacy of tamoxifen in some studies,[11] the debate continues and germ line polymorphisms that affect AI efficacy are still being explored.[13,14] Regardless, the improved outcomes with AIs compared with tamoxifen in postmenopausal women with ER+ breast cancer prompted several trials to be designed to compare these agents in the neoadjuvant setting.

One of the first trials to compare an AI with tamoxifen in the neoadjuvant setting was the P024 trial. This was a randomized, double-blind, multicenter study that randomized 324 postmenopausal women with ER+ and/or progesterone receptor (PgR)-positive breast cancer to letrozole 2.5 mg daily or tamoxifen 20 mg daily for 4 months. At enrollment none of the patients were felt to be candidates for breast-conserving surgery (BCS) and 14% of the patients were inoperable. In the intention-to-treat analysis there was a statistically significant improvement in the overall objective response rate (by clinical palpation) in the letrozole group compared with the tamoxifen group (55% vs 36%; P<.001). All secondary end points were also found to be significant between the 2 groups: ultrasound response, 35% versus 25% (P = .042), mammographic response, 34% versus 16% (P<.001), and BCS, 45% versus 35% (P = .022). Few pathologic complete responses (pCR) were seen in the primary breast lesions in either group with only 2 in the letrozole group and 3 in the tamoxifen group.[6]

The Pre-Operative Arimidex Compared to Tamoxifen (PROACT) trial compared anastrozole with tamoxifen in postmenopausal women with ER+ and/or PgR+ operable or potentially operable invasive breast cancer.[8] This was a randomized, double-blind, double-dummy, multicenter study that randomized 451 patients to 3 months of anastrozole 1 mg daily or tamoxifen 20 mg daily. No significant difference in response rates was observed in the 137 patients who received concomitant neoadjuvant chemotherapy. After excluding those patients who received chemotherapy, similar response rates were seen in the anastrozole (36.2%) and tamoxifen (26.5%) groups (P = .07). The objective response rates for anastrozole and tamoxifen were 48.6% and 35.8% (caliper-measured; P = .04), respectively, and 36.6% and 24.2% (ultrasound-measured; P = .03) in patients who were not eligible for BCS or were inoperable at baseline. Improvement in actual surgery occurred in 43% of anastrozole-treated patients and 31% of tamoxifen-treated patients (P = .04).[8]

Another neoadjuvant endocrine therapy trial, the Immediate Preoperative Anastrozole, Tamoxifen, or Combined with Tamoxifen (IMPACT) trial, was a phase III randomized, double-blind, double-dummy, multicenter trial that randomized patients to anastrozole 1 mg and tamoxifen placebo daily, tamoxifen 20 mg and anastrozole placebo daily, or a combination of tamoxifen 20 mg and anastrozole 1 mg daily for 12 weeks before surgery.[7] There were 330 postmenopausal women with invasive

ER+, nonmetastatic, and operable or locally advanced potentially operable breast cancer included in the study. Objective response rates were 37%, 36%, and 39%, respectively, based on caliper measurement and 24%, 20%, and 28%, respectively, on ultrasound. These differences were not statistically significant. Of the patients felt to be candidates for BCS by their surgeons, a statistically significant number received anastrozole compared with tamoxifen (46% vs 22%, P = .03). There was a trend toward improved numbers of BCS in patients in the anastrozole arm compared with the tamoxifen arm, although this was not significant (44% vs 31%, P = .23).[7]

A phase II study by the Austrian Breast and Colorectal Cancer Study Group (ABCSG) evaluated exemestane in 80 postmenopausal women with ER+ and/or PgR+ operable breast cancer. After 4 months of treatment they found a clinical objective response rate of 34%, pCR rate of 3%, and BCS rate of 76%.[15] These results are similar to those reported in randomized trials of nonsteroidal AIs.

A multicenter trial in the United States enrolled 150 (106 evaluable) postmenopausal women with ER+ or PgR+ breast cancer (>2 cm) to receive 16 to 24 weeks of preoperative letrozole 2.5 mg daily. The overall clinical response rate was 62%, which is comparable with the rate of 55% seen in the P024 trial.[16] On multivariate analysis, several factors predicted for mastectomy rather than BCS: baseline T size (T3/4 vs T2), baseline surgical status (marginal candidate for breast conservation vs mastectomy/operable) and posttreatment clinical stage (T2–4 vs T1/0). Overall, 50% of the patients underwent BCS, including 30 of 46 who were initially marginal for BCS and 15 of 39 who were not candidates for BCS. In addition, all 11 patients who were initially felt to be inoperable were able to undergo surgical resection of their tumors. Nineteen percent of mastectomy patients were found to have a pathologic T1 tumor and therefore could have been candidates for BCS. The investigators concluded that these patients may have been upstaged with current preoperative imaging techniques, and that those patients who seem to have a good clinical response should have BCS attempted.[16]

These trials demonstrate the benefit of AIs over tamoxifen in the neoadjuvant setting. A meta-analysis of 4 trials, the P024, IMPACT, PROACT, and the exemestane trials, was able to reconcile some of the variability in outcomes between the trials.[17] The pooled analysis found a statistically significant improvement in the clinical objective response rate, the ultrasound objective response rate, and the BCS rate with the AIs compared with tamoxifen.[17] A randomized trial (ACOSOG Z1031) comparing 3 AIs directly is underway, but results have not yet been reported (**Fig. 1**).

NEOADJUVANT CHEMOTHERAPY VERSUS ENDOCRINE THERAPY

It is well known that adjuvant endocrine therapy is the most effective adjuvant treatment of ER+ breast cancer in postmenopausal women.[18] Several studies examining

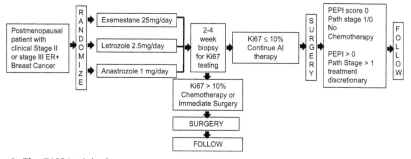

Fig. 1. The Z1031 trial schema.

the gene signatures of ER+ breast tumors have shown that there is a subgroup of patients that gain little from chemotherapy.[19] Therefore, patients who are not responsive to chemotherapy in the adjuvant setting would not likely be responsive to chemotherapy in the neoadjuvant setting. Yet, there has been concern about the use of neoadjuvant endocrine therapy because of the low pCR rates seen in the neoadjuvant endocrine studies (<5%). However, in ER+ patients receiving neoadjuvant chemotherapy, there is also a low pCR rate.[20–23] In a retrospective trial of 372 patients with locally advanced breast cancer who received 4 cycles of neoadjuvant doxorubicin-containing chemotherapy, there was a significant correlation between ER status and pCR rate. ER− tumors and those with a higher nuclear grade were more likely to have a pCR of the primary tumor and axillary lymph nodes that was independent of the initial tumor size (P<.01). There was a significant difference in the pCR rate for ER+ tumors compared with ER− tumors (3% vs 17%; P<.01)[20] demonstrating the ineffectiveness of chemotherapy in ER+ patients. Another retrospective study evaluating 435 patients who received neoadjuvant anthracycline or non–anthracycline-containing regimens correlated pCR rate and overall survival with ER status. They also found a lower pCR rate in ER+ tumors compared with ER− tumors (8.1% vs 21.6%; P<.001). Although there was improved overall survival in all patients who achieved a pCR in this study, the difference was not significant in ER+ patients who achieved a pCR compared with those who did not (93% vs 79%; P = .3).[21] These studies all highlight that ER+ tumors are less responsive to chemotherapy, and therefore may need to be approached differently when planning neoadjuvant treatment.

The only study comparing neoadjuvant endocrine therapy to chemotherapy was a phase II study that randomized 239 postmenopausal women with ER+ and/or PgR+ breast cancer to endocrine therapy with either anastrozole 1 mg daily or exemestane 25 mg daily for 3 months or to chemotherapy with doxorubicin 60 mg/m^2 and paclitaxel 200mg/m^2 every 3 weeks for 4 cycles. All patients were felt to be ineligible for BCS initially and had T2N1-2, T3N0-1, or T4N0M0 disease. They found no statistically significant difference in the primary end point, overall objective response rate (by palpation), for endocrine therapy (anastrozole, 62%; exemestane, 67%) compared with chemotherapy (63%, P>.5). The pCR rates were not statistically different between the hormonal and chemotherapy groups (3% vs 6%; P>.05). The responses as determined by mammography and ultrasound were not statistically different between the hormonal and chemotherapy groups (60% vs 63%; P>.5 and 40% vs 46%; P>.5). In addition, there was a trend toward higher rates of BCS in the endocrine therapy group (33% vs 24%; P = .58). There was also a trend toward higher objective response rates and BCS among patients with strongly ER+ tumors (defined as Allred score ≥6) in the endocrine therapy group compared with the chemotherapy group (43% vs 24%; P = .054).[24] This study at least demonstrates a similar efficacy of neoadjuvant endocrine therapy and chemotherapy in postmenopausal women with ER-expressing tumors. In addition, it suggests that there may be improved responses and BCS rates in patients receiving endocrine therapy compared with chemotherapy. More randomized studies are necessary to clarify this further.

BIOMARKER EVALUATION IN THE NEOADJUVANT ENDOCRINE SETTING TO PREDICT LONG-TERM OUTCOME

Neoadjuvant chemotherapy studies have used pCR as a means to demonstrate response to a regimen. However, this end point is less useful in patients with ER+, human epidermal growth factor receptor 2 (HER2)− disease treated with endocrine therapy because pCRs are infrequently seen and do not necessarily correlate with long-term outcome. Expression of the proliferative antigen Ki67 after a short-term of drug exposure has been proposed in assessing tumor response to endocrine therapy in the neoadjuvant setting. This marker may be suppressed after only a short duration of treatment, thereby making it a tool to predict which patients are most likely to respond to further endocrine treatment.

In the P024 trial, pretreatment biopsies were compared with surgical specimens after 4 months of treatment with either letrozole or tamoxifen. Letrozole was found to produce greater suppression of Ki67 compared with tamoxifen (87% inhibition of geometric mean Ki67 vs 75%; $P = .0009$). This decrease in Ki67 was found to be significantly greater in responders than nonresponders ($P = .025$).[25] Similarly in the IMPACT study, biopsies taken at 2 and 12 weeks showed a significantly greater mean suppression of Ki67 with anastrozole (76% and 81.6%) than with tamoxifen (59.5% and 61.9%). Unlike the P024 trial, a significant correlation between the degree of Ki67 suppression and clinical response was not found. A trend toward greater suppression of Ki67 at 2 and 12 weeks in patients downstaged from mastectomy to BCS was evident.[26] However, not all tumors that respond to endocrine therapy have significant decreases in Ki67, and tumors with suppression of Ki67 do not all have significant responses.[27]

To identify other posttreatment factors that might predict breast cancer survival after neoadjuvant endocrine therapy, a multivariate analysis was performed on the P024 trial. Four factors were found to have independent prognostic value for relapse-free survival and breast cancer–specific survival: pathologic tumor size (T1/2 vs T3/4), pathologic node status (positive or negative), and 2 biomarkers in the surgical resection specimen, the normal log of the Ki67 value and the ER status of the tumor. A prognostic score, the preoperative endocrine prognostic index (PEPI), was developed, which weighs each of these factors according to the magnitude of their hazard ratios (**Table 1**). Three risk groups were formed (score 0, 1–3, and ≥ 4) that were associated with relapse risks of 10%, 23%, and 48% ($P<.001$). For breast cancer death the corresponding risks were 2%, 11%, and 17% ($P<.001$). The PEPI was then validated in an independent data set from the IMPACT trial. In both trials relapses were not seen in patients with pathologic stage 0 or 1 disease with a PEPI score of 0.[28] The PEPI score has become a useful tool to identify patients who are sensitive to estrogen inhibition that integrates multiple biologic variables.

On-therapy biomarkers (ER and Ki67) along with the PEPI score obtained at 2 weeks and 4 months after neoadjuvant endocrine therapy, respectively, have been incorporated in the ACOSOG Z1031 trial for clinical decision making. Patients with a high Ki67 proliferation index (>10%) in a 2- to 4-week on-treatment biopsy will be recommended to switch from neoadjuvant endocrine therapy to neoadjuvant chemotherapy, because these tumors are exhibiting endocrine therapy resistance.[29] The pCR rate to chemotherapy in this situation will be assessed to evaluate their responsiveness to chemotherapy (see **Fig. 1**). Postoperatively, patients in the pathologic stage 1/0 PEPI 0 category will be advised against adjuvant chemotherapy, as they are unlikely to benefit from additional treatment. If this approach to tailoring neoadjuvant endocrine therapy is feasible, a larger, more definitive study will be considered.

RECEPTOR, HER2 STATUS AND SENSITIVITY TO ENDOCRINE THERAPY

In the P024 trial, enrollment in the study required biopsy specimens to have at least 10% nuclear staining for ER and/or PgR on immunohistochemistry (IHC). Yet in a pre-planned central biomarker analysis, 12% of tumors were found to be ER−, demonstrating the variability of IHC methods between institutions. For this reason,

Table 1
The preoperative endocrine prognostic index (PEPI)[a]

Pathology, Biomarker Status	RFS		BCSS	
	HR	Points	HR	Points
Tumor size				
T1/2	–	0	–	0
T3/4	2.8	3	4.4	3
Node status				
Negative	–	0	–	0
Positive	3.2	3	3.9	3
Ki67 level				
0–2.7% (0–1†)	–	0	–	0
>2.7–7.3% (1–2†)	1.3	1	1.4	1
>7.3–19.7% (2–3†)	1.7	1	2.0	2
>19.7–53.1% (3–4†)	2.2	2	2.7	3
>53.1% (>4†)	2.9	3	3.8	3
ER status, Allred score				
0–2	2.8	3	7.0	3
3–8	–	0	–	0

[a] To obtain the PEPI score, risk points for relapse-free survival (RFS) and breast cancer-specific survival (BCSS) were assigned depending on the hazard ratio (HR) defined in the P024 analysis.[28] The total PEPI score assigned to each patient is the sum of the risk points derived from the pT stage, pN stage, Ki67 level, and ER status of the surgical specimen. An HR in the range of 1 to 2 receives 1 risk point; an HR in the 2 to 2.5 range, 2 risk points; an HR greater than 2.5, 3 risk points. The total risk point score for each patient is the sum of all the risk points accumulated from the 4 factors in the model. For example, a patient with a T1N0 tumor, a Ki67 staining percentage of 1%, and an ER Allred score of 6 will have no risk points assigned. In contrast, a patient with a T3 N1 tumor, a Ki67 staining percentage of 25%, and an ER Allred score of 2, will have a total relapse score of 3+3+2+3 = 11.

Data from Ellis M, Tao Y, Luo J, et al Outcome prediction for estrogen receptor–positive breast cancer based on postneoadjuvant endocrine therapy tumor characteristics. J Natl Cancer Inst 2008;100:1380–88.

a standardized method of determining ER expression, using the ER Allred expression score, was implemented to more accurately evaluate the relationship between ER status and response to treatment. Using this approach it was found that there was a linear relationship between the ER Allred score and odds of response for tamoxifen ($P = .0061$) and letrozole ($P = .0013$). Also, letrozole response rates were superior to those of tamoxifen in every ER Allred category from 3 to 8. For unclear reasons, a similar linear relationship was not seen for PgR Allred expression levels because maximum response rates for both agents occurred at intermediate levels of expression.[6]

In the IMPACT study, the definition of ER positivity was only 1% nuclear staining. There was a significant difference in degree of suppression of Ki67 with anastrozole compared with tamoxifen, at all levels of ER, but especially in patients with low levels of ER expression. In contrast to the P024 trial, there was a correlation between PgR and Ki67 expression. Ki67 was suppressed more substantially in PgR+ tumors compared with PgR– tumors in all 3 treatment groups. In addition, at 2 weeks there was a significant suppression of Ki67 and PgR levels in the anastrozole group ($P = .003$) but a decrease in Ki67 and an increase in PgR for the tamoxifen group ($P = .027$).[28]

HER2 status and response were also examined in these trials. In the P024 trial, 15.2% of tumors expressed HER1 and/or HER2 based on IHC. Tumors that were HER1+ and/or HER2+ were found to be more responsive to letrozole compared with tamoxifen (response rate, 88% vs 21%; P = .0004).[30] Fluorescence in situ hybridization (FISH) analysis was done on 305 samples of an expanded P024 cohort that included 106 additional samples from patients treated with preoperative letrozole. HER2 gene amplification was detected in 9.2% of the samples. A higher pretreatment Ki67 (P = .005) and higher histologic grade (P = .0088) were seen in HER2+ tumors by FISH compared with those that were HER2−. Tamoxifen-treated patients who were HER2 FISH+ had lower response rates by clinical examination (33% vs 49%; P = .49) and mammography (11% vs 24%; P = .68), but this was not statistically significant.[31] Interpretation of the data is limited because of the small number of patients. In the letrozole group, there was no significant difference between response rates in HER2 FISH+ and HER2 FISH− groups by clinical examination (71% vs 71%; P = .98), ultrasound (47% vs 54%; P = .61), and mammography (44% vs 47%; P = .79). The Ki67 geometric mean at baseline and after treatment were compared in both the HER2 FISH− and HER2 FISH+ groups. In the letrozole-treated patients there was significantly less suppression of Ki67 in the HER2 FISH+ group compared with the HER2 FISH− group (P = .0001). A similar trend of Ki67 suppression was seen in the smaller tamoxifen group, however, it was not statistically significant. Another interesting finding was that letrozole was only able to induce complete cell cycle arrest in 12% of HER2+ tumors compared with 60% of HER2− tumors (P = .0001). A similar finding was seen in tamoxifen-treated tumors, with only 11% cell cycle inhibition in HER2+ tumors compared with 48% of HER2− tumors. These data suggest that despite the lesser degree of Ki67 suppression and cell cycle inhibition in HER2+ tumors, there does seem to be a similar clinical response to letrozole in HER2+ and HER2− tumors.

In the BIG I-98 study 8010 premenopausal patients were randomized to adjuvant treatment with letrozole alone for 5 years, tamoxifen alone for 5 years, or sequential therapy (letrozole for 2 years followed by tamoxifen for 3 years or tamoxifen for 2 years followed by tamoxifen for 3 years). Time to distant recurrence was greater with tamoxifen compared with letrozole (P = .05) after a median follow-up of 76 months.[10] A central review of 4399 specimens from the BIG I-98 trial evaluated ER, PR, and HER2 status. This analysis found that patients with ER+ and HER2+ tumors had inferior disease-free survival (DFS) compared with HER2− tumors in all treatment groups . In contrast, PgR status did not seem to affect DFS regardless of treatment group.[32] These adjuvant data seem to confirm what has been suggested in the P024 trial: patients with ER+ HER2+ tumors have inferior DFS compared with ER+ HER2− tumors.

WHICH AI IS SUPERIOR?

No published studies thus far have directly compared AIs in the neoadjuvant treatment of breast cancer. A phase III study has been designed by the American College of Surgeons Oncology Group (ACOSOG) to address this question (see **Fig. 1**). The Z1031 trial is a randomized study comparing 16 weeks of neoadjuvant endocrine therapy with exemestane 25 mg daily, letrozole 2.5 mg daily, or anastrozole 1 mg daily in postmenopausal women with clinical stage II and III ER+ breast cancer. The goal is to accrue 375 patients and assess response by tumor measurements on clinical examination, mammography, and ultrasound at baseline and before surgery. Tumor biopsies and serum will be collected at baseline and before surgery for genomic and proteomic predictive marker analysis. The primary end point is to compare the activity of these agents in the neoadjuvant setting. The 3 agents will also be compared based on improvement in surgical outcome, radiographic response (mammogram and ultrasound by central review), safety, pathologic tumor size, pCR, rate of complete cell cycle response (Ki67 staining of 1% or less in the posttreatment sample), incidence of metastatic lymph node involvement at the end of therapy, and 5-year local recurrence rates.

PATIENT SELECTION FOR NEOADJUVANT CHEMOTHERAPY

By examining tumors at the molecular level, we are now finding clues that may help us to select which patients will benefit from neoadjuvant endocrine therapy. A 21-gene signature has been developed to give prognostic information to patients with ER+, node-negative breast cancer treated with adjuvant tamoxifen. The degree of expression of each of these genes is used to calculate a recurrence score that subdivides patients into low, intermediate, or high risk of disease relapse at 10 years.[33] Recently, preliminary results of the Southwest Oncology Group 8814 study were presented that used this 21-gene recurrence score in a group of hormone receptor–positive and node-positive patients randomized to adjuvant treatment with cyclophosphamide, doxorubicin, and fluorouracil (CAF) followed by tamoxifen or tamoxifen alone. The results suggested that patients found to have a low risk of recurrence did not benefit from CAF chemotherapy, yet had a 40% risk of relapse at 10 years. In addition, there seemed to be no benefit with CAF in patients with ER+, HER2− disease with high Allred scores (≥ 7; $P = .052$), although this group only consisted of 15 patients.[34] These data point to the existence of a subgroup of ER+ patients who do not benefit from adjuvant chemotherapy, and also have a high risk of relapse despite treatment with hormonal therapy. This is one example of using genomic profiling to help identify a group of patients who may respond to a particular therapy.

Another method of genomic profiling of breast tumors is to separate them into their intrinsic subtypes. Breast cancers have been described in terms of 5 intrinsic subtypes: luminal A, luminal B, HER2-enriched, basal-like, and normal-like. Luminal A tumors are mostly ER+ and low grade, whereas luminal B tumors may express lower levels of hormone receptors and are usually high-grade tumors.[35] The PAM50 gene expression assay uses quantitative real-time-polymerase chain reaction (qRT-PCR) to provide a continuous risk of recurrence score based on the similarity of each sample to the 5 intrinsic subtypes in ER+, tamoxifen-treated women.[36] Intrinsic subtyping has also been used to demonstrate tumor changes after neoadjuvant endocrine therapy. Loss of tumor ER expression after treatment with neoadjuvant endocrine therapy has recently been shown to be an independent prognostic marker for relapse ($P = .02$) and death ($P = .0005$) from breast cancer.[36] The PAM50 was applied to a group of tumors from a phase II study of neoadjuvant letrozole before treatment and during treatment. Three false hormone receptor–positive tumors were identified in the pretreatment samples. In addition, the on-treatment analysis revealed 8 additional samples that were previously ER+ by IHC and transitioned to ER− after treatment with letrozole. Of the 8 relapses that occurred in this study population, 3 patients had tumors that transitioned from ER+ to ER− and 2 had tumors that were falsely ER+. These tumors were found to behave more aggressively clinically and demonstrated resistance to endocrine therapy.[37] Furthermore, in a study by Rouzier and colleagues,[38] molecular subtyping was done in 82 patients who received neoadjuvant chemotherapy with paclitaxel followed by 5-fluorouracil, doxorubicin, and cyclophosphamide. Of the 28 tumors classified as luminal A or B, only 2 had a pCR, suggesting that luminal-type tumors are less responsive to neoadjuvant chemotherapy.

In an effort to identify the characteristics of the subgroup of ER+ patients who do not respond to neoadjuvant endocrine therapy, tumor specimens of patients enrolled in the Z1031 trial will undergo gene expression profiling to identify a recurrence score based on the 21-gene signature and will be classified according to an intrinsic subtype based on the PAM50. In addition, tumor genomic DNA at baseline will undergo microarray-based genome hybridization to look for chromosomal abnormalities that may point to estrogen-independent cell growth leading to AI resistance. The correlative studies in the Z1031 trial will help to define the patient population that will respond best to neoadjuvant endocrine therapy and identify tests that will select responsive patients early in the treatment course.

NEW COMBINATIONS WITH ENDOCRINE THERAPY IN THE NEOADJUVANT SETTING

The therapeutic effects of endocrine treatments are believed to depend on an inhibitory or cytostatic effect on the tumor cell cycle.[28] Indeed, unlike cytotoxic chemotherapy, it has never been clearly demonstrated that endocrine interventions promote cell death through apoptosis, perhaps explaining why maintenance therapy is necessary and there is a high frequency of delayed recurrence.[39] The pCR rate with endocrine therapy alone is extremely low, which supports this. Thus, other agents have been added to AIs to create a synergistic effect that produces a cytotoxic rather than cytostatic effect on ER+ breast cancer, to improve the pCR rate, and to prevent endocrine resistance by blocking other growth-promoting pathways. Phase II randomized studies of endocrine therapy and signal transduction inhibitor combinations have recently been reported for gefitinib and anastrozole[40,41] and the rapamycin analogue, RAD001, with letrozole.[42] None of these studies have shown a marked improvement in efficacy with the combinations or an increase in the pCR rate. This suggests that these agents are ineffective in combination with endocrine therapy or only modestly add to the antiproliferative effects associated with endocrine treatment.

Another area of active study in ER+ breast cancers is the inhibition of the phosphinositide 3-kinase (PI3K) signaling pathway in the setting of estrogen deprivation. It has been suggested that constitutive activation of the PI3K signaling, as a result of upstream growth factor receptor signaling or genetic/epigenetic abnormalities of PI3K pathway components, is present in most breast cancers.[43] Preclinical data indicate that agents that target PI3K catalytic subunits promote cell death of ER+ breast cancer under estrogen-deprived conditions or in the presence of an anti-estrogen. In these initial experiments, the simultaneous inhibition of PI3K and ER activates cell death through apoptosis, which is reversed by the addition of estrogen, revealing a synthetic lethal mechanism that is dependent on estrogen deprivation.[44] The search for agents that have a synergistic effect with endocrine therapy in the neoadjuvant setting continues to be an active area of research.

SUMMARY

Neoadjuvant endocrine therapy with AIs has been shown to be an effective treatment to downsize ER+ tumors in postmenopausal women and improve operability and breast conservation. AIs seem to give improved outcomes in terms of breast conservation rates compared with tamoxifen, yet it is not known whether there are differences in efficacy between these agents. Current research is focused on identifying the molecular basis for response to endocrine therapy, biomarkers that predict response to endocrine therapy, tumor subtypes that are resistant to endocrine manipulation, and agents that can be used in combination with endocrine therapy to improve pCR rates and help prevent the development of endocrine resistance.

REFERENCES

1. Ma CX, Ellis MJ. Neoadjuvant endocrine therapy for locally advanced breast cancer. Semin Oncol 2005;33:650–6.
2. Fentiman IS, Christiaens MR, Paridaens R, et al. Treatment of operable breast cancer in the elderly: a randomized clinical trial EORTC 10851 comparing tamoxifen alone with modified radical mastectomy. Eur J Cancer 2003;39(3):309–16.
3. Mouridsen H, Gershanovich M, Sun Y, et al. Superior efficacy of letrozole versus tamoxifen as first-line therapy for postmenopausal women with advanced breast cancer: results of a phase III study of the International Letrozole Breast Cancer Group. J Clin Oncol 2001;19:2596–606.
4. Nabholtz JM, Buzdar A, Pollak M, et al. Anastrozole is superior to tamoxifen as first-line therapy for advanced breast cancer in postmenopausal women: results of a North American multicenter randomized trial. J Clin Oncol 2000;18(22): 3758–67.
5. Bonneterre J, Buzdar A, Nabholtz JA, et al. Anastrozole is superior to tamoxifen as first-line therapy in hormone receptor positive advanced breast carcinoma: results of two randomized trials designed for combined analysis. Cancer 2001; 92(9):2247–58.
6. Eiermann W, Paepke S, Appfelstaedt J, et al. Preoperative treatment of postmenopausal breast cancer patients with letrozole: a randomized double-blind multicenter study. Ann Oncol 2001;12:1527–32.
7. Smith IE, Dowsett M, Ebbs SR, et al. Neoadjuvant treatment of postmenopausal breast cancer with anastrozole, tamoxifen, or both in combination: the immediate preoperative anastrozole, tamoxifen, or combined with tamoxifen (impact) multicenter double-blind randomized trial. J Clin Oncol 2005;23:5108–16.
8. Cataliotti L, Buzdar AU, Noguchi S, et al. Comparison of anastrozole versus tamoxifen as preoperative therapy in postmenopausal women with hormone receptor-positive breast cancer: the pre-operative "arimidex" compared to tamoxifen (PROACT) trial. Cancer 2006;106:2095–103.
9. Howell A, Cuzick J, Baum M, et al. Results of the ATAC (Arimidex, Tamoxifen, Alone or in Combination) trial after completion of 5 years' adjuvant treatment for breast cancer. Lancet 2005;365:60–2.
10. Mouridsen H, Giobbie-Hurder A, Goldhirsch A, et al. Letrozole therapy alone or in sequence with tamoxifen in women with breast cancer. N Engl J Med 2009; 361(8):766–76.
11. Lash TL, Lien EA, Sorensen HT, et al. Genotype-guided tamoxifen therapy: time to pause for reflection? Lancet Oncol 2009;10:825–33.
12. Ingle JN. Pharmacogenetics and pharmacogenomics of endocrine agents for breast cancer. Breast Cancer Res 2008;10(4):S17.
13. Garcia-Casado Z, Guerrero-Zotano A, Llombart-Cussac A, et al. A polymorphism at the 3'-UTR region of the aromatase gene defines a subgroup of postmenopausal breast cancer patients with poor response to neoadjuvant letrozole. BMC Cancer 2010;10:36.
14. Colomer R, Monzo M, Tusquets I, et al. A single-nucleotide polymorphism in the aromatase gene is associated with the efficacy of the aromatase inhibitor letrozole in advanced breast carcinoma. Clin Cancer Res 2008;14:811–6.
15. Mlineritsch B, Tausch C, Singer C, et al. Exemestane as primary systemic treatment for hormone receptor positive post-menopausal breast cancer patients: a phase II trial of the Austrian Breast and Colorectal Cancer Study Group (ABCSG-17). Breast Cancer Res Treat 2008;112:203–13.

16. Olson JA Jr, Budd GT, Carey LA, et al. Improved surgical outcomes for breast cancer patients receiving neoadjuvant aromatase inhibitor therapy: results from a multicenter phase II trial. J Am Coll Surg 2009;208:906–14.

17. Seo JH, Kim YH, Kim JS. Meta-analysis of pre-operative aromatase inhibitor versus tamoxifen in postmenopausal woman with hormone receptor-positive breast cancer. Cancer Chemother Pharmacol 2009;63:261–6.

18. Early Breast Cancer Trialists' Collaborative Group. Effects of chemotherapy and hormonal therapy for early breast cancer on recurrence and 15-year survival: an overview of the randomized trials. Lancet 2005;365(9472):1687–717.

19. Paik S, Tang G, Shak S, et al. Gene expression and benefit of chemotherapy in women with node-negative, estrogen receptor-positive breast cancer. J Clin Oncol 2006;24:3726–34.

20. Kuerer HM, Newman LA, Smith TL, et al. Clinical course of breast cancer patients with complete pathologic primary tumor and axillary lymph node response to doxorubicin-based neoadjuvant chemotherapy. J Clin Oncol 1999;17(2):460–9.

21. Ring AE, Smith IE, Ashley S, et al. Oestrogen receptor status, pathological complete response and prognosis in patients receiving neoadjuvant chemotherapy for early breast cancer. Br J Cancer 2004;91(12):2012–7.

22. Bonadonna G, Veronesi U, Brambilla C, et al. Primary chemotherapy to avoid mastectomy in tumors with diameters of three centimeters or more. J Natl Cancer Inst 1990;82(19):1539–45.

23. Mauriac L, Durand M, Avril A, et al. Effects of primary chemotherapy in conservative treatment of breast cancer patients with operable tumors larger than 3 cm: results of a randomized trial in a single centre. Ann Oncol 1991;2(5):347–54.

24. Semiglazov VF, Semiglazov VV, Dashyan GA, et al. Phase 2 randomized trial of primary endocrine therapy versus chemotherapy in postmenopausal patients with estrogen receptor-positive breast cancer. Cancer 2007;110(2): 244–54.

25. Ellis MJ, Coop A, Singh B, et al. Letrozole inhibits tumor proliferation more effectively than tamoxifen independent of HER1/2 expression status. Cancer Res 2003;63:6523–31.

26. Dowsett M, Ebbs SR, Dixon JM, et al. Biomarker changes during neoadjuvant anastrozole, tamoxifen, or the combination: influence of hormonal status and HER-2 in breast cancer–a study from the IMPACT trialists. J Clin Oncol 2005; 23:2477–92.

27. Miller WR, Anderson TJ, White S, et al. Aromatase inhibitors: cellular and molecular effects. J Steroid Biochem Mol Biol 2005;95:83–9.

28. Ellis MJ. Improving outcomes for patients with hormone receptor-positive breast cancer: back to the drawing board. J Natl Cancer Inst 2008;100:159–61.

29. Dowsett M, Smith IE, Ebbs SR, et al. Prognostic value of Ki67 expression after short-term presurgical endocrine therapy for primary breast cancer. J Natl Cancer Inst 2007;99:167–70.

30. Ellis MJ, Coop A, Singh B, et al. Letrozole is more effective neoadjuvant endocrine therapy than tamoxifen for ErbB-1- and/or ErbB-2-positive, estrogen receptor-positive primary breast cancer: evidence from a phase III randomized trial. J Clin Oncol 2001;19:3808–16.

31. Ellis MJ, Tao Y, Young O, et al. Estrogen-independent proliferation is present in estrogen-receptor HER2-positive primary breast cancer after neoadjuvant letrozole. J Clin Oncol 2006;24:3019–25.

32. Viale G, Regan M, Dell'Orto P, et al. Central review of ER, PgR and HER-2 in BIG I-98 evaluating letrozole vs. tamoxifen as adjuvant endocrine therapy for postmenopausal women with receptor-positive breast cancer [abstract 44]. Breast Cancer Res Treat 2005;94(Suppl 1):S13.

33. Paik S, Shak S, Tang G, et al. A multigene assay to predict recurrence of tamoxifen-treated, node-negative breast cancer. N Engl J Med 2004;351: 2817–26.

34. Albain K, Barlow W, Shak S, et al. Southwest Oncology Group and The Breast Cancer Intergroup of NA, San Antonio, TX 8814: Prognostic and predictive value of the 21-gene recurrence score assay in post-menopausal, node-positive, ER-positive breast cancer (S INT0100) [abstract]. Breast Cancer Res Treat 2007; 106:A10.

35. Perou CM, Sorlie T, Eisen MB, et al. Molecular portraits of human breast tumours. Nature 2000;406(6797):47–52.

36. Ellis MJ, Tao Y, Luo J, et al. Outcome prediction for clinical stage II and III ER+ breast cancer based on treatment response, pathological stage, tumor grade, Ki67 proliferation index, and estrogen receptor status after neoadjuvant endocrine therapy [abstract 62]. J Natl Cancer Inst 2007;16(Suppl 1):S16.

37. Ellis MJ, Tao Y, Luo J, et al. A poor prognosis ER and HER2-negative, nonbasal, breast cancer subtype identified through postneoadjuvant endocrine therapy tumor profiling [abstract 502]. J Clin Oncol 2008;26.

38. Rouzier R, Perou CM, Symmans WF, et al. Breast cancer molecular subtypes respond differently to preoperative chemotherapy. Clin Cancer Res 2005; 11(16):5678–85.

39. Dowsett M, Smith IE, Ebbs SR, et al. Proliferation and apoptosis as markers of benefit in neoadjuvant endocrine therapy of breast cancer. Clin Cancer Res 2006;12:1024s–30.

40. Polychronis A, Sinnett HD, Hadjiminas D, et al. Preoperative gefitinib versus gefitinib and anastrozole in postmenopausal patients with oestrogen-receptor positive and epidermal-growth-factor-receptor-positive primary breast cancer: a double-blind placebo-controlled phase II randomised trial. Lancet Oncol 2005;6:383–91.

41. Smith IE, Walsh G, Skene A, et al. A phase II placebo-controlled trial of neoadjuvant anastrozole alone or with gefitinib in early breast cancer. J Clin Oncol 2007; 25:3816–22.

42. Baselga J, Semiglazov V, van Dam P, et al. Phase II randomized study of neoadjuvant everolimus plus letrozole compared with placebo plus letrozole in patients with estrogen receptor-positive breast cancer. J Clin Oncol 2009;27:2630–7.

43. Crowder RJ, Ellis MJ. Treating breast cancer through novel inhibitors of the phosphatidylinositol 3'-kinase pathway. Breast Cancer Res 2005;7:212–4.

44. Crowder RJ, Phommaly C, Tao Y, et al. PIK3CA and PIK3CB inhibition produce synthetic lethality when combined with estrogen deprivation in estrogen receptor-positive breast cancer. Cancer Res 2009;69:3955–62.

Adjuvant Hormonal Therapy for Early-Stage Breast Cancer

Harold J. Burstein, MD, PhD[a],*, Jennifer J. Griggs, MD, MPH[b,c,d]

KEYWORDS

- Adjuvant endocrine therapy • Tamoxifen
- Aromatase inhibitors • Ovarian suppression

Adjuvant endocrine therapy is critical for reducing the risk of recurrence and promoting survival in women with hormone receptor (estrogen receptor [ER] or progesterone receptor [PgR])–positive breast cancers. Adjuvant endocrine therapy reduces the risk of tumor recurrence by approximately 40%, on average. Because of that substantial effect and because of the prevalence of hormone receptor–positive breast cancer, it is arguable that adjuvant endocrine therapy has had greater impact on reducing mortality from cancer than any other medical therapy. In addition to preventing metastatic recurrence, adjuvant endocrine therapy reduces the risk of in-breast or regional recurrences and lowers the risk of contralateral breast cancer.[1] In light of these benefits, adjuvant endocrine therapy is recommended for nearly all patients with hormone receptor–positive breast cancer irrespective of tumor size or nodal status.[2–4]

The prerequisite of benefit from treatment with adjuvant endocrine therapy is tumor expression of the ER or PgR. In the absence of tumor expression of these hormone receptors, adjuvant endocrine therapy is not of clinical benefit.[5] This observation leads to the clinical requirement of high-quality hormone receptor testing on all newly diagnosed breast cancers.[6] A variety of prognostic factors have emerged that are associated with recurrence risk of ER-positive breast cancer (**Box 1**). These markers can inform the likelihood of tumor recurrence and, based on the assumption of proportional risk reduction associated with adjuvant endocrine treatment, may serve to estimate the absolute magnitude of treatment effect. To date, however, no single marker

[a] Breast Oncology Center, Dana-Farber Cancer Institute, Harvard Medical School, 44 Binney Street, Boston, MA 02115, USA
[b] Hematology and Oncology Division, Department of Internal Medicine, University of Michigan, Ann Arbor, MI, USA
[c] Department of Health Management and Policy, University of Michigan, Ann Arbor, MI, USA
[d] Breast Cancer Survivorship Program, Comprehensive Cancer Center, University of Michigan, Ann Arbor, MI, USA
* Corresponding author.
E-mail address: hburstein@partners.org

Surg Oncol Clin N Am 19 (2010) 639–647
doi:10.1016/j.soc.2010.03.006
1055-3207/10/$ – see front matter © 2010 Elsevier Inc. All rights reserved.

surgonc.theclinics.com

Box 1
Prognostic factors in hormone receptor–positive breast cancer

Tumor size (T)

Nodal status (N)

Tumor grade

Quantitative levels of hormone receptor expression

HER2 expression status

Lymphovascular invasion

Proliferative markers, such as Ki-67

Multigene prognostic signatures, such as the 21-gene recurrence score (Oncotype DX assay, Genomic Health Inc, Redwood City, CA, USA)

---

aside from expression of the hormone receptors themselves is adequate for identifying which patients might, or might not, benefit from adjuvant endocrine therapy. Similarly, no single marker can identify which endocrine treatment strategy might be optimal for a given patient.

It is now appreciated that ER-positive breast cancers have a different pattern of tumor recurrence from other forms of breast cancer. In the absence of adjuvant endocrine therapy, there is a peak of recurrences in years 2 through 5 and then a steady persistent risk of recurrence through at least 15 years after diagnosis.[7] Introduction of adjuvant endocrine therapy dramatically reduces the incidence of early recurrences in the first 10 years after diagnosis.[8] Endocrine therapy is also associated with a carry-over effect, such that patients who have had 5 years of therapy continue to have a lower risk of recurrence through at least 15 years of follow-up after breast cancer diagnosis. With longer passage of time, second breast cancers and non–breast cancer mortality contribute a greater percentage of events in studies of adjuvant endocrine therapy. These observations underscore the need for long-term follow-up of patients receiving adjuvant endocrine therapy.

TAMOXIFEN

Tamoxifen, a selective ER modulator, has been the historic standard for adjuvant endocrine therapy.[9] Multiple prospective, randomized, clinical trials of adjuvant tamoxifen therapy have been analyzed as part of the Early Breast Cancer Trialists' Group overview analysis.[10] Five years of tamoxifen therapy lowers the risk of breast cancer recurrence by approximately 40% and lowers the risk of breast cancer mortality by approximately 20%. The benefits of tamoxifen are seen regardless of patient age or menopausal status. The optimal duration of tamoxifen therapy seems to be a total of 5 years. Published studies that have examined continuation of tamoxifen treatment beyond 5 years have not demonstrated a significant clinical benefit for additional therapy.[11] Preliminary studies from the large Adjuvant Tamoxifen Treatment Offers More? (ATTOM) and Adjuvant Tamoxifen—Longer Against Shorter (ATLAS) trials have raised anew questions regarding the optimal duration of tamoxifen treatment; however, at present, 5 years remains the standard for women taking tamoxifen alone.

The side effects of tamoxifen have been well characterized (**Table 1**). Common side effects include menopausal symptoms, such as hot flashes and night sweats, and in premenopausal women, menstrual irregularities. Tamoxifen is associated with a low

Table 1
Side effects of adjuvant endocrine therapy

	Tamoxifen	Aromatase Inhibitors	Ovarian Suppression
Gynecologic	Vaginal discharge or dryness/atrophy; increased risk of vaginal bleeding and uterine cancer	Vaginal dryness/atrophy	Vaginal dryness/atrophy
Menstrual function	Irregular menstrual cycles or amenorrhea	Not applicable	Amenorrhea
Menopausal symptoms	Hot flashes, night sweats	Hot flashes, night sweats	Hot flashes, night sweats
Musculoskeletal health	Mixed effects on bone density	Osteopenia, osteoporotic fractures; musculoskeletal (arthralgia) syndrome	Osteopenia
Cardiovascular health	Increased risk of deep vein thrombosis	Increased risk of hypercholesterolemia, hypertension	Unknown

but increased risk of uterine cancer and deep venous thrombosis, particularly in postmenopausal women. Quality-of-life studies suggest that most women on tamoxifen have a well-preserved quality of life in all functional domains and that most women are reasonably adherent with treatment.

ADJUVANT ENDOCRINE THERAPY FOR POSTMENOPAUSAL WOMEN WITH HORMONE RECEPTOR–POSITIVE EARLY-STAGE BREAST CANCER

The introduction of aromatase inhibitors (AIs) has defined a new era of adjuvant endocrine treatment for postmenopausal women with hormone receptor–positive breast cancer. AIs function by blocking the conversion of androgens into estrogens through the aromatase enzyme.[12] The consequence of such therapy for postmenopausal women is profound estrogen deprivation—circulating estrogen levels are typically depleted by 90% from baseline.[13] It is presumed that the resultant estrogen deprivation causes the antineoplastic effects of AI therapy. Because premenopausal women have residual ovarian function and the capacity to up-regulate aromatase expression in ovarian tissues in response to estrogen deprivation, AIs are contraindicated in premenopausal women.

AIs have been studied in several contexts as adjuvant endocrine treatment for postmenopausal women. Because the historical standard for adjuvant therapy has been 5 years of tamoxifen, most of the major adjuvant trials have compared AI-based treatment with 5 years of tamoxifen. The development of AIs as adjuvant treatment has included studies of primary endocrine therapy, which used AIs as initial treatment instead of tamoxifen; sequential endocrine therapy, which integrated AIs as adjuvant treatment after several (typically, 2 to 3) years of tamoxifen; and extended adjuvant therapy, which explored AI-based treatment after 5 years of adjuvant tamoxifen. **Table 2** identifies the major adjuvant trials that have reported in the past decade on the role of AIs in the adjuvant setting.

Collectively, these trials have demonstrated important observations. First, incorporation of an AI during the first 5 years of adjuvant endocrine treatment, or as extended therapy after 5 years of tamoxifen, is associated with a reduction in the risk of breast

Table 2
Major trials of AI therapy as adjuvant treatment of postmenopausal, early-stage, hormone receptor–positive breast cancer

	Study Name	Schema	Total Duration of Therapy (y)	AI	References
Primary endocrine therapy	ATAC	TAM versus AI versus TAM + AI	5	ANA	30,31
	BIG 1-98	TAM → AI versus AI → TAM versus TAM versus AI	5	LET	32,33
	ABCSG 12	TAM versus AI premenopausal at diagnosis; all patients receive ovarian suppression	5	ANA	34
	TEAM	AI versus TAM → AI	5	EXE	35
Sequential endocrine therapy (after 2–3 years of TAM)	IES	TAM versus TAM → AI	5	EXE	36
	ARNO 95, ABCSG 8, Italian	TAM versus TAM → AI	5	ANA	37,38
Extended endocrine therapy (after 5 years of TAM)	MA 17	AI versus placebo	10	LET	39
	ABCSG 6a	AI versus placebo	7	ANA	40
	NSABP B-22	AI versus placebo	10	EXE	41

Abbreviations: ABCSG, Austrian Breast and Colorectal Cancer Study Group; ANA, anastrozole; ARNO 95, Arimidex-Nolvadex; EXE, exemestane; IES, Intergroup Exemestane Study; LET, letrozole; NSABP, National Surgical Adjuvant Breast and Bowel Project; TAM, tamoxifen.

cancer recurrence. This reduction in risk is approximately a 15% to 20% proportionate risk reduction compared with tamoxifen alone. Because of the generally favorable prognosis for most postmenopausal women with early-stage breast cancer, the absolute difference in breast cancer events associated with AI-based therapy compared with tamoxifen is approximately 2% to 3%. The improvement in breast cancer outcomes includes reduction in the risk of distant metastatic recurrence as well as reduction in local/in-breast events and contralateral breast cancer.[14] These modest gains are noted in comparing initial use of an AI with tamoxifen or in comparing tamoxifen alone with a sequence of tamoxifen followed by an AI.[15] To date, studies have not reported a significant survival advantage for initial use of an AI compared with a sequential treatment program of tamoxifen and an AI. Compared with treatment with tamoxifen alone, sequential use of an AI may confer a modest survival advantage.

Second, it seems that a variety of treatment strategies yield similar outcomes, provided that an AI is incorporated at some point. Direct comparisons of results between initial use of an AI and a sequential program of a tamoxifen followed by an AI show equivalent rates of tumor recurrence in the Breast International Group (BIG) 1-98 and Tamoxifen Exemestane Adjuvant Multicentre (TEAM) trials. In the Arimidex, Tamoxifen Alone or in Combination (ATAC) study, the combination of an AI with tamoxifen was not superior to tamoxifen alone.

These findings support the recommendation for consideration of an AI at some point during adjuvant endocrine treatment in postmenopausal women.[16] The optimal timing of AI therapy vis-à-vis tamoxifen remains unknown. It is also unknown whether or not a longer total duration of treatment, accomplished with extended therapy using tamoxifen followed by an AI, would differ from initial use of an AI. Another persistent question remains the best duration of AI treatment itself. Different studies used different durations of AI therapy. As primary treatment, data show equivalence for 2.5 or 5 years of AI therapy. Ongoing trials are examining whether or not longer-term use of an AI in excess of 5 years' total duration is safe and effective. No studies reported to date have directly compared the cancer outcomes for one AI with another as adjuvant treatment. In broad terms, the findings with each of the commercially available AIs (anastrozole, exemestane, and letrozole) seem qualitatively similar; thus, it seems likely that the benefits seen with AI treatment represent a class effect. Ongoing trials are comparing directly one AI with another.

Clinical experience with in the adjuvant setting has identified common side effects of AI treatment (see **Table 1**). Patients taking AIs are at greater risk for musculoskeletal health problems, including accelerated osteoporosis and fractures, than are women taking tamoxifen.[17] Bisphosphonate therapy seems to mitigate AI-associated loss of bone mineral density.[18,19] AIs are associated with a unique arthralgia syndrome, characterized by muscle and joint stiffness and achiness, which is common although usually of modest intensity.[20] AIs are also associated with a slightly greater risk of hypertension and hypercholesterolemia; the long-term cardiac consequences of these effects are not yet well characterized.[21]

There remains considerable interest in efforts to tailor specific adjuvant endocrine treatment options for individual patients based on tumor characteristics or biomarkers or based on consideration of pharmacogenetic studies. These retrospective efforts remain inconclusive. At present, it does not seem that there are sufficient data for using CYP2D6 genotyping for deciding whether or not tamoxifen is a suitable treatment option for specific women.[22] A variety of pathologic and other biomarker studies confirm prognostic markers for patients treated with AIs.[23,24] These measures lack sufficient data, however, for predicting which treatment strategy (tamoxifen alone, AI alone, or a sequence of tamoxifen and an AI) would be best for a given woman.

Currently, the recommendation for initial treatment choices should be informed by the available data on efficacy, side-effect profiles, and patient preferences in postmenopausal women.

ADJUVANT ENDOCRINE THERAPY FOR PREMENOPAUSAL WOMEN WITH HORMONE RECEPTOR–POSITIVE EARLY-STAGE BREAST CANCER

Tamoxifen, which is effective irrespective of menopausal status, remains the adjuvant endocrine treatment standard for pre- or perimenopausal women with ER-positive breast cancer. AIs (discussed previously) are contraindicated in women with residual ovarian function. Young women who received adjuvant chemotherapy may experience treatment-related amenorrhea. Because these women may recover ovarian function over time, they are not appropriate candidates for initial AI therapy and should receive tamoxifen as the adjuvant endocrine treatment of choice.[25]

The seminal issue in the management of premenopausal women with early-stage, hormone receptor–positive breast cancer is the role of ovarian suppression in addition to tamoxifen. Ovarian suppression, achieved through administration of gonadotropin-releasing hormone analogues or oophorectomy, is an effective adjuvant treatment for women with ER-positive breast cancer.[10] Its role in modern management is unclear, however. This uncertainty arises because of the confounding effects of chemotherapy-induced amenorrhea in younger women who receive adjuvant chemotherapy. It also arises because the design of major clinical studies in the 1990s analyzed the impact of ovarian suppression as an alternative to chemotherapy or tamoxifen but typically not in addition to other endocrine therapy (namely, tamoxifen). Thus, there is persistent debate as to the value of ovarian suppression in addition to tamoxifen for pre- or perimenopausal patients.[26]

Several lines of indirect data suggest that patients with ER-positive breast cancer may benefit from ovarian suppression in addition to tamoxifen. Ovarian suppression, by itself or as a consequence of chemotherapy, improves outcomes for premenopausal breast cancer patients. The addition of ovarian suppression and tamoxifen improves outcomes in young women compared with chemotherapy alone.[27] Women who receive both chemotherapy and tamoxifen and who experience treatment-induced amenorrhea have a superior outcome compared with women who do not go into menopause with therapy.[28] A meta-analysis of ovarian suppression trials suggests that gonadotropin-releasing hormone analogues might reduce the risk of cancer recurrence.[29] This collective work invites the possibility that adding ovarian suppression might lower the risk of breast cancer recurrence in addition to tamoxifen in premenopausal women. The data are not definitive, however. It is hoped that the Suppression of Ovarian Function Trial, a randomized study run by the International Breast Cancer Study Group that compares tamoxifen alone with tamoxifen plus ovarian suppression with ovarian suppression plus an AI, will resolve this question.

Women who experience ovarian suppression as part of a program of adjuvant therapy seem to suffer more intensive menopausal side effects than women receiving tamoxifen alone. This includes greater severity of hot flashes, night sweats, and other climacteric symptoms and osteoporosis.

SUMMARY

Adjuvant endocrine treatment is an essential component in therapy for women with hormone receptor–positive breast cancer. In postmenopausal patients, options include tamoxifen, AIs, or a sequence of these agents. It seems that incorporating an AI at some point in the treatment program improves outcomes compared with tamoxifen alone. Tamoxifen and AIs have distinctive side-effect profiles that clinicians should understand. Among premenopausal women, tamoxifen remains the standard treatment. The role of ovarian suppression in addition to tamoxifen is still under investigation. Indirect data suggest there may be a role for ovarian suppression, but this is not yet a standard treatment option. Questions about the duration of adjuvant endocrine therapy, the use of biomarkers for treatment selection and prognosis, and the management of side effects of adjuvant endocrine therapy remain key areas of ongoing investigation.

REFERENCES

1. Fisher B, Bryant J, Dignam JJ, et al. Tamoxifen, radiation therapy, or both for prevention of ipsilateral breast tumor recurrence after lumpectomy in women with invasive breast cancers of one centimeter or less. J Clin Oncol 2002; 20(20):4141–9.
2. National Institutes of Health Consensus Development Conference statement: adjuvant therapy for breast cancer, November 1–3, 2000. J Natl Cancer Inst Monogr 2001;30:5–15.
3. Goldhirsh A, Ingle JN, Gelber RD. Thresholds for therapies: highlights of the St Gallen International Expert Consensus on the primary therapy of early breast cancer 2009. Ann Oncol 2009;20(8):1319–29.
4. Carlson RW, Allred DC, Anderson BO, et al. Breast cancer. Clinical practice guidelines in oncology. J Natl Compr Canc Netw 2009;7(2):122–92.
5. Fisher B, Anderson S, Tan-Chiu E, et al. Tamoxifen and chemotherapy for axillary node-negative, estrogen receptor-negative breast cancer: findings from National Surgical Adjuvant Breast and Bowel Project B-23. J Clin Oncol 2001;19(4): 931–42.
6. Allred DC, Carlson RW, Berry DA, et al. NCCN task force report: estrogen receptor and progesterone receptor testing in breast cancer by immunohisto-chemistry. J Natl Compr Canc Netw 2009;7(Suppl 6):S1–21.
7. Saphner T, Tormey DC, Gray R. Annual hazard rates of recurrence for breast cancer after primary therapy. J Clin Oncol 1996;14(10):2738–46.
8. Love RR, Van Dinh N, Quy TT, et al. Survival after adjuvant oophorectomy and tamoxifen in operable breast cancer in premenopausal women. J Clin Oncol 2008;26:253–7.
9. Osborne CK. Tamoxifen in the treatment of breast cancer. N Engl J Med 1998; 339:1609–18.
10. Early Breast Cancer Trialists' Collaborative Group (EBCTCG). Effects of chemotherapy and hormonal therapy for early breast cancer on recurrence and 15-year survival: an overview of the randomised trials. Lancet 2005;365:1687–717.
11. Fisher B, Dignam J, Bryant J, et al. Five versus more than five years of tamoxifen for lymph node-negative breast cancer: updated findings from the National Surgical Adjuvant Breast and Bowel Project B-14 randomized trial. J Natl Cancer Inst 2001;93(9):684–90.
12. Smith IE, Dowsett M. Aromatase inhibitors in breast cancer. N Engl J Med 2003; 348(24):2431–42.
13. Geisler J, Helle H, Ekse D, et al. Letrozole is superior to anastrozole in suppressing breast cancer tissue and plasma estrogen levels. Clin Cancer Res 2008; 14(19):6330–5.

14. Hudis CA, Barlow WE, Costantino JP, et al. Proposal for standardized definitions for efficacy end points in adjuvant breast cancer trials: the STEEP system. J Clin Oncol 2007;25:2127–32.

15. Dowsett M, Cuzick J, Ingle J, et al. Meta-analysis of breast cancer outcomes in adjuvant trials of aromatase inhibitors versus tamoxifen. J Clin Oncol 2010; 28(3):509–18.

16. Winer EP, Hudis C, Burstein HJ, et al. American Society of Clinical Oncology technology assessment on the use of aromatase inhibitors as adjuvant therapy for postmenopausal women with hormone receptor-positive breast cancer: status report 2004. J Clin Oncol 2005;23:619–29.

17. Eastell R, Adams JE, Coleman RE, et al. Effect of anastrozole on bone mineral density: 5-year results from the anastrozole, tamoxifen, alone or in combination trial 18233230. J Clin Oncol 2008;26:1051–7.

18. Brufsky A, Bundred N, Coleman R, et al. Integrated analysis of zoledronic acid for prevention of aromatase inhibitor-associated bone loss in postmenopausal women with early breast cancer receiving adjuvant letrozole. Oncologist 2008; 13(5):503–14.

19. Van Posnack C, Hannon RA, Mackey JR, et al. Prevention of aromatase inhibitor-induced bone loss using risedronate: the SABRE trial. J Clin Oncol 2010; 28(No 6):967–75.

20. Burstein HJ, Winer EP. Aromatase inhibitors and arthralgias: a new frontier in symptom management for breast cancer survivors. J Clin Oncol 2007;25:3797–9.

21. Mouridsen H, Keshaviah A, Coates AS, et al. Cardiovascular adverse events during adjuvant endocrine therapy for early breast cancer using letrozole or tamoxifen: safety analysis of BIG 1-98 trial. J Clin Oncol 2007;25:5715–22.

22. Higgins MJ, Rae JM, Flockhart DA, et al. Pharmacogenetics of tamoxifen: who should undergo CYP2D6 genetic testing? J Natl Compr Canc Netw 2009;7(2): 203–13.

23. Mauriac L, Keshaviah A, Debled M, et al. Predictors of early relapse in postmenopausal women with hormone receptor-positive breast cancer in the BIG 1-98 trial. Ann Oncol 2007;18:859–67.

24. Dowsett M, Cuzick J, Wale C, et al. Prediction of risk of distant recurrence using the 21-gene recurrence score in node-negative and node-positive postmenopausal patients with breast cancer treated with anastrozole or tamoxifen: a Trans-ATAC study. J Clin Oncol 2010;28(11):1829–34.

25. Smith IE, Dowsett M, Yap YS, et al. Adjuvant aromatase inhibitors for early breast cancer after chemotherapy-induced amenorrhoea: caution and suggested guidelines. J Clin Oncol 2006;24:2444–7.

26. Parton M, Smith IE. Controversies in the management of patients with breast cancer: adjuvant endocrine therapy in premenopausal women. J Clin Oncol 2008;26(5):745–52.

27. Davidson NE, O'Neill AM, Vukov AM, et al. Chemoendocrine therapy for premenopausal women with axillary lymph node-positive, steroid hormone receptor-positive breast cancer: results from INT 0101 (E5188). J Clin Oncol 2005;23(25): 5973–82.

28. International Breast Cancer Study Group, Colleoni M, Gelber S, et al. Tamoxifen after adjuvant chemotherapy for premenopausal women with lymph node-positive breast cancer: International Breast Cancer Study Group Trial 13-93. J Clin Oncol 2006;24(9):1332–41.

29. LHRH-agonists in Early Breast Cancer Overview group 3, Cuzick J, Ambroisine L, et al. Use of lueinising-hormone-releasing hormone agonists as adjuvant

treatment in premenopausal patients with hormone-receptor positive breast cancer: a meta-analysis of individual patient data from randomized adjuvant trials. Lancet 2007;369:1711–23.

30. Baum M, Budzar AU, Cuzick J, et al. Anastrozole alone or in combination with tamoxifen versus tamoxifen alone for adjuvant treatment of postmenopausal women with early breast cancer: first results of the ATAC randomised trial. Lancet 2003;359:2131–9.

31. Forbes JF, Cuzick J, Buzdar A, et al. Effect of anastrozole and tamoxifen as adjuvant treatment for early-stage breast cancer: 100-month analysis of the ATAC trial. Lancet Oncol 2008;9:45–53.

32. Breast International Group (BIG) 1-98 Collaborative Group, Thürlimann B, Keshaviah A, et al. A comparison of letrozole and tamoxifen in postmenopausal women with early breast cancer. N Engl J Med 2005;353(26):2747–57.

33. Mouridsen H, Giobbie-Hurder A, Goldhirsch A, et al. Letrozole therapy alone or in sequence with tamoxifen in women with breast cancer. N Engl J Med 2009;361: 766–76.

34. Gnant M, Mlineritsch B, Schippinger W, et al. Endocrine therapy plus zoledronic acid in premenopausal breast cancer. N Engl J Med 2009;360:679–91.

35. Bliss JM, Kilburn LS, Coleman RE, et al. Disease related outcome with long term follow-up: an updated analysis of the Intergroup Exemestaine Study (IES). Presented at the 2009 San Antonio Breast Cancer Symposium. December, 2009.

36. Coombes RC, Hall E, Gibson LJ, et al. A randomized trial of exemestane after two to three years of tamoxifen therapy in postmenopausal women with primary breast cancer. N Engl J Med 2004;350:1081–92.

37. Jakesz R, Jonat W, Gnant M, et al. Switching of postmenopausal women with endocrine-responsive early breast cancer to anastrozole after 2 years' adjuvant tamoxifen: combined results of ABCSG trial 8 and ARNO 95 trial. Lancet 2005; 366:455–62.

38. Boccardo F, Rubagotti A, Puntoni M, et al. Switching to anastrozole versus continued tamoxifen treatment of early breast cancer: preliminary results of the Italian Tamoxifen Anastrozole Trial. J Clin Oncol 2005;23:5138–47.

39. Goss PE, Ingle JN, Martino S, et al. A randomized trial of letrozole in postmenopausal women after five years of tamoxifen therapy for early-stage breast cancer. N Engl J Med 2003;349:1793–802.

40. Jakesz R, Greil R, Gnant M, et al. Extended adjuvant therapy with anastrozole among postmenopausal breast cancer patients: results from the randomized Austrian Breast and Colorectal Cancer Study Group Trial 6a. J Natl Cancer Inst 2007;99(24):1845–53.

41. Mamounas EP, Jeong JH, Wickerham DL, et al. Benefit from exemestane as extended adjuvant therapy after 5 years of adjuvant tamoxifen: intention-to-treat analysis of the National Surgical Adjuvant Breast and Bowel Project B-33 trial. J Clin Oncol 2008;26:1965–71.

Adjuvant Chemotherapy in Early-Stage Breast Cancer: What, When, and for Whom?

Catherine M. Kelly, MD, MSc (ClinEpi)[a], Gabriel N. Hortobagyi, MD[b],*

KEYWORDS

• Early-stage breast cancer • Adjuvant chemotherapy
• Anthracyclines • Taxanes

Breast cancer mortality has been falling in the United States over the last several decades.[1] This trend has been attributed to early detection as a result of the widespread adoption of screening mammography and the use of effective adjuvant therapies.[2] Nevertheless, despite recent advances breast cancer remains a considerable public health issue. Globally it is estimated that 1.5 million women will be diagnosed with breast cancer in 2010.[3] In the United States, 192,370 new breast cancer diagnoses (comprising 27% of all incident cancers in females) and 40,000 breast cancer deaths were estimated for 2009.[1] Better adjuvant therapies are needed to reduce the burden of illness caused by breast cancer.

Adjuvant chemotherapy is directed at treating occult micrometastatic disease, thereby reducing the risk of recurrence. Chemotherapy works most effectively when the tumor volume is small and still in the linear growth phase.[4] This rationale led to some of the first adjuvant clinical trials of polychemotherapy versus observation in lymph node–positive breast cancer that showed improved disease-free survival (DFS) and overall survival (OS).[5] Subsequently in 1988, based on the early results of several randomized trials evaluating systemic therapy in lymph node–negative breast cancer, the US National Cancer Institute (NCI) issued a "clinical alert" that resulted in the recommendation by the 2000 National Institutes of Health (NIH) Consensus Conference that chemotherapy should be considered in all women with tumors greater than 1 cm or positive lymph nodes.[6–10]

[a] Department of Breast Medical Oncology, University of Texas M.D. Anderson Cancer Center, 1155 Herman P Pressler, Houston, TX 77030-1439, USA
[b] Department of Breast Medical Oncology, University of Texas M.D. Anderson Cancer Center, 1515 Holcombe Boulevard, Unit 1354, Houston, TX 77030-4009, USA
* Corresponding author.
E-mail address: ghortoba@mdanderson.org

Surg Oncol Clin N Am 19 (2010) 649–668
doi:10.1016/j.soc.2010.03.007
1055-3207/10/$ – see front matter © 2010 Elsevier Inc. All rights reserved.

The Early Breast Cancer Trialists' Collaborative Group (EBCTCG) meta-analyses (Oxford Overview, *Overview Analyses*) have provided extensive evidence illustrating the efficacy of adjuvant chemotherapy in early breast cancer.[11,12] The EBCTCG was established in 1984 to 1985 and conducts 5-yearly worldwide meta-analyses of centrally collected data from every individual patient enrolled in all randomized trials already running for at least 5 years. The most recent publication in 2005 reports the 2000 meta-analyses and was based on data from 60 randomized trials initiated before 1995 comparing polychemotherapy to none, and included 29,000 women of whom 10,000 died.[11] At 15 years there was a significant reduction in the absolute risk of recurrence and breast cancer mortality for polychemotherapy compared with none (**Fig. 1**). The absolute benefits at 10 or 15 years were 3 times greater for younger compared with older women. In younger women adjuvant polychemotherapy reduced the annual risk of relapse and death by 37% and 30%, respectively, and the absolute

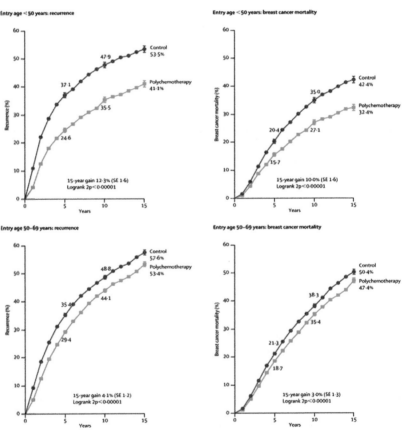

Fig. 1. Polychemotherapy versus no polychemotherapy (Control), by entry age younger than 50 or 50 to 69 years: 15-year probabilities of recurrence and of breast cancer mortality. Younger women, 35% node-positive; older women, 70% node-positive. Error bars are ±1 SE. (*Reprinted from* Early Breast Cancer Trialists' Collaborative Group (EBCTCG). Effects of chemotherapy and hormonal therapy for early breast cancer on recurrence and 15-year survival: an overview of the randomized trials. Lancet 2005;365:1687–717; Copyright 2005; with permission from Elsevier.)

gain in survival was twice as great at 15 years as it was at 5 years (10% vs 4.7%). In older women (50–69 years) the annual risk of relapse and breast cancer mortality was reduced by 19% and 12%, respectively, and translated into an absolute gain of 4.1% and 3.0%, respectively, at 15 years.[11,13] The proportional reductions in recurrence and breast cancer mortality were similar in node-negative and node-positive patients. However, the absolute benefit was greater in node-positive patients. The *Overview Analyses* also indicate that the greatest effect of adjuvant chemotherapy occurs in the initial few years after therapy; however, the effects last for long periods of time, exceeding 15 to 20 years.

Further subgroup analysis showed that adjuvant chemotherapy was effective in both estrogen receptor (ER)-negative and ER-positive breast cancer. However, the *Overview Analyses* and data from several Cancer and Leukemia Group B (CALGB) trials in patients with node-positive breast cancer indicate greater chemotherapy benefit in ER-negative compared with ER-positive disease.[11,14] The first report from the 2005-2006 *Overview Analyses* specifically considered the benefit of chemotherapy in ER-negative tumors. In this analysis there were 20,000 women with ER-negative breast cancer randomized to polychemotherapy versus none.[15] Significant reductions were observed in the absolute risk of recurrence and cancer-specific mortality of 12.3% and 9.2%, and 8.6% and 6.1% for patients younger than 50 years and between 50 and 69 years, respectively. These data are based on clinical trials conducted with older regimens, and it is expected the proportional reductions observed for recurrence and mortality would be greater with contemporary chemotherapy.

Decisions regarding adjuvant chemotherapy have been based predominately on anatomic stage (tumor size [T], the status of the surrounding lymph nodes [N], and the presence of distant metastases [M]). The American Joint Committee on Cancer (AJCC) developed the TNM classification in 1959 when less was known about the influence of tumor biology on prognosis.[16] Fifty years later the TNM classification continues to provide essential prognostic information; however, there has been a conceptual shift. Breast cancer is no longer considered as a single disease entity but rather a group of molecularly distinct subtypes each with different prognoses, natural histories, and chemotherapeutic sensitivities, all of which factor into decisions regarding adjuvant chemotherapy.[17] This review considers the questions: (1) Who should be offered adjuvant chemotherapy? (2) What adjuvant chemotherapy should be given? and (3) When should chemotherapy be given?

WHO SHOULD BE CONSIDERED FOR ADJUVANT CHEMOTHERAPY?
Prognostic Markers

Decisions regarding adjuvant chemotherapy are based on prognosis, that is, risk of breast cancer recurrence, and on the likelihood of benefiting from treatment. A risk of distant recurrence of 10% or more is often used as the threshold at which systemic adjuvant chemotherapy is recommended.

Tumor size and nodal status are important independent prognostic factors for survival for early stage breast cancer (**Fig. 2**). Other important prognostic factors include histologic grade (based on morphologic features of the tumor), ER, PR (progesterone receptor), HER2 (human epidermal growth factor receptor 2), and the presence of lymphovascular invasion. Several consensus and evidence-based guidelines produced by the National Comprehensive Cancer Network (NCCN),[18] the NIH Consensus Development criteria,[10] and the St Gallen expert opinion criteria[19] provide recommendations on the use of adjuvant chemotherapy in early breast cancer based on clinical data and tumor characteristics.

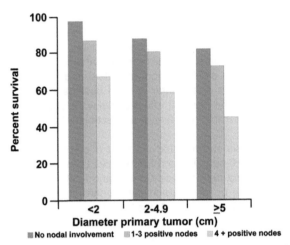

Fig. 2. Percent survival at 5 years by size of primary tumor and number of nodes involved. (*From* Breast. In: Edge SB, Byrd DR, Compton CC, editors. AJCC cancer staging manual. 7th edition. New York: Springer; 2009. p. 437; with permission.)

Adjuvant! Online (www.adjuvantonline.com) is a widely used freely available web-based tool. It considers multiple clinical and pathologic factors and produces estimates for recurrence and mortality. In addition, this program incorporates the effect of comorbid conditions in the determination of prognosis and benefit from various therapeutic interventions. Adjuvant! Online has been independently validated by Canadian investigators, and the concordance with actual recurrence and mortality rates was within 1% of predictions based on this model.[20,21]

Genomic Tests

Several prognostic tests have been developed recently using gene expression profiling. The most widely used commercially available test in the United States is Oncotype Dx (Genomic Health Inc, Redwood City, CA, USA). This reverse transcriptase-polymerase chain reaction (RT-PCR) assay is intended for use in hormone receptor (HR)-positive node-negative breast cancer patients who will receive 5 years of tamoxifen. It measures the gene expression of 16 cancer-related genes (including ER, PR, HER2, and Ki67) in paraffin-embedded tumor tissue and, using a regression model, calculates a recurrence score (RS) that is an estimate of the risk of developing a distant metastases at 10 years. Two suggested cut-off points categorize patients into low (RS <18), intermediate (RS ≥18 <31) and high (RS ≥31) risk groups corresponding to 6.8%, 14.3%, and 30.5% risk of distant recurrence at 10 years after 5 years of tamoxifen therapy, respectively. These risk estimates represent the range of distant recurrence rates for HR-positive, node-negative breast cancers treated with 5 years of tamoxifen.[22]

Recent studies have examined the assay in patients treated with aromatase inhibitors and patients with HR-positive node-positive breast cancer.[23,24] Other studies have assessed the RS as a tool to predict the risk of locoregional recurrence,[25] the response to neoadjuvant therapy,[26] and finally to predict chemotherapy benefit (specifically for CMF [cyclophosphamide, methotrexate, fluorouracil] and CAF [cyclophosphamide, doxorubicin, fluorouracil]).[24,27] The ongoing TAILORx (Trial Assigning Individualized Options for Treatment) trial is randomizing patients with HR-positive, node-negative breast cancer and an intermediate RS to chemotherapy and endocrine therapy versus endocrine therapy only. A similar trial for patients with HR-positive, node-positive breast cancer was recently proposed.

Traditional Markers Presented as a Combined Score

Preliminary but very interesting data presented at San Antonio Breast Cancer Symposium 2009 showed that a composite prognostic profile using traditional immunohistochemical markers but measured centrally could provide quantitatively equivalent information as Oncotype DX to clinical information.[28] These data require validation using independent cohorts; nevertheless, they are interesting and highlight the importance of analytical validity and clinical utility for traditional and newer generation prognostic and predictive markers.

The Food and Drug Administration–approved 70-gene signature (Mammaprint, Agendia) was developed at The Netherlands Cancer Institute from a retrospective series of 78 patients younger than 55 years who received no adjuvant systemic therapy and had, node-negative breast cancer of less than 5 cm. This assay stratifies patients into good and poor risk groups according to the risk of developing a distant metastasis.[29,30] In a study comparing it to Adjuvant! Online, almost 30% of patients had discordant results and for these cases Mammaprint was more accurate at predicting outcome. The prospective multicenter randomized MINDACT (Microarray In Node-negative Disease May Avoid Chemotherapy) trial will test the clinical utility of Mammaprint in selecting patients with node-negative, HR-positive or -negative breast cancer for adjuvant chemotherapy.[31]

There are multiple tools for estimating risk of treatment failure, with and without the use of adjuvant systemic therapies, and some may also predict the magnitude of benefit from endocrine or chemotherapy. All require determination of their clinical utility in prospective trials; while all of them seem to predict outcome, it is uncertain whether there is a "best" predictor.

WHAT ADJUVANT CHEMOTHERAPY?

Adjuvant chemotherapy regimens contain non–cross-resistant agents with differing targets and mechanisms of action. There are many regimens considered "standard," and most were evaluated in clinical trials before the last decade when breast cancer when was considered a single disease entity (**Table 1**). Selecting the optimum chemotherapy regimen takes into consideration the tumor biology (ER, PR, and HER2 status) and patient factors such as the presence of a comorbidities, for example, congestive heart failure, and peripheral neuropathy. The side effects and toxicities of modern adjuvant chemotherapy are largely transient and reversible; chronic, irreversible side effects (cardiomyopathy, acute myelogenous leukemia, myelodysplastic syndrome) are rare. The following section considers (1) the role of anthracyclines and taxanes in the adjuvant treatment of early breast cancer and (2) how increasingly tumor biology informs chemotherapy choices.

Anthracyclines in the Adjuvant Treatment of Early Breast Cancer

Classic CMF (cyclophosphamide, methotrexate, fluorouracil) was one of the first adjuvant polychemotherapy regimens to significantly improve DFS and OS compared with observation in patients with node-positive breast cancer, and remains a widely used regimen.[5] The anthracycline antibiotics (doxorubicin and epirubicin) have been

Table 1
Selected standard chemotherapeutic regimens listed in descending order of efficacy according to comparative randomized trials

Regimen	Selected Standard Chemotherapy Regimens
Dose-dense AC-T	Doxorubicin 60 mg/m^2, cyclophosphamide 600 mg/m^2 IV day 1 every 14 days for 4 cycles Followed by Paclitaxel 175 mg/m^2 IV day 1 every 14 days for 4 cycles Granulocyte colony stimulating factor (GCSF) days 3–10 or peg-filgrastim day 2 cycles 1–8
TAC	Docetaxel 75 mg/m^2 IV, doxorubicin 50 mg/m^2, cyclophosphamide 500 mg/m^2 IV day 1 every 21 days for 6 cycles. GCSF days 3–10 or peg-filgrastim day 2 cycles 1–8
T+(FAC)[32]	Paclitaxel 80 mg/m^2 IV weekly for 12 weeks Followed by Fluorouracil 500 mg/m^2, doxorubicin 50 mg/m^2, cyclophosphamide 500 mg/m^2 IV day 1 every 21 days for 4 cycles
FEC + Docetaxel	Fluorouracil 500 mg/m^2, epirubicin 100 mg/m^2, cyclophosphamide 500 mg/m^2 IV day 1 every 21 days for 3 cycles Followed by Docetaxel 100 mg/m^2 day 1 every 21 days for 3 cycles
CEF (Canadian)	Cyclophosphamide 75 mg/m^2 PO days 1–14, epirubicin 60 mg/m^2 IV days 1 and 8, fluorouracil 500 mg/m^2 IV days 1 and 8 every 28 days for 6 cycles With cotrimoxazole support
CAF	Cyclophosphamide 100 mg/m^2 day 1, doxorubicin 30 mg/m^2 IV day 1 & 8, fluorouracil 500 mg/m^2 IV day 1 & 8 every 28 days for 6 cycles
AC-T	Doxorubicin 60 mg/m^2 IV day 1, cyclophosphamide 600 mg/m^2 IV day 1 Followed by Paclitaxel 80 mg/m^2 IV weekly for 12 weeks
TC	Docetaxel 75 mg/m^2 IV day 1, cyclophosphamide 600 mg/m^2 IV day 1 every 21 days for 4 cycles
AC	Doxorubicin 60 mg/m^2, cyclophosphamide 600 mg/m^2 IV day 1 every 21 days for 4 cycles
Oral (classic) CMF	Cyclophosphamide 100 mg/m^2 PO days 1–14, methotrexate 40 mg/m^2 days 1–8, fluorouracil 600 mg/m^2 days 1–8 days every 28 days for 6 cycles
IV CMF	Cyclophosphamide 100 mg/m^2 IV day 1, methotrexate 40 mg/m^2 IV day 1 and fluorouracil 600 mg/m^2 day 1 IV every 21 days for 9–12 cycles

Data *from* National Comprehensive Cancer Network. NCCN Clinical Practice Guidelines in Oncology; Breast Cancer. V.I.2010. Available at: http://www.nccn.org/professionals/physician_gls/PDF/breast.pdf. Accessed January 19, 2010.

extensively studied in the adjuvant setting beginning in the 1980s mostly in comparison with CMF.[33,34] The EBCTCG meta-analyses of randomized trials showed that anthracycline-containing regimens were superior to first-generation nonanthracycline-containing regimens such as CMF.[11] Anthracycline-based regimens given for approximately 6 months were shown to reduce the annual breast cancer death rates by approximately 38% for women younger than 50 years at diagnosis and by approximately 20% for women aged between 50 and 69 years at diagnosis.

The effect of anthracycline dose escalation was studied in the Cancer and Leukemia Group B (CALGB) 9344 trial. At doxorubicin doses of 60 mg/m^2, 75 mg/m^2 and 90 mg/m^2 there was increased toxicity but no improvement in outcome with higher doses.[35] The optimum doses of doxorubicin and epirubicin are considered to be 60 mg/m^2 and 100 mg/m^2, respectively.[36] Anthracycline-induced cardiac toxicity has been well described. The incidence of congestive heart failure with cumulative doxorubicin doses of 240 to 360 mg/m^2 is between 1.6% and 2.1%. Data from adjuvant breast cancer trials indicate that the risk of congestive cardiac failure is low for women treated with an anthracycline.[37,38]

Anthracyclines in HER2-Positive Breast Cancer

Over the past 15 years many studies have indicated that the incremental benefit from anthracycline-based therapy is largely confined to HER2-positive breast cancer.[39–42] A recent meta-analysis reported significant benefit for anthracycline-based regimens in HER2-positive breast cancer in terms of DFS compared to HER2-negative disease.[43] Coamplification of topoisomerase-II-α (TOP2A) and HER2 has been proposed as the mechanism underlying anthracycline sensitivity in HER2-positive beast cancer. TOP2A is one of several targets for anthracyclines and lies in close proximity to HER2 on chromosome 17. Amplification or deletion of TOP2A appears to occur predominately in HER2-positive breast cancer.[44–46]

Preliminary data from the Breast Cancer International Research Group (BCIRG) 006 trial, which randomized HER2-positive patients to a trastuzumab-containing regimen that contained an anthracycline or did not, reported similar efficacy for both, but fewer cardiac events and secondary leukemias in the nonanthracycline-containing arm.[47] These data have prompted considerable debate regarding the role of anthracyclines in the management of early breast cancer. However, due to the presence of conflicting data and the known existence of unpublished negative studies, HER2 and TOP2A are not considered ready for use in selecting patients for anthracycline therapy.[48,49] Although there is interest in developing validated and reproducible assays that would help select the most effective drugs or combinations for individual patients, at this time anthracycline-based regimens continue to be the standard of care.

Taxanes in the Adjuvant Treatment of Early Breast Cancer

Activity in the metastatic setting led to clinical trials designed to determine whether the addition of a taxane (paclitaxel or docetaxel) to anthracycline-containing regimens could improve outcome in the adjuvant treatment of breast cancer. These studies have examined sequential and concurrent taxane administration and taxanes as a substitute for an anthracycline. Several meta-analyses have shown small but statistically significant improvements in DFS and OS (approximately 5% and 3% absolute benefit, respectively) favoring the inclusion of a taxane compared with standard anthracycline-containing regimens. Improvements in outcome appear independent of the type of taxane, schedule of administration, hormone receptor, and nodal status.[50–52]

Randomized Controlled Trials of Taxanes in Early Breast Cancer

The CALGB 9344 trial studied doxorubicin and cyclophosphamide (AC) for 4 cycles followed by paclitaxel (175 mg/m^2 intravenously [IV] every 3 weeks) in node-positive breast cancer compared with AC alone.[35] Improvement in both DFS and OS was observed. The National Surgical Adjuvant Breast and Bowel Project (NSABP) B-28 studied sequential paclitaxel (225 mg/m^2 IV every 3 weeks) after 4 cycles of AC in a similar population and observed improved DFS but not OS.[53] Neoadjuvant docetaxel given sequentially with AC was studied in the NSABP B-27 trial and no difference in DFS or OS was observed.[54] However, this trial was underpowered to detect the observed differences with statistical significance.

Several randomized trials examined the efficacy of replacing part of a regimen with a taxane instead of continuing the anthracycline portion. Protocol Adjuvant dans le Cancer du Sein (PACS) 01 trial randomized 1999 node-positive women to 6 cycles of FEC (fluorouracil 500 mg/m^2, epirubicin 100 mg/m^2, and cyclophosphamide 500 mg/m^2) or 3 cycles of FEC followed by 3 cycles of docetaxel (100 mg/m^2 IV 3 weekly).[55] The addition of docetaxel was associated with an improvement in DFS (hazard ratio, 0.82; 95% CI 0.69–0.99) and OS (hazard ratio, 0.73; 95% CI 0.56–0.94).[55] The GEICAM 9906 study compared 6 cycles of FEC to 4 cycles of FEC followed by paclitaxel for 8 weeks at 100 mg/m^2.[56] An improvement in DFS (hazard ratio of relapse, 0.77; 95% CI 0.62–0.95; $P = .022$) and a trend toward improvement in the risk of death (adjusted hazard ratio, 0.78; 95% CI 0.57–1.06; $P = .110$) in FEC-P compared to FEC was reported.[56]

By contrast, the recently reported UK TACT (Taxotere as Adjuvant Chemotherapy) trial did not report improved outcome with the addition of a taxane.[57] The study randomized more than 4000 pre- and postmenopausal, node-positive or high-risk node-negative patients with operable early breast cancer to FEC (fluorouracil 600 mg/m^2, epirubicin 60 mg/m^2, cyclophosphamide 600 mg/m^2 every 3 weeks) for 4 cycles followed by docetaxel (100 mg/m^2 every 3 weeks) for 4 cycles compared with FEC for 8 cycles or epirubicin (100 mg/m^2 every 3 weeks) for 4 cycles followed by CMF (cyclophosphamide 600 mg/m^2, methotrexate 40 mg/m^2, and fluorouracil 600 mg/m^2 every 4 weeks) for 4 cycles. There was no benefit observed with the addition of a taxane in terms of DFS (hazard ratio, 0.95; 95% CI 0.85–1.08; $P = .44$). Suboptimal anthracycline dosing before the delivery of docetaxel may have factored in the lack of reported benefit.

The BCIRG 001 trial compared 6 cycles of FAC to 6 cycles of TAC (docetaxel 75 mg/m^2 IV, doxorubicin 50 mg/m^2 IV, cyclophosphamide 500 mg/m^2 every 3 weeks).[58] Improvement in DFS and OS supporting the replacement of a docetaxel instead of fluorouracil was observed. In the Eastern Cooperative Oncology Group (ECOG) 2197 trial patients were randomized to 4 cycles of AC or 4 cycles AT and no difference in DFS or OS was reported.[59] More recently, studies have examined substituting a taxanes for an anthracycline. The US Oncology clinical trials group compared 4 cycles of AC to 4 cycles of TC and observed a benefit in DFS and OS for TC over AC.[60] An ongoing US Oncology/NSABP clinical trial is currently comparing 6 cycles of TC to 6 cycles of TAC and to 6 cycles of TC plus bevacizumab for 1 year. The NSABP B-30 trial compared (1) 4 cycles of AC followed by 4 cycles of docetaxel (100 mg/m^2) every 3 weeks, versus (2) 4 cycles of AT every 3 weeks versus (3) 4 cycles of TAC every 3 weeks.[61] Results from this trial were presented at the 2008 San Antonio Breast Cancer Symposium and demonstrated the superiority of the sequential anthracycline/taxane regimen over the 2 combination regimens.[62] The shorter duration of the combination regimens in the B-30 trial (each 4 cycles total) may have accounted for their inferiority as a similar BCIRG trial that compared 4 cycles of AC followed by 4 cycles of docetaxel (100 mg/m^2) every 3 weeks, versus 6 cycles of TAC showed no difference between the two treatment groups.[63]

Preliminary data from the EBCTCG overview analysis, which included more than 20,000 women randomized to a taxane compared with nontaxane-containing regimen, found an improvement in recurrence-free survival (hazard ratio, 0.83, $P<.00001$) with the addition of a taxane to adjuvant chemotherapy. As with anthracyclines, there is considerable interest in identifying a subgroup particularly sensitive to these agents. Several retrospective studies have observed greater benefit from taxane administration in patients with HER2-positive breast cancer; however, others have not.[54,56,64] At this time HER2 status is not used to decide whether a taxane is included or omitted from the adjuvant chemotherapy regimen. Based on the known mechanism of action of taxanes, several other biomarkers have been proposed as potential predictors of response or resistance, for example, overexpression of p-glycoprotein, a drug efflux pump,[65] and alterations in the structure of β-tubulin[66–68] and microtubule associated proteins (MAP), (eg, MAP-Tau). At present no established single gene markers exist that could identify a patient population that is particularly sensitive to these agents.

Taxane Scheduling

The ECOG 1199 study provided evidence that the scheduling of taxane treatment is important.[69] In this study almost 5000 patients with node-positive breast cancer were randomized in a 2-by-2 factorial design to 4 different taxane regimens—(1) 4 cycles of paclitaxel 175 mg/m^2 every 3 weeks, (2) 12 cycles of paclitaxel 80 mg/m^2 given weekly, (3) 4 cycles of docetaxel 100 mg/m^2 every 3 weeks, or (4) 12 cycles of docetaxel 35 mg/m^2 given weekly—after completion of 4 cycles of AC. The DFS rates were 76.9% for 3-weekly paclitaxel; 81.5% for weekly paclitaxel; 81.2% for 3-weekly docetaxel; and 77.6% for weekly docetaxel. Improvements in OS were observed for weekly paclitaxel and 3-weekly docetaxel in comparison with paclitaxel given every 3 weeks. Toxicities in the weekly docetaxel arm, in particular hematological, led to administration of fewer cycles of treatment.

Dose Density

Gompertzian growth kinetics display increased doubling time and decreased growth fraction as a function of time, and provide the rationale for dose-dense chemotherapy. The Norton-Simon hypothesis argues that smaller rapidly dividing tumors are more sensitive to cytotoxic chemotherapy, and that by shortening the interval between each cycle of chemotherapy there is less time for tumor regrowth and therefore greater fraction of cell kill per cycle.[4,70] This strategy has been studied in several randomized controlled trials.[71,72] The CALGB 9741 randomized, 2005 node-positive patients to standard doses of sequential A, T, C, or concurrent AC followed by T in a 2-by-2 factorial design. Each regimen was administered every 3 weeks or at dose-dense intervals every 2 weeks with granulocyte colony-stimulating factor support. The same number of drug cycles and the same cumulative dose of each drug were administered to all patients.[73] An improvement in DFS and OS was observed with the dose-dense strategy. In the NCIC MA.21 study at a median follow-up of 30 months, AC-T given every 3 weeks was inferior to both dose-dense EC-T and CEF for 6 cycles. Dose-dense AC-T has been compared with TAC in the NSABP B-38 trial.[61] These results are not available as yet.

TUMOR BIOLOGY AND CHOICE OF ADJUVANT CHEMOTHERAPY

Important differences in the clinical behavior of ER-positive and negative breast cancers have been recognized for a long time.[74] Gene expression profiling studies have identified at least 4 distinct molecular subtypes of breast cancer; basal-like, HER2-enriched, luminal A, and luminal B. In addition to differing biologic and clinical behaviors they also have unique chemosensitivities.[17,75] Gene expression profiling is not routinely performed so immunohistochemical surrogates are commonly used to determine subtype. Although at this time there is no consensus as to the specific panel of immunohistochemical (IHC) markers that define each subtype, in general the basal-like and HER2-positive subtypes are predominately ER-negative, whereas the luminal subtypes are ER-positive. In the clinic the triple negative phenotype is used to identify basal-like cancers; however, this misclassifies up to 30% of basal-like cancers.[76]

Chemotherapy for ER-Positive Breast Cancer

HR-positive breast cancer comprises about 75% of all invasive breast cancers. Chemotherapy in addition to endocrine therapy is associated with an improvement in DFS and OS compared with endocrine therapy alone.[77] However, the overall benefit from chemotherapy is modest. Substantial molecular differences exist between good and poor risk ER-positive tumors, and this has facilitated the development several gene expression-based prognostic predictors, for example, Oncotype DX and Mammaprint. Luminal A cancers (Oncotype Dx "low RS," Mammaprint "good risk") are characterized by high expression of ER and ER-related genes, have low expression of proliferative markers such as Ki67, and are typically low grade. These patients have a good prognosis and high likelihood of benefit from endocrine therapy. In contrast "luminal B" (Oncotype DX "high RS," Mammaprint "poor risk") cancers are characterized by lower expression of ER and ER-related genes, high expression of proliferation markers, are typically high grade, and have a poorer prognosis. Standard chemotherapeutic regimens and endocrine therapy should be considered for these patients (see **Table 1**).

Chemotherapy and Trastuzumab for HER2-Positive Breast Cancer

Between 20% to 25% of breast cancers are HER2-positive. Overexpression of HER2 is generally regarded as a poor prognostic marker.[78,79] It is also predictive for response to trastuzumab (Herceptin; Genentech, South San Francisco, CA, USA), a humanized monoclonal antibody that targets the extracellular domain of the HER2 receptor. Given in the preoperative setting pathologic complete response rates of up to 65% have been reported with trastuzumab in combination with chemotherapy,[80,81] the administration of chemotherapy in combination with 1 year of trastuzumab is associated with a 50% relative reduction in the risk of recurrence and about a 30% relative reduction in the risk of death.[82,83] On the basis of several large randomized controlled trials, 1 year of adjuvant trastuzumab has become a standard of care in for HER2-positive breast cancers (**Table 2**).

The largest of these studies was HERA (Herceptin Adjuvant), an international study that randomized 5102 women with HER2-positive breast cancer to observation versus 1 or 2 years of trastuzumab after completion of at least 4 cycles of chemotherapy. In this study over half of the women accrued had node-positive disease and only 26% of patients in this study received both an anthracycline and a taxane.[82] At a median follow-up of 23.5 months, 1 year of adjuvant trastuzumab was associated with a reduced risk of breast cancer recurrence (hazard ratio, 0.64; 95% CI 0.54–0.76;

Table 2
Summary of the randomized clinical trials evaluating the clinical efficacy of trastuzumab in the treatment of HER2-positive early-stage breast cancer

Trial (References)	N	Chemotherapy	Median Follow-up (mo)	HR for DFS	95% CI	P value	OS	95% CI	P value
HERA[82]	5102	Any CT → Observation Any CT → T (1 y) Any CT → T (2 y)	23.5	0.64	0.54–0.76	<.0001	0.66	0.47–0.91	.0115
NSABP B-31	2,043	AC × 4 → [a]P × 4 vs AC × 4 → P × 4 + T (1 y)	34.8	0.48	0.41–0.57	<.0001	0.65	0.51–0.84	.0007
Intergroup N9831[83]	2,766	AC × 4 → P versus AC × 4 → P → T (1 y) or AC × 4 → P + [b]T (1 y)							
BCIRG 006[47]	3,222	AC × 4 → D × 4 vs AC × 4 → D + [c]T (1 y) D + Cb × 6 + [c]T (1 y)	65	1 0.64 0.75	0.53–0.78 0.63–0.90	<.001 .04	0.63 0.77	0.48–0.81 0.60–0.99	<.001 .038
FINHER[84]	232	V or D × 3 ± T for 6 wk → FEC × 3	36	0.42	0.21–0.83	.01	0.41	0.16–1.08	.07
PACS 04[85]	528	FEC × 6 or ET × 6 FEC × 6 or ET × 6→T	47	0.86	0.61–1.22	.41	1.27	0.68–2.38	NR

Abbreviations: AC, doxorubicin, cyclophosphamide; Cb, carboplatin; 95% CI, 95% confidence interval; CT, chemotherapy; D, docetaxel; DFS, disease-free survival; ET, epirubicin and docetaxel; FEC, fluorouracil, epirubicin, cyclophosphamide; NR, not reported; OS, overall survival; P, paclitaxel; T, trastuzumab; V, vinorelbine.
[a] P, given 3-weekly.
[b] T starts concurrently with weekly P for 12 weeks.
[c] T starts concurrently with D.

$P<.0001$) and risk of death (hazard ratio, 0.66; 95% CI 0.47–0.91; $P = .0115$) compared with observation alone.

The North Central Cancer Treatment Group trial (N9831) and NSABP B-31 examined the efficacy of adding trastuzumab to AC followed by paclitaxel.[83] In a somewhat unusual step a combined analysis of the 3968 women included in the concurrent paclitaxel-trastuzumab and AC-P observation groups was performed. At a median follow-up of 2.9 years, AC followed by concurrent paclitaxel trastuzumab resulted in a significant reduction in the risk of breast cancer recurrence (hazard ratio, 0.48; 95% CI 0.41–0.57; $P<.0001$) and death (hazard ratio, 0.65; 95% CI 0.51–0.84; $P = .0007$) compared with AC followed by paclitaxel alone.

A slightly different approach was taken by BCIRG 006. In this international multicenter open-label trial, 3222 women with HER2-positive, predominately node-positive disease were randomized to receive AC followed by docetaxel, or the same but with trastuzumab concurrent with docetaxel or a nonanthracycline-containing regimen consisting of docetaxel (T), carboplatin (C), trastuzumab (H) (TCH) given for 6 cycles every 3 weeks. Trastuzumab was given for 1 year in both trastuzumab-containing arms. The third efficacy analysis at a median follow-up of 65 months demonstrated an improvement in DFS (75%, 84%, and 81% for ACT, ACTH, and TCH, respectively) and OS (87%, 92%, and 91% for ACT, ACTH, and TCH, respectively) in both trastuzumab-containing arms.[47]

The Finland Herceptin (FinHer) multicenter, open-label, study has raised the question of what is the optimum duration of trastuzumab therapy.[84] This study was designed to examine 3-weekly docetaxel compared with weekly vinorelbine followed by FEC in node-positive or high-risk node-negative patients. Patients with HER2-positive disease (n = 232) were randomized to receive 9 weeks of weekly trastuzumab administered with docetaxel of vinorelbine versus chemotherapy alone. At a median follow-up of 3 years there was a reduction in recurrence (hazard ratio, 0.42; 95% CI 0.21–0.83; $P = .01$) and a trend toward improved survival (hazard ratio, 0.41; 95% CI 0.16–1.08; $P = .07$) in the group receiving trastuzumab compared with those who did not. At the present time 1 year of treatment is the standard of care; however, a shorter course as observed in the FinHER study may be adequate. There are currently 4 prospective studies addressing this question by randomizing women with HER2-positive breast cancer to 1 year versus 6 months (PHARE and PERSEPHONE) or 1 year versus 2 months (SOLD and SHORTER).[61]

The recently reported Protocol Adjuvant dans le Cancer du Sein (PACS) 04 study enrolled 3010 lymph node–positive patients and was designed to compare 6 cycles of FEC100 to 6 cycles of epirubicin given concurrently with docetaxel.[85] Patients with HER2-positive disease (n = 528) were randomized a second time to received trastuzumab after completion of chemotherapy or to observation alone after chemotherapy. Results at a median follow-up of 4 years show no significant difference in the DFS or OS for the trastuzumab-containing compared with nontrastuzumab-containing arms. The absence of benefit in this study is in contrast to most other studies and may reflect small sample size, early discontinuation of trastuzumab, and that about 10% of patients randomized to receive trastuzumab did not receive it. Alternatively, it may be that concomitant rather than sequential trastuzumab is better; this would be consistent with the results of the interim analysis of N9831 that showed an improved DFS for concurrent trastuzumab-taxane therapy compared with sequential trastuzumab.[86] However, this was an unplanned analysis, follow-up is short, and the number of events is small.

Data are lacking regarding the benefit of trastuzumab in small (<1 cm) HER2-positive node-negative tumors. Retrospective analyses from trastuzumab-untreated patient cohorts with T1abN0 HER2-positive tumors showed an increased risk of recurrence by two- to fivefold, with absolute risks through approximately 5 years of follow-up of 10% to 23%.[87,88] The NCCN guidelines recommend consideration of trastuzumab and chemotherapy for T1b or larger HER2-positive tumors. However, T1a-b,N0.M0 breast cancers overall have a good prognosis and therefore an awareness of the potential harms of therapy is essential.[18]

Considerable advances have been made in the treatment of HER2-positive breast cancer. Ongoing studies evaluating the role of lapatinib, a small tyrosine kinase inhibitor molecule targeting HER2 and epidermal growth factor receptor (EGFR) in the adjuvant/neoadjuvant setting (ALTTO, Neo-ALTTO, NSABP B-41, CALGB 40601, and TEACH), will provide further insight into the efficacy, resistance, and sensitivity of HER2-targeted agents.[61]

Chemotherapy for Triple-Negative Breast Cancer

Triple-negative breast cancers are highly proliferative and carry a worse prognosis than other breast cancer subtypes.[17,89,90] This subtype is uniquely sensitive to standard chemotherapy.[75,91] At present, DNA-damaging agents are being tested in this subgroup to exploit the strong association between these tumors and the presence of BRCA1 mutations.[92,93] Homologous recombination, a high-fidelity DNA repair pathway, relies on functioning BRCA1 and when this pathway is dysfunctional the poly(ADP-ribose) polymerase (PARP) DNA repair mechanisms take over. PARP inhibitors have been investigated in two phase 2 studies for triple negative and BRCA1/2-deficient cancers, and results to date are promising.[94,95] Epothilones, antiangiogenic agents, EGFR inhibitors, and agents that induce DNA double-strand breaks such as platinum agents are being tested in clinical trials.

ADJUVANT CHEMOTHERAPY WHEN?

Adjuvant chemotherapy is equally effective up to 12 weeks after definitive surgery, but may be compromised by delays of more than 12 weeks after definitive surgery.[96] Administering chemotherapy before primary surgery (neoadjuvant or preoperative) with the same chemotherapy regimen has the same therapeutic effects. Preoperative chemotherapy was initially introduced as a strategy to downstage patients with inoperable breast cancer and enable successful local treatment. Subsequently, it was studied in patients with operable disease. Several phase 2 studies and 8 randomized controlled trials have observed no difference in DFS or OS between adjuvant and neoadjuvant therapy. There are, however, increased rates of breast-conserving therapy with the latter approach.[97,98]

Delivering chemotherapy in the preoperative setting allows the effects of treatment on the tumor burden to be directly observed, which is important for several reasons. First, it can provide important prognostic information; patients who achieve a pathologic complete response have improved overall outcomes.[99] Second, therapy can be altered based on tumor response and exposure to ineffective agents can be minimized. Finally, preoperative chemotherapy provides an opportunity to examine the relationship between molecular markers and chemotherapy response. There are number of unresolved issues with this approach, such as the timing of the sentinel lymph node biopsy (before or after preoperative chemotherapy) and whether a patient should receive postmastectomy irradiation if found to have 3 or fewer lymph nodes involved with metastases at the time of surgery. These issues are subject of ongoing research.

SUMMARY

Multiple randomized controlled trials over the last several decades have shown significant reductions in recurrence and mortality as a result of effective adjuvant chemotherapy. The greatest effects of chemotherapy occur in the first year or two after treatment and the effects persist for beyond 10 years. In general the proportional benefit of adjuvant chemotherapy regimens is the same regardless of the prognostic group; however, more recent analyses suggest greater benefit for HR-negative and high-grade cancers. The administration of adjuvant chemotherapy regimens beyond 6 to 8 cycles imparts no incremental benefit. Adjuvant chemotherapy is tailored to some degree according to breast cancer subtype, defined at this time predominately by IHC markers. Patients with HR-positive breast cancer benefit from chemotherapy in addition to endocrine therapy. Routinely tested IHC markers guide treatment; in some instances a genomic test can provide additional information, particularly in clinically "intermediate" cases. Patients with HER2-positive breast cancer of any hormone receptor or menopausal status should receive chemotherapy and trastuzumab for 1 year. Ongoing studies will establish the optimum duration and timing of trastuzumab in addition to the role of lapatinib in the adjuvant setting. At this time there is no reliable or reproducible marker of anthracycline sensitivity that would serve to identify the patients most and least likely to benefit from these agents. Patients with the triple-negative breast cancer should receive standard chemotherapy regimens that include an anthracycline, cyclophosphamide and a taxane. DNA-damaging agents, nonanthracycline-containing regimens, and antiangiogenic agents are some of the agents being tested in the adjuvant/neoadjuvant setting for this tumor subtype. Major advances have been made in the treatment of early breast cancer over the last decade. The results of current trials will determine whether more precise prognostic determination and prediction of patients most likely or least likely to benefit from specific therapies can improve the efficacy and reduce the toxicity of systemic treatments.

REFERENCES

1. Jemal A, Siegel R, Ward E, et al. Cancer statistics, 2009. CA Cancer J Clin 2009; 59:225–49.
2. Berry DA, Inoue L, Shen Y, et al. Modeling the impact of treatment and screening on U.S. breast cancer mortality: a Bayesian approach. J Natl Cancer Inst Monogr 2006;36:30–6.
3. Anderson BO, Yip CH, Smith RA, et al. Guideline implementation for breast healthcare in low-income and middle-income countries: overview of the breast health global initiative global summit 2007. Cancer 2008;113:2221–43.
4. Norton L. A Gompertzian model of human breast cancer growth. Cancer Res 1988;48:7067–71.
5. Bonadonna G, Brusamolino E, Valagussa P, et al. Combination chemotherapy as an adjuvant treatment in operable breast cancer. N Engl J Med 1976;294:405–10.
6. Fisher B, Redmond C, Dimitrov NV, et al. A randomized clinical trial evaluating sequential methotrexate and fluorouracil in the treatment of patients with node-negative breast cancer who have estrogen-receptor-negative tumors. N Engl J Med 1989;320:473–8.
7. Mansour EG, Gray R, Shatila AH, et al. Survival advantage of adjuvant chemotherapy in high-risk node-negative breast cancer: ten-year analysis—an intergroup study. J Clin Oncol 1998;16:3486–92.

8. Fisher B, Jeong JH, Dignam J, et al. Findings from recent national surgical adjuvant breast and bowel project adjuvant studies in stage I breast cancer. J Natl Cancer Inst Monogr 2001;30:32–6.
9. Fisher B, Dignam J, Wolmark N, et al. Tamoxifen and chemotherapy for lymph node-negative, estrogen receptor-positive breast cancer. J Natl Cancer Inst 1997;89:1673–82.
10. National Institutes of Health Consensus Development Panel. Adjuvant therapy for breast cancer. NIH Consensus Statement 2000;17:1–35.
11. Early Breast Cancer Trialists' Collaborative Group. Effects of chemotherapy and hormonal therapy for early breast cancer on recurrence and 15-year survival: an overview of the randomised trials. Lancet 2005;365:1687–717.
12. Early Breast Cancer Trialists' Collaborative Group. Polychemotherapy for early breast cancer: an overview of the randomised trials. Lancet 1998; 352:930–42.
13. Clarke M. Meta-analyses of adjuvant therapies for women with early breast cancer: the Early Breast Cancer Trialists' Collaborative Group overview. Ann Oncol 2006;17(Suppl 10):59–62.
14. Berry DA, Cirrincione C, Henderson IC, et al. Estrogen-receptor status and outcomes of modern chemotherapy for patients with node-positive breast cancer. JAMA 2006;295:1658–67.
15. Clarke M, Coates AS, Darby SC, et al. Adjuvant chemotherapy in oestrogen-receptor-poor breast cancer: patient-level meta-analysis of randomised trials. Lancet 2008;371:29–40.
16. Edge SB, Compton DR, April CC, et al. AJCC Cancer Staging Manual. 7th edition. New York: Springer; 2009.
17. Perou CM, Sorlie T, Eisen MB, et al. Molecular portraits of human breast tumours. Nature 2000;406:747–52.
18. National Comprehensive Cancer Network. NCCN Clinical Practice Guidelines in Oncology. Breast Cancer. V.I. 2010. Available at: http://www.nccn.org/professionals/physician_gls/PDF/breast.pdf. Accessed January 19, 2010.
19. Goldhirsch A, Ingle JN, Gelber RD, et al. Thresholds for therapies: highlights of the St Gallen International Expert Consensus on the primary therapy of early breast cancer 2009. Ann Oncol 2009;20:1319–29.
20. Ravdin PM, Siminoff LA, Davis GJ, et al. Computer program to assist in making decisions about adjuvant therapy for women with early breast cancer. J Clin Oncol 2001;19:980–91.
21. Olivotto IA, Bajdik CD, Ravdin PM, et al. Population-based validation of the prognostic model ADJUVANT! for early breast cancer. J Clin Oncol 2005;23: 2716–25.
22. Paik S, Shak S, Tang G, et al. A multigene assay to predict recurrence of tamoxifen-treated, node-negative breast cancer. N Engl J Med 2004;351:2817–26.
23. Dowsett M, Cuzick, J, Wales, C et al. Risk of recurrence using Oncotype DX in postmenopausal primary breast cancer patients treated with anastrozole or tamoxifen: a TransATAC study. Presented at the 31st San Antonio Breast Cancer Symposium. San Antonio (TX), December 10–14, 2008.
24. Albain K, Barlow WE, Shak S, et al. Prognostic and predictive value of the 21-gene recurrence score assay in postmenopausal women with node-positive, oestrogen-receptor-positive breast cancer on chemotherapy: a retrospective analysis of a randomised trial. Lancet Oncol 2010;11(1):55–65.
25. Mamounas E, Tang G, Fisher B, et al. Association between the 21-gene recurrence score assay and risk of locoregional recurrence in node-negative, estrogen

receptor-positive breast cancer: results from NSABP B-14 and NSABP B-20. J Clin Oncol 2010;28(10):1677–83.

26. Gianni L, Zambetti M, Clark K, et al. Gene expression profiles in paraffin-embedded core biopsy tissue predict response to chemotherapy in women with locally advanced breast cancer. J Clin Oncol 2005;23:7265–77.

27. Paik S, Tang G, Shak S, et al. Gene expression and benefit of chemotherapy in women with node-negative, estrogen receptor-positive breast cancer. J Clin Oncol 2006;24:3726–34.

28. Cuzick J, Dowsett M, Wale C, et al. Prognostic value of a combined ER, PgR, Ki67, HER2 Immunohistochemical (IHC4) Score and Comparison with the GHI Recurrence Score -Results from TransATAC [abstract 74]. Cancer Res 2009; 69(Suppl).

29. van 't Veer LJ, Dai H, van de Vijver MJ, et al. Gene expression profiling predicts clinical outcome of breast cancer. Nature 2002;415:530–6.

30. Buyse M, Loi S, van't Veer L, et al. Validation and clinical utility of a 70-gene prognostic signature for women with node-negative breast cancer. J Natl Cancer Inst 2006;98:1183–92.

31. Cardoso F, Van't Veer L, Rutgers E, et al. Clinical application of the 70-gene profile: the MINDACT trial. J Clin Oncol 2008;26:729–35.

32. Green MC, Buzdar AU, Smith T, et al. Weekly paclitaxel improves pathologic complete remission in operable breast cancer when compared with paclitaxel every 3 weeks. J Clin Oncol 2005;23(25):5983–92.

33. Fisher B, Brown AM, Dimitrov NV, et al. Two months of doxorubicin-cyclophosphamide with and without interval reinduction therapy compared with 6 months of cyclophosphamide, methotrexate, and fluorouracil in positive-node breast cancer patients with tamoxifen-nonresponsive tumors: results from the National Surgical Adjuvant Breast and Bowel Project B-15. J Clin Oncol 1990;8:1483–96.

34. Fisher B, Anderson S, Tan-Chiu E, et al. Tamoxifen and chemotherapy for axillary node-negative, estrogen receptor-negative breast cancer: findings from National Surgical Adjuvant Breast and Bowel Project B-23. J Clin Oncol 2001;19:931–42.

35. Henderson IC, Berry DA, Demetri GD, et al. Improved outcomes from adding sequential Paclitaxel but not from escalating doxorubicin dose in an adjuvant chemotherapy regimen for patients with node-positive primary breast cancer. J Clin Oncol 2003;21:976–83.

36. Trudeau M, Charbonneau F, Gelmon K, et al. Selection of adjuvant chemotherapy for treatment of node-positive breast cancer. Lancet Oncol 2005;6:886–98.

37. Zambetti M, Moliterni A, Materazzo C, et al. Long-term cardiac sequelae in operable breast cancer patients given adjuvant chemotherapy with or without doxorubicin and breast irradiation. J Clin Oncol 2001;19:37–43.

38. Jones LW, Haykowsky MJ, Swartz JJ, et al. Early breast cancer therapy and cardiovascular injury. J Am Coll Cardiol 2007;50:1435–41.

39. Dressler LG, Berry DA, Broadwater G, et al. Comparison of HER2 status by fluorescence in situ hybridization and immunohistochemistry to predict benefit from dose escalation of adjuvant doxorubicin-based therapy in node-positive breast cancer patients. J Clin Oncol 2005;23:4287–97.

40. Muss HB, Thor AD, Berry DA, et al. c-erbB-2 expression and response to adjuvant therapy in women with node-positive early breast cancer. N Engl J Med 1994;330:1260–6.

41. Paik S, Bryant J, Park C, et al. erbB-2 and response to doxorubicin in patients with axillary lymph node-positive, hormone receptor-negative breast cancer. J Natl Cancer Inst 1998;90:1361–70.

42. Pritchard KI, Shepherd LE, O'Malley FP, et al. HER2 and responsiveness of breast cancer to adjuvant chemotherapy. N Engl J Med 2006;354:2103–11.
43. Dhesy-Thind B, Pritchard KI, Messersmith H, et al. HER2/neu in systemic therapy for women with breast cancer: a systematic review. Breast Cancer Res Treat 2008;109:209–29.
44. Jarvinen TA, Liu ET. HER-2/neu and topoisomerase IIalpha in breast cancer. Breast Cancer Res Treat 2003;78:299–311.
45. Beser AR, Tuzlali S, Guzey D, et al. HER-2, TOP2A and chromosome 17 alterations in breast cancer. Pathol Oncol Res 2007;13:180–5.
46. Slamon DJ, Press MF. Alterations in the TOP2A and HER2 genes: association with adjuvant anthracycline sensitivity in human breast cancers. J Natl Cancer Inst 2009;101:615–8.
47. Slamon D, Eiermann W, Robert N, et al. BCIRG 006 Phase III trial comparing AC→T with AC→TH and with TCH in the adjuvant treatment of HER2-amplified early breast cancer patients: third planned efficacy analysis. Presented at San Antonio Annual Breast Cancer symposium. San Antonio (TX), December 10–13, 2009.
48. Esteva FJ, Hortobagyi GN. Topoisomerase II{alpha} amplification and anthracycline-based chemotherapy: the jury is still out. J Clin Oncol 2009;27: 3416–7.
49. Pritchard KI. Are HER2 and TOP2A useful as prognostic or predictive biomarkers for anthracycline-based adjuvant chemotherapy for breast cancer? J Clin Oncol 2009;27:3875–6.
50. Bria E, Nistico C, Cuppone F, et al. Benefit of taxanes as adjuvant chemotherapy for early breast cancer: pooled analysis of 15,500 patients. Cancer 2006;106: 2337–44.
51. Ferguson T, Wilcken N, Vagg R, et al. Taxanes for adjuvant treatment of early breast cancer. Cochrane Database Syst Rev 2007;4:CD004421.
52. De Laurentiis M, Cancello G, D'Agostino D, et al. Taxane-based combinations as adjuvant chemotherapy of early breast cancer: a meta-analysis of randomized trials. J Clin Oncol 2008;26:44–53.
53. Mamounas EP, Bryant J, Lembersky B, et al. Paclitaxel after doxorubicin plus cyclophosphamide as adjuvant chemotherapy for node-positive breast cancer: results from NSABP B-28. J Clin Oncol 2005;23:3686–96.
54. Bear HD, Anderson S, Smith RE, et al. Sequential preoperative or postoperative docetaxel added to preoperative doxorubicin plus cyclophosphamide for operable breast cancer: National Surgical Adjuvant Breast and Bowel Project Protocol B-27. J Clin Oncol 2006;24:2019–27.
55. Roche H, Fumoleau P, Spielmann M, et al. Sequential adjuvant epirubicin-based and docetaxel chemotherapy for node-positive breast cancer patients: the FNCLCC PACS 01 Trial. J Clin Oncol 2006;24:5664–71.
56. Martin M, Rodriguez-Lescure A, Ruiz A, et al. Randomized phase 3 trial of fluorouracil, epirubicin, and cyclophosphamide alone or followed by paclitaxel for early breast cancer. J Natl Cancer Inst 2008;100:805–14.
57. Ellis P, Barrett-Lee P, Johnson L, et al. Sequential docetaxel as adjuvant chemotherapy for early breast cancer (TACT): an open-label, phase III, randomised controlled trial. Lancet 2009;373:1681–92.
58. Martin M, Pienkowski T, Mackey J, et al. Adjuvant docetaxel for node-positive breast cancer. N Engl J Med 2005;352:2302–13.
59. Goldstein LO, Sparano A. J. E2197:Phase III AT (doxorubicin/docetaxel) vs. AC (doxorubicin/cyclophosphamide) in the adjuvant treatment of node positive and high risk node negative breast cancer. J Clin Oncol 2005;23(16S):A512.

60. Jones F, Shaughnessy J. Extended follow-up and analysis by age of the U.S Oncology Adjuvant trial 9735: docetaxel/cyclophosphamide is associated with an overall survival benefit compared to doxorubicin/cyclophosphamide and is well-tolerated in women 65 or older. Breast Cancer Res Treat 2007; 106(S1):A12.

61. ClinicalTrials.gov. Available at: http://clinicaltrials.gov/ct2/home. Accessed January 25, 2010.

62. Swain SM, Jeong JH, Geyer CE, et al. NSABP B-30: definitive analysis of patient outcome from a randomized trial evaluating different schedules and combinations of adjuvant therapy containing doxorubicin, docetaxel and cyclophosphamide in women with operable, node-positive breast cancer. Presented at the 31st Annual San Antonio Breast Cancer Symposium. San Antonio (TX), December 10–14, 2008.

63. Eiermann W, Pienkowski T, Crown J, et al. BCIRG 005 main efficacy analysis: a phase III randomized trial comparing docetaxel in combination with doxorubicin and cyclophosphamide (TAC) versus doxorubicin and cyclophosphamide followed by docetaxel (ACT) in women with Her-2/neu negative axillary lymph node positive early breast cancer. Presented at the 31st Annual San Antonio Breast Cancer Symposium. San Antonio (TX), December 10–14, 2008.

64. Hayes DF, Thor AD, Dressler LG, et al. HER2 and response to paclitaxel in node-positive breast cancer. N Engl J Med 2007;357:1496–506.

65. Szakacs G, Paterson JK, Ludwig JA, et al. Targeting multidrug resistance in cancer. Nat Rev Drug Discov 2006;5:219–34.

66. Giannakakou P, Sackett DL, Kang YK, et al. Paclitaxel-resistant human ovarian cancer cells have mutant beta-tubulins that exhibit impaired paclitaxel-driven polymerization. J Biol Chem 1997;272:17118–25.

67. Kamath K, Wilson L, Cabral F, et al. BetaIII-tubulin induces paclitaxel resistance in association with reduced effects on microtubule dynamic instability. J Biol Chem 2005;280:12902–7.

68. Rouzier R, Rajan R, Wagner P, et al. Microtubule-associated protein tau: a marker of paclitaxel sensitivity in breast cancer. Proc Natl Acad Sci U S A 2005;102:8315–20.

69. Sparano JA, Wang M, Martino S, et al. Weekly paclitaxel in the adjuvant treatment of breast cancer. N Engl J Med 2008;358:1663–71.

70. Norton L. Theoretical concepts and the emerging role of taxanes in adjuvant therapy. Oncologist 2001;6(Suppl 3):30–5.

71. Venturini M, Del Mastro L, Aitini E, et al. Dose-dense adjuvant chemotherapy in early breast cancer patients: results from a randomized trial. J Natl Cancer Inst 2005;97:1724–33.

72. Bonadonna G, Zambetti M, Valagussa P. Sequential or alternating doxorubicin and CMF regimens in breast cancer with more than three positive nodes. Ten-year results. JAMA 1995;273:542–7.

73. Citron ML, Berry DA, Cirrincione C, et al. Randomized trial of dose-dense versus conventionally scheduled and sequential versus concurrent combination chemotherapy as postoperative adjuvant treatment of node-positive primary breast cancer: first report of Intergroup Trial C9741/Cancer and Leukemia Group B Trial 9741. J Clin Oncol 2003;21:1431–9.

74. Hess KR, Pusztai L, Buzdar AU, et al. Estrogen receptors and distinct patterns of breast cancer relapse. Breast Cancer Res Treat 2003;78:105–18.

75. Rouzier R, Perou CM, Symmans WF, et al. Breast cancer molecular subtypes respond differently to preoperative chemotherapy. Clin Cancer Res 2005;11: 5678–85.

76. Bertucci F, Finetti P, Cervera N, et al. How basal are triple-negative breast cancers? Int J Cancer 2008;123:236–40.
77. Fisher B, Jeong JH, Bryant J, et al. Treatment of lymph-node-negative, oestrogen-receptor-positive breast cancer: long-term findings from National Surgical Adjuvant Breast and Bowel Project randomised clinical trials. Lancet 2004;364: 858–68.
78. Slamon DJ, Clark GM, Wong SG, et al. Human breast cancer: correlation of relapse and survival with amplification of the HER-2/neu oncogene. Science 1987;235:177–82.
79. Slamon DJ, Godolphin W, Jones LA, et al. Studies of the HER-2/neu proto-oncogene in human breast and ovarian cancer. Science 1989;244:707–12.
80. Buzdar AU, Ibrahim NK, Francis D, et al. Significantly higher pathologic complete remission rate after neoadjuvant therapy with trastuzumab, paclitaxel, and epirubicin chemotherapy: results of a randomized trial in human epidermal growth factor receptor 2-positive operable breast cancer. J Clin Oncol 2005; 23:3676–85.
81. Buzdar AU, Valero V, Ibrahim NK, et al. Neoadjuvant therapy with paclitaxel followed by 5-fluorouracil, epirubicin, and cyclophosphamide chemotherapy and concurrent trastuzumab in human epidermal growth factor receptor 2-positive operable breast cancer: an update of the initial randomized study population and data of additional patients treated with the same regimen. Clin Cancer Res 2007;13:228–33.
82. Piccart-Gebhart MJ, Procter M, Leyland-Jones B, et al. Trastuzumab after adjuvant chemotherapy in HER2-positive breast cancer. N Engl J Med 2005;353:1659–72.
83. Romond EH, Perez EA, Bryant J, et al. Trastuzumab plus adjuvant chemotherapy for operable HER2-positive breast cancer. N Engl J Med 2005;353:1673–84.
84. Joensuu H, Kellokumpu-Lehtinen PL, Bono P, et al. Adjuvant docetaxel or vinorelbine with or without trastuzumab for breast cancer. N Engl J Med 2006;354: 809–20.
85. Spielmann M, Roche H, Delozier T, et al. Trastuzumab for patients with axillary-node-positive breast cancer: results of the FNCLCC-PACS 04 trial. J Clin Oncol 2009;27:6129–34.
86. Perez E, Suman VJ, Davidson NE, et al. Interim cardiac safety analysis of NCCTG N9831 Intergroup adjuvant trastuzumab trial [abstract 556]. J Clin Oncol 2005; 23:17s.
87. Gonzalez-Angulo AM, Litton JK, Broglio KR, et al. High risk of recurrence for patients with breast cancer who have human epidermal growth factor receptor 2-positive, node-negative tumors 1 cm or smaller. J Clin Oncol 2009;27:5700–6.
88. Curigliano G, Viale G, Bagnardi V, et al. Clinical relevance of HER2 overexpression/amplification in patients with small tumor size and node-negative breast cancer. J Clin Oncol 2009;27:5693–9.
89. Sotiriou C, Neo SY, McShane LM, et al. Breast cancer classification and prognosis based on gene expression profiles from a population-based study. Proc Natl Acad Sci U S A 2003;100:10393–8.
90. Dent R, Trudeau M, Pritchard KI, et al. Triple-negative breast cancer: clinical features and patterns of recurrence. Clin Cancer Res 2007;13:4429–34.
91. Carey LA, Dees EC, Sawyer L, et al. The triple negative paradox: primary tumor chemosensitivity of breast cancer subtypes. Clin Cancer Res 2007;13:2329–34.
92. Foulkes WD, Brunet JS, Stefansson IM, et al. The prognostic implication of the basal-like (cyclin E high/p27 low/p53+/glomeruloid-microvascular-proliferation+) phenotype of BRCA1-related breast cancer. Cancer Res 2004;64:830–5.

93. Foulkes WD, Stefansson IM, Chappuis PO, et al. Germline BRCA1 mutations and a basal epithelial phenotype in breast cancer. J Natl Cancer Inst 2003;95:1482–5.
94. Fong PC, Boss DS, Yap TA, et al. Inhibition of poly(ADP-ribose) polymerase in tumors from BRCA mutation carriers. N Engl J Med 2009;361:123–34.
95. O'Shaughnessy JO, Pippen C. Efficacy of BSI-201, a poly (ADP-ribose) polymerase-1 (PARP1) inhibitor, in combination with gemcitabine/carboplatin (G/C) in patients with metastatic triple negative breast cancer (TNBC): Results of a randomized phase II trial [abstract 3]. J Clin Oncol 2009;27:18s (Suppl).
96. Lohrisch C, Paltiel C, Gelmon K, et al. Impact on survival of time from definitive surgery to initiation of adjuvant chemotherapy for early-stage breast cancer. J Clin Oncol 2006;24:4888–94.
97. Green MC, Esteva FJ, Hortobagyi GN. Neoadjuvant chemotherapy. Breast Dis 2009;21:23–31.
98. Mieog JS, van der Hage JA, van de Velde CJ. Neoadjuvant chemotherapy for operable breast cancer. Br J Surg 2007;94:1189–200.
99. Hortobagyi GN, Ames FC, Buzdar AU, et al. Management of stage III primary breast cancer with primary chemotherapy, surgery, and radiation therapy. Cancer 1988;62:2507–16.

Targeted Therapies in Early-Stage Breast Cancer: Achievements and Promises

George W. Sledge Jr, MD*, Aparna C. Jotwani, MD, Lida Mina, MD

KEYWORDS

• Breast cancer • Targeted therapy • HER2 • Chemotherapy

One of the most impressive changes in the therapeutic landscape of breast cancer in the past decade has been the advent of targeted therapies for specific subtypes. This article discusses the meaning of targeted therapy and examines the genomic basis for targeted therapy as it has emerged over the past decade. Human epidermal growth factor receptor 2 (HER2)–targeted therapy, the principle example of targeted therapy to enter the adjuvant arena in the past decade, is described in depth. Novel targeted therapies under development, many currently being examined in the adjuvant setting, are also explored, including anti–vascular endothelial growth factor therapy, poly (ADP ribose) polymerase (PARP) inhibition for triple-negative breast cancers, and agents targeting site-specific metastasis to the bone (receptor activator of NF-κB [RANK] ligand [RANKL] inhibition). Chemotherapy, the epitome of nonspecific anticancer therapy, is in the process of becoming targeted therapy as understanding of breast cancer biology improves.

WHAT IS MEANT BY TARGETED THERAPY?

The meaning of the term *targeted therapy* is open to wide interpretation. At its most basic level, targeted therapy might simply imply that a drug has a specific molecular target, but this is a very low-level definition, because all therapeutic agents have molecular targets.[1] Saying that a taxane targets microtubules and is therefore targeted therapy renders the concept essentially trivial and meaningless.

Indiana University, Simon Cancer Center, Indiana Cancer Pavilion, RT-473, 535 Barnhill Drive, Indianapolis, IN 46202, USA
* Corresponding author.
E-mail address: gsledge@iupui.edu

Surg Oncol Clin N Am 19 (2010) 669–679
doi:10.1016/j.soc.2010.04.005
1055-3207/10/$ – see front matter

Instead, the authors previously suggested that targeted therapy should have a broader and more inclusive meaning.[1] Useful elements in defining targeted therapy might include the following:

1. The drug has a specific molecular target, which is the lowest level of meaning for targeted therapy. However, the idea is implied that the target should be a relatively specific one (ie, the more promiscuous the agent in its molecular targets, the less it should be considered a targeted therapy.
2. The target is biologically relevant (eg, part of the malignant phenotype) for specific cancers. The estrogen receptor (ER) is biologically relevant to the growth of specific human breast cancers, as is HER2. Replicating DNA is relevant to the malignant phenotype but is nonspecific (rendering most chemotherapeutics poor examples of targeted therapy).
3. The target is reproducibly measurable in individual patients. Tamoxifen is useful because estrogen receptor can be measured. Trastuzumab is useful because HER2 can be measured with some reliability using immunohistochemistry or fluorescence in situ hybridization. The robustness of the ability to assay a target therefore becomes of crucial importance. However, this does not necessarily imply that the target must always be measured. For instance, the presence of a B-cell lymphoma or of a chronic myelogenous leukemia routinely indicates the presence of the molecular target for these tumors.
4. The presence of that measurable target correlates with clinical benefit when the therapy is used. A targeted therapy used for every patient with breast cancer by definition cannot be targeted in any meaningful sense. Hormonal therapy only benefits patients who are estrogen receptor–positive, and trastuzumab's real benefits are (probably) confined to patients with HER2-positive cancers.

TARGETED THERAPY IN THE CONTEXT OF GENOMICS

One of the profound revolutions in the understanding of breast cancer occurred in the past decade, with the realization that breast cancer was not a single disease but rather several diseases that happened to arise from the same organ.[2,3] The new technology of cDNA microarrays allowed the examination of large numbers of expressed genes in human breast cancer. Bioinformatic exploration of relatively large patient cohorts for outcome end points such as disease-free and overall survival in the context of gene expression followed rapidly.[4]

It became obvious breast cancer was, from a genetic standpoint, a collection of diseases. Unsupervised cluster analysis defined luminal, basal, cerbB2+, and "normal" breast subtypes (though the "normal" subtype may prove to have been artifactual).[2] The luminal cancers (so called because their expression profile resembled that of luminal cells of milk ducts) were further divisible into A and B subtypes. These subtypes paralleled clinical subtypes long recognized by physicians. Luminal cancers show substantial overlap with ER-positive tumors, and, in their A and B subtypes, relatively hormone-sensitive and -insensitive ER-positive breast cancers. Basal cancers, in contrast, overlap with what so-called triple-negative" breast cancers (ER-, progesterone receptor [PR]-, and HER2-negative), and c-erbB2- (HER2) positive tumors were self-explanatory. Although clinicians might believe that unsupervised cluster analysis "told us what we already knew," when these studies first became available physicians rarely considered basal tumors a biologically distinct subset, nor were they aware of distinct genomic subsets within the luminal (ER-positive) subgroup.

From a therapeutic standpoint, and for the point of this article, this genomic clustering offers an underlying biologic rationale for the basic approaches to systemic therapies in breast cancer, and more specifically for targeted therapy of breast cancer. We will not focus on hormonal therapy as a targeted therapy (although ER-targeted therapies are arguably the first targeted therapy in all of cancer medicine), but will instead focus on other existing and novel molecular targets with potential adjuvant benefits for early-stage breast cancer.

HER2-TARGETED THERAPY

The HER family of receptor tyrosine kinases plays an important role in breast cancer biology. These transmembrane receptor tyrosine kinases have a standard motif comprising an external (ligand-binding) domain, a transmembrane domain, and an internal tyrosine kinase domain.[5] HER2 particularly has long attracted the attention of scientists because of its profound effect on tumor biology in the tumors in which it is amplified (approximately 15%–20% of patients with breast cancer). HER2 drives growth, invasion, and metastasis of breast cancers, and in the past its presence in a primary breast cancer was associated with increased risk for, and early death from, breast cancer.[6–8]

In the mid-1990s, the concurrent development of reliable assays for HER2 overexpression (using immunohistochemistry) and amplification (using fluorescence in situ hybridization), and the development of the first agent targeting HER2 (the humanized monoclonal antibody trastuzumab), led to the first clinical trials specifically targeting HER2 in the metastatic setting. In a pivotal phase III trial in the front-line metastatic breast cancer setting, Slamon and colleagues[9] showed that addition of trastuzumab to standard chemotherapy regimens improved both progression-free and overall survival.

This demonstration of the benefits of targeted therapy for HER2-positive metastatic disease led rapidly to the development of adjuvant therapy trials for HER2-positive early-stage breast cancer. Several large trials testing HER2-targeted therapy in the adjuvant setting have been presented, and provide stunning confirmation for the benefits of targeted therapy in the context of HER2-positive breast cancer. Two North American studies, the National Surgical Adjuvant Breast and Bowel Project (NSABP) B-31 trial and the North Central Cancer Treatment Group (NCCTG)–coordinated Intergroup trial N9831, merged their chemotherapy control arms (doxorubicin and cyclophosphamide followed by paclitaxel) in a comparison with the same regimens plus a year of trastuzumab for a joint analysis. They reported a highly significant 49% reduction in the risk for disease recurrence with sequential trastuzumab (4-year disease-free survival, 86% vs 73%; hazard ratio [HR], 0.51) and a 37% reduction in the risk of death (4-year overall survival, 93% vs 89%; HR, 0.63).[10]

These results were confirmed by the Herceptin Adjuvant (HERA) trial, in which 5090 women with HER2-positive (node-negative or -positive) early breast cancer underwent standard adjuvant chemotherapy and then were randomly assigned to either observation or the addition of trastuzumab for 1 or 2 years after completion of the cytotoxic chemotherapy regimen chosen by their oncologist. A significant reduction in disease-free survival (36%) and a significant improvement in overall survival (34%) was reported.[11]

Subsequently, the BCIRG 006 study examined the role of non–anthracycline-based chemotherapy in combination with trastuzumab. Patients receiving trastuzumab in the context of anthracycline-based chemotherapy clearly experience an increased risk for congestive heart failure, and preclinical studies have suggested that non–anthracycline-based combinations had significant activity. The Breast Cancer International Research Group (BCIRG) 006 trial compared two anthracycline-containing regimens (doxorubicin/cyclophosphamide [AC] followed by docetaxel with or without trastuzumab) versus a non–anthracycline trastuzumab combination (carboplatin plus docetaxel and trastuzumab [CTH]) in 3222 women with HER2-positive early breast cancer. Both trastuzumab-containing arms were superior to the non-trastuzumab arm, and no significant efficacy difference between the 2 trastuzumab-containing arms was observed (with an HR for disease-free survival of 0.67 and 0.61 for AC/docetaxel/trastuzumab and TCH, respectively).[12]

The debate regarding the benefit of anthracyclines in HER2-positive breast cancer continues to vex oncologists. It was first hypothesized that HER2-positive tumors are more sensitive to anthracyclines. However this was not confirmed in the preclinical setting. Pegram and colleagues[13] tested the sensitivity of HER2-overexpressing cell lines to doxorubicin and found that HER2 overexpression alone did not predict for doxorubicin sensitivity. More recently, the topoisomerase II alpha gene amplification was also studied, given anthracyclines' principle role as topoisomerase II alpha inhibitors. The topoisomerase II alpha gene is located on the long arm of chromosome 17 near the HER2 gene. Topoisomerase II alpha amplification correlates strongly with HER2 overexpression.[12] Several retrospective studies in the metastatic setting suggested that topoisomerase II alpha amplification is a predictor of anthracycline response, and results of the control arm of the BCIRG 006 adjuvant trial (ie, in the absence of trastuzumab) seemed to confirm this.[12] Because BCIRG 006 was not powered to compare anthracycline and non–anthracycline trastuzumab-containing regimens, no solid prospective data show which approach (if either) is preferred. Both anthracycline and non-anthracycline approaches fall within the current standard of care.

The proper duration of treatment in the adjuvant setting remains unanswered. The four larger clinical trials (NSABP B-31, N9831, HERA, and BCIRG 006) have used at least 1 year of adjuvant trastuzumab. The results of the HERA trial arms of 1 versus 2 years of adjuvant trastuzumab are awaited. In contrast, the smaller FinHer trial suggested that as little as 9 weeks might provide the same efficacy with less toxicity, which in turn has led to trials examining a shorter duration of therapy.[14] Current practice uses a standard 1-year regimen.

Although trastuzumab-based regimens remain the standard of care in the adjuvant HER2 setting, newer agents have entered the HER2 arena. Lapatinib is an oral small molecule receptor tyrosine kinase inhibitor of both epidermal growth factor receptor and HER2. Preclinical data suggest that it is synergistic with trastuzumab against HER2-positive breast cancer. It was recently approved for advanced HER2-positive metastatic breast cancer, because it showed activity in trastuzumab-refractory metastatic disease in combination with capecitabine in a large phase III randomized trial.[15] Lapatinib's role is currently being examined in the adjuvant setting in the international, multi-group Adjuvant Lapatinib and/or Trastuzumab Treatment Optimisation (ALTTO) trial, which randomizes patients undergoing standard chemotherapy approaches to receive either trastuzumab, lapatinib, the combination of the two drugs, or their sequential use.

NOVEL APPROACHES: ANTI–VASCULAR ENDOTHELIAL GROWTH FACTOR THERAPY

Evidence for a role of angiogenesis (new blood vessel formation) in breast cancer is derived from several independent lines of evidence. Beginning in the early 1990s, evidence emerged that tumor microvessel density in human breast cancers was associated with an increased risk for relapse and death. Proangiogenic factors are readily measurable in early breast cancers, and vascular endothelial growth factor (VEGF) in particular is associated with an increased risk for recurrence and death in patients with early-stage breast cancer.[16] Increased VEGF production by breast cancers is also associated with an increased risk for brain and visceral metastasis. HER2 amplification is also associated with increased VEGF production in human breast cancers, suggesting this important breast cancer subtype as a particular target of interest.[17,18]

The improved understanding of VEGF biology suggested several potential means of targeting the VEGF system.[19,20] The VEGFs are a family of five related glycoproteins (VEGFA, VEGFB, VEGFC, VEGFD, and placental growth factor) that act through three type III receptor tyrosine kinases (VEGFR-1, VEGFR2, VEGFR-3); in addition the neuropilins (NP1 and NP2) act as coreceptors for the VEGFRs, increasing the binding affinity of VEGF to VEGFR tyrosine kinase receptor. The functional effects of VEGF depend on which ligand-receptor complex is activated.

The VEGF axis may be attacked in multiple ways, including (among FDA-approved agents) ligand-binding agents (eg, bevacizumab), agents interfering with the VEGF receptor tyrosine kinase (eg, sunitinib, sorafenib), agents interfering with downstream effectors of VEGF activity (eg, mammalian target of rapamycin [mTOR] inhibitors), and agents that indirectly affect angiogenesis through modulation of VEGF production (eg, HER2-targeting agents).

Of these approaches, ligand inhibition with bevacizumab is currently the only FDA- and European Medicines Agency (EMEA)–approved agent for metastatic breast cancer. This approval is based on two randomized controlled trials. E2100 randomized women to receive paclitaxel alone or in combination with bevacizumab as front-line therapy for HER2-negative metastatic disease,[21] and the AVADO trial randomized a similar patient population to receive docetaxel alone or in combination with bevacizumab at one of two doses.[22] Both trials showed a statistically significant improvement in progression-free survival. Neither showed a significant improvement in overall survival, although both were relatively poorly powered to show a survival advantage. Other phase II metastatic trials have suggested that patients HER2-positive advanced breast cancer might benefit from the combination of anti-VEGF therapies with anti-HER2 therapies.[23,24]

Based on the results in advanced disease, adjuvant trials have been initiated in both HER2-negative and HER2-positive populations. E5103 randomizes women with lymph node–positive and high-risk lymph node–negative disease to receive either a backbone chemotherapy regimen (AC followed by paclitaxel) alone or in combination with bevacizumab (administered either for the duration of chemotherapy or for a total of a year of therapy). The BEvacizumab and Trastuzumab Adjuvant Therapy in HER2-positive Breast Cancer (BETH) trial randomizes patients with HER2-positive breast cancer to undergo either a standard chemotherapy/trastuzumab combination or the same with bevacizumab. Both are large, well-powered trials with primary disease-free survival end points and secondary overall survival end points.

Whether bevacizumab (or other VEGF-targeting agents) can legitimately be called targeted therapy is currently uncertain. Although the molecular target (VEGF) is well defined and readily measurable, a specific subpopulation benefiting from anti-VEGF therapy cannot currently be defined. Early investigations suggested that specific single nucleotide polymorphism variants of VEGF may be associated with clinical benefit in the metastatic setting, an observation that is currently being examined as part of the large E5103 adjuvant bevacizumab proof-of-concept trial.[25]

Concerns have been raised regarding the potential benefits of anti-VEGF therapy in the adjuvant setting. The vasculature of micrometastases and overt metastases may differ significantly, and therefore benefits seen in the overt metastatic setting may not translate to the adjuvant setting. Preclinical studies in some animal models of micrometastatic disease have suggested that anti-VEGF therapy may actually promote the development of metastases, although these models are open to question on several grounds.[26] Finally, the adjuvant colorectal NSABP C-08 trial failed to show a statistically significant clinical benefit regarding its primary disease-free survival end point. The results of ongoing adjuvant bevacizumab trials are therefore awaited with some trepidation.

NOVEL APPROACHES: CHEMOTHERAPY AS TARGETED THERAPY

Although chemotherapeutic agents have specific molecular targets (typically DNA or microtubules), their relative nonspecificity has argued against defining them as targeted agents. Modern genomic analyses are well on their way to changing this perception. The identification of genomic subgroups within the luminal breast cancers allows subpopulations with specifically greater or lesser benefit with adjuvant chemotherapy to be defined. In general, patients with ER-positive breast cancer experiencing benefit (across several genomic classification platforms) are characterized by relatively high proliferation rates and relatively lower ER concentrations.[27] This finding has allowed clinicians (using commercially available assays such as Oncotype DX and Mammaprint) to offer adjuvant chemotherapy as targeted therapy for early-stage disease and, more importantly, to avoid toxic therapies when the therapeutic target (rapidly proliferating cancer cells) is not present.[28] More recently, the initial observations seen in lymph node–negative breast cancer have been extended to the lymph node–positive, ER-positive setting.[29]

The first-generation genomic tests (eg, Oncotype DX, Mammaprint) define the role of relatively generic chemotherapy regimens as targeted therapy. Future developments in this arena will undoubtedly identify individual chemotherapy agents as targeted therapies based on their genomic or proteomic characteristics.

NOVEL APPROACHES: PARP INHIBITION FOR TRIPLE-NEGATIVE (BASAL) BREAST CANCER

Genomic analyses showed the existence of a genomically distinct subpopulation of breast cancers now called *basal* or *triple-negative* breast cancer (the latter based on the lack of ER, ER, and HER2). This population of patients constitutes approximately 15% of those with newly diagnosed breast cancer, and is clinically significant both because of its relative aggressiveness and the lack of available targeted therapies.[30] This subpopulation represents the common "home" for *BRCA*-1 mutated breast cancers. In addition, many non–*BRCA*-mutated breast cancers have a *BRCA*-like phenotype.

These observations have led to the development of the first targeted therapeutics for triple-negative breast cancers. The most promising targeted therapy currently being examined is PARP inhibition in triple-negative and *BRCA*-mutated cancers. PARPs are DNA-binding proteins involved in detection and repair of single-stranded DNA breaks. Triple-negative and *BRCA*-deficient cancers have impaired homologous double-stranded DNA repair mechanisms. In this setting, a compensatory pathway of DNA repair known as *base excision repair* (BER), which is dependent on the function of PARP, allows the cancer cell to recover from DNA damage by upregulation of PARP.[31,32]

Multiple PARP inhibitors are under development, two of which (BSI-201 and olaparib) have shown promising results in phase II studies presented at the 2010 American Society of Clinical Oncology meetings. O'Shaughnessy and colleagues[33] reported the results of a randomized phase II trial of chemotherapy (carboplatin/

gemcitabine) with or without BSI-201 in 123 women with triple-negative metastatic breast cancer. The overall response rate was 16% in the group of patients treated with chemotherapy alone and 48% among those who underwent chemotherapy plus BSI-201 ($P = .002$). A striking improvement was also seen in progression-free and overall survivals in patients treated with BSI-201 (progression-free survival, 3.3 vs 6.3 months, $P<.0001$; overall survival, 5.7 vs 9.2 months; $P = .0005$). Surprisingly, the addition of BSI-201 was not reported to be associated with additional toxicity.

Tutt and colleagues[34] reported a single-arm phase II study of olaparib in 54 patients with metastatic breast cancer carrying a *BRCA* mutation. Impressive results were reported, with response rates as high as 41% and median progression-free survival of 5.7 months when olaparib was given at a dose of 400 mg orally twice daily. Again, toxicity was very tolerable. These remarkable results are currently being confirmed in ongoing phase III trials.

If the results of the first phase III trials with PARP inhibition in metastatic disease confirm earlier phase II findings, they will be followed with phase III trials in the adjuvant setting for patients with triple-negative breast cancers. Pilot trials examining novel combinations and schedules in the adjuvant setting are underway. The presence of distinct molecular targets (*BRCA* mutations) that are clinically measurable suggests the possibility that PARP inhibition my also find a place in the breast cancer prevention setting, a concept being examined in pilot studies currently being developed under the auspices of the National Cancer Institute.

NOVEL APPROACHES: TARGETING SITE-SPECIFIC BONE METASTASIS

Breast cancer has long been characterized by the presence of site-specific metastasis, with bone metastasis being the most common specific site. In patients with metastatic breast cancer, the incidence of bone metastases is 73%.[35,36] In addition, bone health and maintenance of bone integrity are important issues for clinicians treating breast cancer patients.[37] Treatment considerations include local (eg, surgery, radiation) and systemic disease control (eg, chemotherapy; biologic and endocrine therapy).

Systemic therapies can be associated with late effects that impact bone health. An estimated 50% to 70% of premenopausal women who have undergone adjuvant chemotherapy will develop permanent ovarian failure or early menopause. Chemotherapy-induced ovarian failure is considered a high-risk factor for bone loss.[38] Adjuvant hormonal therapies that decrease circulating estrogen levels also place breast cancer patients at increased risk for osteoporosis. Recently, aromatase inhibitors have been found to improve progression-free survival and have fewer adverse effects compared with tamoxifen, the historical standard, in postmenopausal women with hormone receptor–positive, early-stage breast cancer.

Bone is a dynamic tissue that is continually undergoing formation through osteoblastic activity and resorption through osteoclastic activity. This system is tightly controlled and balanced by many factors, but the dominant pathway that controls normal bone remodeling is the RANK/RANKL/osteoprotegerin (OPG) signaling triad.[39] Osteoblasts and bone marrow stromal cells secrete RANKL and OPG. Binding of RANKL to its receptor RANK on the surface of osteoclast precursors stimulates osteoclastogenesis. OPG is a soluble decoy receptor for RANKL. Through binding to RANKL, OPG prevents the interaction between RANKL and RANK to regulate excessive bone resorption.[40] Estrogen effects bone through decreasing osteoclasts and stimulating osteoblastic activity.[41] Thus, estrogen deficiency leads to increased bone resorption and rapid bone loss.[41]

The mechanism of bone metastases involves bone destruction, which is mediated by osteoclasts. Osteoclasts require the RANKL for their maturation, function, and survival.[42–44] Binding of RANKL to the osteoclasts stimulate increased bone resorption and the release of other growth factors that trigger a cycle of bone destruction and tumor cell proliferation, in addition to the migration of tumor cells to the bone.[45,46]

Denosumab is a fully human monoclonal antibody that specifically inhibits RANKL and therefore inhibits osteoclast function and bone resorption.[47–50] Given subcutaneously, a single dose was shown to suppress bone turnover for up to 6 months in postmenopausal women with low bone mass.[47] In a small, randomized, double-blind study to determine the safety and efficacy of denosumab in patients with radiologically confirmed bone metastases from either breast cancer (n = 29) or multiple myeloma (n = 25), denosumab was found to suppress bone turnover for up to 84 days and was well tolerated.[49]

Promising results in phase II trials of denosumab led to a larger phase III study involving more than 2000 patients.[51] This trial randomized patients with metastatic breast cancer to either subcutaneous denosumab and intravenous placebo (n = 1026) or subcutaneous placebo and intravenous zoledronic acid (n = 1020). Preliminary reports indicate that denosumab was superior to zoledronic acid in delaying the time to first on-study skeletal-related event (SRE), and overall survival and time to progression were similar in both arms.

Although denosumab is not yet approved for use in the United States for the management of bone metastases from breast cancer, these studies define it as a potential new targeted therapy for metastatic breast cancer. In the near future, denosumab will be studied in the adjuvant setting for patients with breast cancer. Denosumab is also under investigation for the treatment of bone loss associated with aromatase inhibitors. A randomized, double-bind, placebo-controlled phase III trial in postmenopausal women with ER-positive breast cancer undergoing adjuvant hormonal therapy with an aromatase inhibitor plus calcium and vitamin D supplementation compared placebo (n = 125) with subcutaneous denosumab (n = 127) every 6 months.[52] The twice-yearly administration of denosumab led to significant increases in bone mineral density, with similar overall adverse effect rates.

Although denosumab is arguably the first therapy for site-specific bone metastasis with a specific molecular target, it is not the first approach to site-specific bone metastasis. Several phase III trials have examined the role of bisphosphonate therapies for bone metastasis in breast cancer, and several of these trials indicate that the use of bisphosphonates may reduce the incidence of bone (and other) metastases.

SUMMARY

Targeted therapy in the adjuvant setting is now a clinical reality. Targeted therapies have a basis in the underlying genomics of breast cancer, with genomic subpopulations of breast cancer paralleling (to greater or lesser extent) existing therapeutic categories for the disease. Although targeting of ER and HER2 have led the way, newer targeted therapies are rapidly advancing toward the clinic in the adjuvant setting. Although not all of these may arrive, the future certainly seems promising. The ability to identify specific lesions at the molecular and cellular levels, together with the increasing availability of agents targeting these specific lesions, will increasingly dominate breast cancer therapeutics. These agents should improve outcomes of all patients with early-stage breast cancer, and simultaneously diminish the toxicity experienced.

REFERENCES

1. Sledge G. What is targeted therapy? J Clin Oncol 2005;23:1614–5.
2. Sorlie T, Perou C, Tibshirani R, et al. Gene expression patterns of breast carcinomas distinguish tumor subclasses with clinical implications. Proc Natl Acad Sci U S A 2001;98:10869–74.
3. Perou C, Sorlie T, Eisen M, et al. Molecular portraits of human breast tumours. Nature 2000;406:747–52.
4. van de Vijver M, He Y, van't Veer L, et al. A gene-expression signature as a predictor of survival in breast cancer. N Engl J Med 2002;347:1999–2009.
5. Riese DJ, Stern DF. Specificity within the EGF family/ErbB receptor family signaling network. Bioessays 1998;20(1):41–8.
6. Slamon DJ, Clark GM, Wong SG, et al. Human breast cancer: correlation of relapse and survival with amplification of the HER-2/neu oncogene. Science 1987;235(4785):177–82.
7. Hynes N, Stern D. The biology of erbB-2/neu/HER-2 and its role in cancer. Biochim Biophys Acta 1994;1198:165–84.
8. Ravdin P, Chamness G. The c-erbB-2 proto-oncogene as a prognostic and predictive marker in breast cancer: a paradigm for the development of other macromolecular markers—a review. Gene 1995;159:19–27.
9. Slamon D, Leyland-Jones B, Shak S, et al. Use of chemotherapy plus a monoclonal antibody against HER2 for metastatic breast cancer that overexpresses HER2. N Engl J Med 2001;344:783–92.
10. Romond E, Perez E, Bryant J, et al. Trastuzumab plus adjuvant chemotherapy for operable HER2-positive breast cancer. N Engl J Med 2005;353:1673–84.
11. Piccart-Gebhart M, Proctor M, Leyland-Jones B, et al. Trastuzumab after adjuvant chemotherapy in HER2-positive breast cancer. N Engl J Med 2005;353:1659–72.
12. Slamon D, Eiermann W, Robert N. Phase III randomized trial comparing doxorubicin and cyclophosphamide followed by docetaxel (AC→T) with doxorubicin and cyclophosphamide followed by docetaxel and trastuzumab (AC→TH) with docetaxel, carboplatin and trastuzumab (TCH) in Her2neu positive early breast cancer patients: BCIRG 006 study [abstract-A-62]. Presented at the 32nd Annual San Antonio Breast Cancer Symposium. San Antonio (TX), December 9–13, 2009.
13. Pegram M, Finn R, Arzoo K, et al. The effect of HER-2/neu overexpression on chemotherapeutic drug sensitivity in human breast and ovarian cancers cells. Oncogene 1997;15:537–47.
14. Joensuu H, Kellokumpu-Lehtinen PL, Bono P, et al. Adjuvant docetaxel or vinorelbine with or without trastuzumab for breast cancer. N Engl J Med 2006;354(8):809–20.
15. Geyer C, Forster J, Lindquist D, et al. Lapatinib plus capecitabine for HER2-positive advanced breast cancer. N Engl J Med 2006;355(26):2733–43.
16. Sledge G, Miller K. Angiogenesis and antiangiogenic therapy. Curr Probl Cancer 2002;26:1–60.
17. Konecny G, Meng Y, Untch M, et al. Association between HER-2/neu and vascular endothelial growth factor expression predicts clinical outcome in primary breast cancer patients. Clin Cancer Res 2004;10:1706–16.
18. Linderholm B, Andersson J, Lindh B, et al. Overexpression of c-erbB-2 is related to a higher expression of vascular endothelial growth factor (VEGF) and constitutes an independent prognostic factor in primary node-positive breast cancer after adjuvant systemic treatment. Eur J Cancer 2004;40:33–42.

19. Hicklin D, Ellis L. Role of the vascular endothelial growth factor pathway in tumor growth and angiogenesis. J Clin Oncol 2005;23:1011–27.
20. Ellis L, Hicklin D. VEGF-targeted therapy: mechanisms of anti-tumour activity. Nat Rev Cancer 2008;8:579–91.
21. Miller K, Wang M, Gralow J, et al. Paclitaxel plus bevacizumab versus paclitaxel alone for metastatic breast cancer. N Engl J Med 2007;357:2666–76.
22. Miles D, Chan A, Romieu G, et al. Randomized, double-blind, placebo-controlled, phase III study of bevacizumab with docetaxel or docetaxel with placebo as first-line therapy for patients with locally recurrent or metastatic breast cancer (AVA-DO) [abstract LBA 1011]. J Clin Oncol 2008;26(Suppl 1).
23. Pegram M, Chan D, Dichmann RA, et al. Phase II combined biological therapy targeting the HER2 proto-oncogene and the vascular endothelial growth factor using trastuzumab (T) and bevacizumab (B) as first line treatment of HER2-amplified breast cancer [abstract 301]. Breast Cancer Res Treat Suppl 2006; 100(Suppl 1).
24. Slamon D, Gomez H, Kabbinavar F, et al. Randomized study of pazopanib + lapatinib vs. lapatinib alone in patients with HER2-positive advanced or metastatic breast cancer. Proc Am Soc Clin Oncol 2008;16(155):1016.
25. Schneider B, Wang M, Radovich M, et al. Association of VEGF and VEGFR-2 genetic polymorphisms with outcome in E2100. J Clin Oncol 2008;26:4672–8.
26. Schneider B, Sledge GJ. Anti-VEGF therapy as adjuvant therapy: clouds on the horizon? Breast Cancer Res 2009;11(3):303.
27. Wirapati P, Sotiriou C, Kunkel S, et al. Meta-analysis of gene expression profiles in breast cancer: toward a unified understanding of breast cancer subtyping and prognosis signatures. Breast Cancer Res 2008;10:R65.
28. Paik S, Tang G, Shak S, et al. Gene expression and benefit of chemotherapy in women with node-negative, estrogen receptor-positive breast cancer. J Clin Oncol 2006;24:3726–34.
29. Albain K, Barlow W, Shak S, et al. Prognostic and predictive value of the 21-gene recurrence score assay in postmenopausal women with node-positive, oestrogen-receptor-positive breast cancer on chemotherapy: a retrospective analysis of a randomised trial. Lancet Oncol 2010;11(1):55–65.
30. Schneider B, Winer E, Foulkes W, et al. Triple-negative breast cancer: risk factors to potential targets. Clin Cancer Res 2008;14(24):8010–8.
31. Comen E, Robson M. Inhibition of poly(ADP)-ribose polymerase as a therapeutic strategy for breast cancer. Oncology (Williston Park) 2010;24(1):55–62.
32. Martin S, Lord C, Ashworth A. DNA repair deficiency as a therapeutic target in cancer. Curr Opin Genet Dev 2008;18(1):80–6.
33. O'Shaughnessy B, Osborne J, Pippen M, et al. Final results of a randomized phase II study demonstrating efficacy and safety of BSI-201, a poly (ADP-Ribose) polymerase (PARP) inhibitor, in combination with gemcitabine/carboplatin (G/C) in metastatic Triple Negative Breast Cancer (TNBC) [abstract 3]. Presented at the San Antonio Breast Cancer Symposium. 2009. J Clin Oncol 2009; 27(Suppl):18s.
34. Tutt A. Phase II trial of the oral PARP inhibitor olaparib in BRCA-deficient advanced breast cancer. J Clin Oncol 2009;27:18S.
35. James J, Evans A, Pinder S, et al. Bone metastases from breast carcinoma: histopathological – radiological correlations and prognostic features. Br J Cancer 2003;89:660–5.
36. Coleman R. Clinical features of metastatic bone disease and risk of skeletal morbidity. Clin Cancer Res 2006;12:6243s.

37. Gralow J, Biermann S, Farooki A, et al. NCCN task force report: bone health in cancer care. J Natl Compr Canc Netw 2009;7(3):S1.
38. Hillner B, Ingle J, Chlebowski R, et al. American Society of Clinical Oncology 2003 update on the role of bisphosphonates and bone health issues in women with breast cancer. J Clin Oncol 2003;21:4042–57.
39. Guise T. Breaking down bone: new insight into the site specific mechanisms of breast cancer osteolysis mediated by metalloproteinases. Genes Dev 2009; 23(18):2117.
40. Hofbauer L, Hosla S, Dunstan C, et al. The roles of osteoprotegerin and osteoprotegerin ligand in the paracrine regulation of bone resorption. J Bone Miner Res 2000;15(1):2–12.
41. Harada S, Rodan G. Control of osteoblast function and regulation of bone mass. Nature 2003;423:349–55.
42. Lacey D, Timms E, Tan H, et al. Osteoprotegerin ligand is a cytokine that regulates osteoclast differentiation and activation. Cell 1998;93:165–76.
43. Roodman G. Biology of osteoclast activation in cancer. J Clin Oncol 2001;19: 3562–71.
44. Yasuda H, Shima N, Nakagawa N, et al. Osteoclast differentiation factor is a ligand for osteoprotegerin/osteoclastogenesis-inhibitory factor and is identical to TRANCE/RANKL. Proc Natl Acad Sci U S A 1998;95(7):3597–602.
45. Roodman G. Mechanisms of bone metastasis. N Engl J Med 2004;350(16): 1655–70.
46. Jones DH, Nakashima T, Sanchez O, et al. Regulation of cancer cell migration and bone metastasis by RANKL. Nature 2006;440:692–6.
47. Bekker P, Holloway D, Rasmussen A, et al. A single-dose placebo-controlled study of AMG1 162, a fully human monoclonal antibody to RANKL, in postmenopausal women. J Bone Miner Res 2004;19:1059.
48. McClung M, Lewecki E, Cohen S, et al. Denosumab in postmenopausal women with low bone mineral density. N Engl J Med 2006;354:821–31.
49. Body J, Facon T, Coleman R, et al. A study of the biological receptor activator of nuclear factor-kappaB ligand inhibitor, denosumab, in patients with multiple myeloma or bone metastases from breast cancer. Clin Cancer Res 2006;12:1221.
50. Lipton A, Steger G, Figueroa J, et al. Randomized active-controlled phase II study of denosumab efficacy and safety in patients with breast-cancer related bone metastases. J Clin Oncol 2007;25:4431–7.
51. Stopeck A, Body JJ, Fujiwara Y, et al. Denosumab versus zoledronic acid for the treatment of breast cancer patients with bone metastases: results of a randomized phase 3 study [abstract 14LBA]. Presented at the Joint ECCO 15–34th ESMO Multidisciplinary Congress. Berlin (Germany), September 20–24, 2009.
52. Ellis G, Bone H, Chlebowski R, et al. Randomized trial of denosumab in patients receiving adjuvant aromatase inhibitors for nonmetastatic breast cancer. J Clin Oncol 2008;26:4875–82.

Index

Note: Page numbers of article titles are in **boldface** type.

A

Adjuvant therapy, chemotherapy, in early-stage breast cancer, **649–668**
  patient selection for, 651–653
    genomic tests, 652–653
    prognostic markers, 651–652
    traditional markers in combined score, 653
  regimen selection for, 653–657
    anthracyclines, 653–655
    taxanes, 655–657
  timing of, 661–662
  tumor biology and choice of, 658–661
    ER-positive, 658
    HER2-positive, 658–661
    triple-negative, 661
  hormonal, for early-stage breast cancer, **639–647**
    for postmenopausal women with hormone receptor-positive, 641–644
    for premenopausal women with hormone receptor-positive, 644–645
    tamoxifen, 640–641
American Society of Clinical Oncology, clinical practice guidelines for pharmacologic
  intervention for breast cancer risk reduction, 471
Anthracyclines, in adjuvant treatment of early breast cancer, 653–655
  in HER2-positive cases, 655
Aromatase inhibitors, comparison of, 633–634
  in breast cancer chemoprevention, 470–471
  versus tamoxifen, 628–629
Arzoxifene, in breast cancer chemoprevention, 470
Augmentation, breast, sentinel lymph node surgery after previous, 544
Axillary lymph node dissection (ALND), after positive pretreatment SLN biopsy after
  chemotherapy, 524
  for SLN-positive disease, 496
  safety of avoiding after a negative SLN biopsy after neoadjuvant chemotherapy, 527–529
  SLN surgery after previous, 544–545

B

Bioinformatics, methods for analysis of gene expression in breast cancer, 589–590
Biology, tumor, in selection of adjuvant chemotherapy for early breast cancer, 658–661
Biomarkers, evaluation in neoadjuvant endocrine setting to predict long-term breast cancer
  outcome, 630–631
Biopsy, excisional, SLN surgery after previous, 543
  of SLN in early stage breast cancer, **483–505**

doi:10.1016/S1055-3207(10)00044-X
1055-3207/10/$ – see front matter © 2010 Elsevier Inc. All rights reserved.
surgonc.theclinics.com

Biopsy (*continued*)
   SLN, before or after neoadjuvant chemotherapy, **519–538**
   with internal mammary SNLs, 509–513
      indications, 509–510
      technical considerations, 510–513
Bone metastases, site-specific in breast cancer, targeted therapy of, 675
Breast augmentation, SNL surgery after previous, 544
Breast cancer, early-stage, adjuvant chemotherapy for, **649–668**
      patient selection for, 651–653
      regimen selection for, 653–657
      timing of, 661–662
      tumor biology and choice of, 657–661
   adjuvant hormonal therapy for, **639–647**
      for postmenopausal women with hormone receptor-positive, 641–644
      for premenopausal women with hormone receptor-positive, 644–645
      tamoxifen, 640–641
   chemoprevention, **463–473**
      American Society of Clinical Oncology clinical practice guidelines for, 471
      aromatase inhibitors, 470–471
      arzoxifene, 470
      lasofoxifene, 470
      raloxifene studies, 467–468
      selective estrogen receptor modulators, 464
      tamoxifen and raloxifene trial, 468–469
      tamoxifen trials, 464–467
   extra-axillary sentinel lymph nodes, **507–517**
      internal mammary, 507–513
      other nonaxillary sites, 513–514
   gene expression profiling in, **581–606**
      classifiers developed by other methods, 597–599
      classifiers developed by supervised analysis, 591–597
      clinical usefulness, 600–602
      invasive gene signature, 599–600
      methods for analyzing, 585–588
      methods for bioinformatics analysis of, 589–590
      multiparameter assays compared with integrated clinical information, 597
      process for development of multiparameter assay, 585
      prognostic and predictive markers, 584–585
      prospective clinical trials, 600
      quality control in, 588–589
      regulatory approval of multiparameter assays, 591
      validity, reproducibility, and reporting of microarray studies, 590–591
      wound-response signature, 599
   magnetic resonance imaging and breast-conserving surgery, **475–492**
      for detection of local recurrence, 486–487
      for screening, 476–478
      for treatment selection, 479–486
         effect on long-term cancer outcomes, 484–486
         effect on short-term surgical outcomes, 480–484
   minimal involvement of sentinel lymph nodes in, **493–505**
      axillary lymph node dissection for positive disease, 496–497

clinical trials, 499–500
predictive models, 497–499
what constitutes a positive node, 493–496
neoadjuvant chemotherapy for operable, **607–626**
assessing response to, 614–616
breast conservation *vs.* mastectomy for resection of the primary, 616–617
chemotherapy *vs.* hormonal therapy, 611–612
management of regional lymph nodes with, 617–618
optimal regimen, 613–614
postmastectomy regional/chest wall irradiation after, 618–619
potential benefits, 607–609
pre-therapy assessment and staging, 612–613
predicting response to, 609–611
neoadjuvant endocrine therapy for, **627–638**
aromatase inhibitors *versus* surgery, 628–629
biomarker evaluation to predict long-term outcome, 630–631
comparison of aromatase inhibitors, 633–634
new combinations in adjuvant setting, 635
patient selection for, 634–635
receptor, HER2 status, and sensitivity to, 631–633
tamoxifen *versus* surgery, 627–628
versus neoadjuvant chemotherapy, 629–630
oncoplastic surgery, **567–580**
definition of, 570
historical perspective, 567–570
in the large breast, 575–578
in the small breast, 575
preoperative assessment, 573–574
surgical planning, 574–575
sentinel lymph node biopsy before or after neoadjuvant chemotherapy, **519–538**
accuracy of, after neoadjuvant chemotherapy, 524–525
accuracy with clinically involved nodes before chemotherapy, 525–526
accuracy with clinically negative nodes, 526–527
after, potential advantages of, 521–524
before, potential advantages of, 520–521
choice of approach to obtain most relevant information, 529–531
safety of avoiding axillary lymph node dissection after negative biopsy, 527–529
sentinel lymph node surgery in uncommon clinical circumstances, **539–553**
ductal carcinoma in situ, 541–542
in men, 539–540
in pregnant patients, 540–541
internal mammary SLN surgery, 545
multicentric/multifocal, 542
previous axillary surgery, 544–545
previous breast surgery, 543–544
breast reduction, 544
excisional biopsy, 543
prophylactic mastectomy, 546–547
with neoadjuvant chemotherapy, 542–543
targeted therapies in, **669–679**
anti-vascular endothelial growth factor therapy, 672–674

Breast cancer (*continued*)
    chemotherapy as, 674
    definition, 669–670
    HER2-targeted, 671–672
    in context of genomics, 670–671
    of site-specific bone metastases, 675
  total skin sparing mastectomy, **555–566**
    discussion, 560–564
    literature review, 556–557
    technical considerations, 558–560
      creating skin flaps, 559–560
      incision planning, 559
      patient selection, 559
Breast reduction, SLN surgery after previous, 544
Breast-conserving surgery, magnetic resonance imaging and, **475–492**
    for detection of local recurrence, 486–487
    for screening, 476–478
    for treatment selection, 479–486
      effect on long-term cancer outcomes, 484–486
      effect on short-term surgical outcomes, 480–484
    versus mastectomy after neoadjuvant chemotherapy, 616–617

C

Chemoprevention, of breast cancer, **463–473**
    American Society of Clinical Oncology clinical practice guidelines for, 471
    aromatase inhibitors, 470–471
    arzoxifene, 470
    lasofoxifene, 470
    raloxifene studies, 467–468
    selective estrogen receptor modulators, 464
    tamoxifen and raloxifene trial, 468–469
    tamoxifen trials, 464–467
Chemotherapy, adjuvant, in early-stage breast cancer, **649–668**
    patient selection for, 651–653
      genomic tests, 652–653
      prognostic markers, 651–652
      traditional markers in combined score, 653
    regimen selection for, 653–657
      anthracyclines, 653–655
      taxanes, 655–657
    timing of, 661–662
    tumor biology and choice of, 658–661
      ER-positive, 658
      HER2-positive, 658–661
      triple-negative, 661
  as target therapy for early breast cancer, 674
  neoadjuvant, for operable breast cancer, **607–626**
    assessing response to, 614–616
    breast conservation *vs.* mastectomy for resection of the primary, 616–617
    chemotherapy *vs.* hormonal therapy, 611–612
    management of regional lymph nodes with, 617–618

optimal regimen, 613–614
postmastectomy regional/chest wall irradiation after, 618–619
potential benefits, 607–609
pre-therapy assessment and staging, 612–613
predicting response to, 609–611
SLN biopsy before or after, **519–538**
accuracy of biopsy done after, 524–525
accuracy of biopsy with clinically involved nodes done before, 525–526
accuracy of biopsy with clinically negative nodes, 526–527
biopsy after, potential advantages of, 521–524
biopsy before, potential advantages of, 520–521
choice of approach to obtain most relevant information, 529–531
safety of avoiding axillary lymph node dissection after negative biopsy, 527–529
SLN surgery after, 542–543
Classifiers, in gene expression profiling for breast cancer, 591–597
developed by other methods, 597–599
intrinsic breast cancer subtypes and PAM50, 599
developed by supervised analysis, 591–597
2-gene HOXB13/IL17BR ratio, 593
21-gene assay (oncotype DX recurrence score), 596–597
70-gene assay, 591–593
76-gene assay, 593
genomic grade index, 593–596
Contralateral axillary sentinel lymph nodes, 513
Contralateral cancer, of breast, effect of magnetic resonance imaging on outcome, 485–486

D

Diagnosis, of breast cancer, magnetic resonance imaging in, 486–487
Docetaxel. *See* Taxanes.
Doxorubicin. *See* Anthracyclines.
Ductal carcinoma in situ, SLN surgery for, 541–542

E

Early-stage breast cancer. *See* Breast cancer, early-stage.
Endocrine therapy, adjuvant, for early-stage breast cancer, **639–647**
for postmenopausal women with hormone receptor-positive, 641–644
for premenopausal women with hormone receptor-positive early-stage, 644–645
tamoxifen, 640–641
neoadjuvant, for breast cancer, **627–638**
aromatase inhibitors *versus* surgery, 628–629
biomarker evaluation to predict long-term outcome, 630–631
comparison of aromatase inhibitors, 633–634
new combinations in adjuvant setting, 635
patient selection for, 634–635
receptor, HER2 status, and sensitivity to, 631–633
tamoxifen *versus* surgery, 627–628
versus neoadjuvant chemotherapy, 629–630
Epirubicin. *See* Anthracyclines.

Estrogen receptors (ER), and sensitivity to endocrine therapy, 631–633
    status in choice of adjuvant chemotherapy, 658–661
Excisional biopsy, SLN surgery after previous, 543
Extended radical mastectomy, with internal mammary SLNs, 507–508
Extra-axillary sentinel lymph nodes, in early stage breast cancer, **507–517**
    internal mammary, 507–513
        extended radical mastectomy, 507–508
        implications in current era, 508–509
        is biopsy ever indicated, 509–510
        technical considerations for biopsy of, 510–511
    other nonaxillary sites, 513–514
        contralateral, 514
        intramammary, 513
        Rotter (interpectoral) nodes, 513
        supraclavicular, 513–514

G

Gene expression profiling, in breast cancer, **581–606**
    classifiers developed by other methods, 597–599
    classifiers developed by supervised analysis, 591–597
    clinical usefulness, 600–602
    invasive gene signature, 599–600
    methods for analyzing, 585–588
    methods for bioinformatics analysis of, 589–590
    multiparameter assays compared with integrated clinical information, 597
    process for development of multiparameter assay, 585
    prognostic and predictive markers, 584–585
    prospective clinical trials, 600
    quality control in, 588–589
    regulatory approval of multiparameter assays, 591
    validity, reproducibility, and reporting of microarray studies, 590–591
    wound-response signature, 599
Genomic grade index, in gene expression profiling for breast cancer, 593–596
Genomics, in patient selection for adjuvant chemotherapy for early-stage breast cancer,
    652–653
    targeted therapy of early breast cancer in context of, 670–671

H

HER2 status, adjuvant therapy with anthracyclines in HER2-positive breast cancer, 655
    and sensitivity to endocrine therapy, 631–633
    HER2-targeted therapy, 671–672
Hormonal therapy, adjuvant, for early-stage breast cancer, **639–647**
    for postmenopausal women with hormone receptor-positive, 641–644
    for premenopausal women with hormone receptor-positive, 644–645
    tamoxifen, 640–641
    neoadjuvant, for breast cancer, **627–638**
        aromatase inhibitors *versus* surgery, 628–629
        biomarker evaluation to predict long-term outcome, 630–631
            633–634

new combinations in adjuvant setting, 635
patient selection for, 634–635
receptor, HER2 status, and sensitivity to, 631–633
tamoxifen *versus* surgery, 627–628
versus neoadjuvant chemotherapy, 629–630
versus chemotherapy for early stage breast cancer, 611–612

I

Imaging, magnetic resonance, and breast-conserving surgery, **475–492**
Internal mammary nodes, SLN surgery of, 545
  sentinel, in early stage breast cancer, 507–513
    extended radical mastectomy, 507–508
    implications in current era, 508–509
    is biopsy ever indicated, 509–510
    technical considerations for biopsy of, 510–511
Intramammary sentinel lymph nodes, 512
Irradiation, postmastectomy regional/chest wall, after neoadjuvant chemotherapy,
  618–619

L

Lasofoxifene, in breast cancer chemoprevention, 470
Local recurrence, of breast cancer, effect of magnetic resonance imaging on, 484–485
    magnetic resonance imaging for detection of, 486–487
Lymph nodes, extra-axillary. *See* Extra-axillary lymph nodes.
  regional, management in patients treated with neoadjuvant chemotherapy, 617–618
  sentinel. *See* Sentinel lymph nodes.
Lymphoscintigraphy, preoperative, of internal mammary sentinel lymph nodes, 510–511

M

Magnetic resonance imaging, breast-conserving surgery and, **475–492**
    for detection of local recurrence, 486–487
    for screening, 476–478
    for treatment selection, 479–486
      effect on long-term cancer outcomes, 484–486
      effect on short-term surgical outcomes, 480–484
Markers, in patient selection for adjuvant chemotherapy for early-stage breast cancer,
  651–653
    prognostic, 651–652
    traditional, presented as a combined score, 653
  tumor, gene expression profiling in breast cancer, **581–606**
Mastectomy, extended radical, with internal mammary SLNs, 507–508
  prophylactic, SLN surgery after, 546–547
  skin sparing, with oncoplastic surgery, **567–580**
  total skin sparing (nipple sparing), **555–566**
    discussion, 560–564
    literature review, 556–557
    technical considerations, 558–560
      creating skin flaps, 559–560

Mastectomy (*continued*)
    incision planning, 559
    patient selection, 559
  versus breast-conserving surgery after neoadjuvant chemotherapy, 616–617
Men, breast cancer in, SLN surgery in, 539–540
Menopausal status, in adjuvant hormonal therapy for early-stage breast cancer, 641–645
    in postmenopausal women, 641–644
    in premenopausal women, 644–645
Metastases, site-specific bone, in breast cancer, targeted therapy of, 675
Microarray studies, in gene expression profiling for breast cancer, 590–591
Multicentric breast cancer, SLN surgery for, 542
Multifocal breast cancer, SLN surgery for, 542
Multiparameter assays, in gene expression profiling for breast cancer, 585, 591, 597, 600–602

N

Neoadjuvant therapy, chemotherapy before or after SLN biopsy, **519–538**
    accuracy of biopsy done after, 524–525
    accuracy of biopsy with clinically involved nodes done before, 525–526
    accuracy of biopsy with clinically negative nodes, 526–527
    biopsy after, potential advantages of, 521–524
    biopsy before, potential advantages of, 520–521
    choice of approach to obtain most relevant information, 529–531
    safety of avoiding axillary lymph node dissection after negative biopsy, 527–529
    SLN surgery after, 542–543
  chemotherapy, for operable breast cancer, **607–626**
    assessing response to, 614–616
    breast conservation *vs.* mastectomy for resection of the primary, 616–617
    chemotherapy *vs.* hormonal therapy, 611–612
    management of regional lymph nodes with, 617–618
    optimal regimen, 613–614
    postmastectomy regional/chest wall irradiation after, 618–619
    potential benefits, 607–609
    pre-therapy assessment and staging, 612–613
    predicting response to, 609–611
  endocrine, for breast cancer, **627–638**
    aromatase inhibitors *versus* surgery, 628–629
    biomarker evaluation to predict long-term outcome, 630–631
    comparison of aromatase inhibitors, 633–634
    new combinations in adjuvant setting, 635
    patient selection for, 634–635
    receptor, HER2 status, and sensitivity to, 631–633
    tamoxifen *versus* surgery, 627–628
    versus neoadjuvant chemotherapy, 629–630
Nipple sparing mastectomy, evidence for, **555–566**
    discussion, 560–564
    literature review, 556–557
    technical considerations, 558–560
      creating skin flaps, 559–560
      incision planning, 559
      patient selection, 559

O

Oncoplastic surgery, in breast cancer management, **567–580**
    definition of, 570
    historical perspective, 567–570
    in the large breast, 575–578
    in the small breast, 575
    preoperative assessment, 573–574
    surgical planning, 574–575
Outcomes, of breast cancer, effect of magnetic resonance imaging on long-term, 484–486
    surgical, effect of magnetic resonance imaging on short-term, 480–484
Ovarian suppression, in adjuvant hormonal therapy for early-stage breast cancer, 639–644

P

Paclitaxel. *See* Taxanes.
PARP inhibition, in targeted therapy for triple negative (basal) breast cancer, 674–675
Pregnancy, SLN surgery for breast cancer during, 540–541
Prevention, of breast cancer. *See* Chemoprevention.
Prognostic markers. *See* Markers.
Prophylactic mastectomy, SLN surgery after, 546–547

R

Radiation, postmastectomy regional/chest wall irradiation after neoadjuvant
    chemotherapy, 618–619
Radical mastectomy, extended, with internal mammary SLNs, 507–508
Raloxifene, breast cancer chemoprevention studies with, 467–468
    with tamoxifen, 468–469
Reconstruction, oncoplastic surgery in breast cancer management, **567–580**
Recurrence, local, of breast cancer, effect of magnetic resonance imaging on outcome,
    484–485
    magnetic resonance imaging for detection of, 486–487
Reduction, breast, SLN surgery after previous, 544
Risk reduction, of breast cancer. *See* Chemoprevention.
Rotter sentinel lymph nodes, 512

S

Screening, for breast cancer with magnetic resonance imaging, 476–478
Selective estrogen receptor modulators, chemoprevention of breast cancer with, 464–469
Sentinel lymph nodes (SLN), biopsy before or after neoadjuvant chemotherapy, **519–538**
    accuracy of, after neoadjuvant chemotherapy, 524–525
    accuracy with clinically involved nodes before chemotherapy, 525–526
    accuracy with clinically negative nodes, 526–527
    after, potential advantages of, 521–524
    before, potential advantages of, 520–521
    choice of approach to obtain most relevant information, 529–531
    safety of avoiding axillary lymph node dissection after negative biopsy, 527–529
    extra-axillary, in early stage breast cancer, **507–517**
        internal mammary, 507–513

Sentinel lymph nodes (SLN) (*continued*)
    extended radical mastectomy, 507–508
    implications in current era, 508–509
    is biopsy ever indicated, 509–510
    technical considerations for biopsy of, 510–511
  other nonaxillary sites, 513–514
    contralateral, 514
    intramammary, 513
    Rotter (interpectoral) nodes, 513
    supraclavicular, 513–514
 management of regional nodes in patients treated with neoadjuvant chemotherapy, 617–618
 minimal involvement of, in early stage breast cancer, **493–505**
  axillary lymph node dissection for positive disease, 496–497
  clinical trials, 499–500
  predictive models, 497–499
  what constitutes a positive node, 493–496
 surgery in uncommon clinical circumstances, **539–553**
  ductal carcinoma in situ, 541–542
  in men, 539–540
  in pregnant patients, 540–541
  internal mammary SLN surgery, 545
  multicentric/multifocal, 542
  previous axillary surgery, 544–545
  previous breast surgery, 543–544
   breast reduction, 544
   excisional biopsy, 543
  prophylactic mastectomy, 546–547
  with neoadjuvant chemotherapy, 542–543
Supraclavicular sentinel lymph nodes, 512–513
Surgery, axillary lymph node dissection (ALND), 496, 524, 527–529
    after positive pretreatment SLN biopsy after chemotherapy, 524
    for sentinel node-positive disease, 496
    safety of avoiding after a negative SLN biopsy after neoadjuvant chemotherapy, 527–529
  mastectomy *versus* breast-conserving surgery after neoadjuvant chemotherapy, 616–617
  oncoplastic, in breast cancer management, **567–580**
   definition of, 570
   historical perspective, 567–570
   in the large breast, 575–578
   in the small breast, 575
   preoperative assessment, 573–574
   surgical planning, 574–575
  sentinel lymph node, in uncommon clinical circumstances, **539–553**
   ductal carcinoma in situ, 541–542
   in men, 539–540
   in pregnant patients, 540–541
   internal mammary SLN surgery, 545
   multicentric/multifocal, 542
   previous axillary surgery, 544–545
   previous breast surgery, 543–544

breast reduction, 544
    excisional biopsy, 543
  prophylactic mastectomy, 546–547
  with neoadjuvant chemotherapy, 542–543
total skin sparing (nipple sparing) mastectomy, **555–566**
  discussion, 560–564
  literature review, 556–557
  technical considerations, 558–560
    creating skin flaps, 559–560
    incision planning, 559
    patient selection, 559
versus tamoxifen for breast cancer, 628–629

T

Tamoxifen, adjuvant therapy for early-stage breast cancer, 640–641
  breast cancer chemoprevention trials, 464–467
    with raloxifene, 468–469
  versus surgery for breast cancer, 628–629
Targeted therapy, in early-stage breast cancer, **669–679**
  anti-vascular endothelial growth factor therapy, 672–674
  chemotherapy as, 674
  definition, 669–670
  HER2-targeted, 671–672
  in context of genomics, 670–671
  of site-specific bone metastases, 675
Taxanes, for adjuvant therapy in early breast cancer, 655–657
  dose density, 657
  randomized controlled trials, 656–657
  scheduling, 657
Timing, of adjuvant chemotherapy for early breast cancer, 661–662
Total skin sparing mastectomy, evidence for, **555–566**
  discussion, 560–564
  literature review, 556–557
  technical considerations, 558–560
    creating skin flaps, 559–560
    incision planning, 559
    patient selection, 559
Trastuzumab, chemotherapy and, for HER2-positive breast cancer, 658–661
Triple negative (basal) breast cancer, adjuvant chemotherapy for, 661
  targeted PARP inhibition for, 674–675
Tumor biology, in selection of adjuvant chemotherapy for early breast cancer, 658–661
Tumor markers, gene expression profiling in breast cancer, **581–606**

V

Vascular endothelial growth factor (VEGF), targeted anti-VEGF therapy for early stage
  breast cancer, 672–674

W

Wound-response signature, in breast cancer gene expression profiling, 599